AF701597

Medical Emergencies in Dental Practice

Edited by
Louis F. Rose, D.D.S., M.D.
Medical College of Pennsylvania and the
University of Pennsylvania School of Dental Medicine

Barry H. Hendler, D.D.S., M.D.
Medical College of Pennsylvania and the
University of Pennsylvania School of Dental Medicine

quintessence books

Quintessence Publishing Co., Inc. 1981
Chicago, Berlin, Rio de Janeiro and Tokyo

© 1981 by Quintessence Publishing Co., Inc., Chicago, Illinois.
All rights reserved.

This book or any part thereof must not be reproduced by any means or in any form without the written permission of the publisher.

Lithography: Central Photo Engraving, Chicago
Composition: Beslow, Chicago
Printing and binding: North Central Publishing Co., St. Paul
Printed in U.S.A.

ISBN: 0-931386-39-X

Foreword

This text has arisen from the needs perceived by two astute educators who have led the successful collaboration of a School of Dental Medicine and a School of Medicine in providing a better education for dental and medical students. Drs. Rose and Hendler and their colleagues have offered information in this text which is essential to any practitioner caring for the oral health needs of our society. They have succinctly and cleverly brought together current topics within a single volume, which can be utilized by all members of the dental team. Their teachings at the University of Pennsylvania School of Dental medicine, and the Medical College of Pennsylvania have attracted attention in all areas of the educational community and the Department of Dental Medicine at the Medical College is looked upon as an exemplary model for other institutions to follow.

The clinician who masters the material included in this book will be of greater value to his/her patients. Dr. Rose and Dr. Hendler have made many significant contributions to the literature but their monographs and articles dealing with medical emergencies in dental practice have been extremely well received and are translated into several foreign languages.

The reader is encouraged to explore each of these topics and prepare the staff that cares for his patients to recognize and be ready to treat the problem that can occur on a day-to-day basis.

Congratulations to the authors for a fine contribution to the science of dental medicine.

D. Walter Cohen D.D.S., Dean,
Professor of Periodontics, University of
Pennsylvania School of Dental Medicine

Dedication:

To Claire, David, Michael and
my parents—Louis F. Rose

To Lana, Jason, Jennifer and
Mom and Dad—Barry H. Hendler

Preface

There is a growing consensus within the dental profession that traditional education has left many practitioners unprepared to deal effectively with medical emergencies which may arise during dental treatment. The anxiety and pain often associated with dental therapy may precipitate medical emergencies even in healthy individuals. Such emergencies are even more common, however, among geriatric and medically compromised persons who comprise an even greater proportion of the outpatient dental population. The common use of medications by the elderly, including steroids, anticoagulants, cardiac drugs and immunosuppressive agents requires that dentists formulate a plan of management which reflects a knowledge of both pharmaceuticals themselves, and the diseases for which they were prescribed.

It is indeed unfortunate that many within the private sector of our profession have not dealt more thoroughly with the concepts to be presented. The commonly professed notion that medical emergencies, are, in fact, exceedingly rare within the dental environment, betrays the fact that many such emergencies simply go unrecognized, and hence, untreated. As greater interest in the subject of emergency management is fostered, it is hoped that such neglect may be eliminated.

It is our belief that the dentist has a moral obligation to obtain the knowledge and technical skills needed to recognize, treat, and, where possible, prevent medical emergencies which may arise in the dental office. This should include the management of those emergencies not directly related to dental treatment itself. Since such emergencies will occur in ever greater numbers as medical science prolongs the lives of the chronically ill, it is the responsibility of every dentist and his auxilliary staff to identify those potentially at risk.

This text presents what we consider to be an in-depth overview of emergency evaluation and management. Contributors with disparate backgrounds have purposely been recruited in an effort to avoid nearsightedness which has at times characterized the treatment of this topic by individuals from one specialty. Each contributor has participated in the education of dental students and residents and feels strongly that this material be presented to all practitioners of dentistry.

Although the dental literature is replete with "easy approach" considerations of medical emergencies, our intent has been to treat the subject at a depth which befits the complexity of this material. We feel that this will be of interest to the general practitioner, hospital dentist, or specialist who is concerned not only with the management of emergencies, but also with the basic pathophysiology underlying these events.

We have included a chapter which briefly describes each emergency and outlines in chart form the cause, signs, symptoms and treatment of same. It is strongly recommended that the dentist and his staff periodically study these charts. In addition, it would be a far-sighted preventive measure to actually practice emergency procedures, such as the administration of oxygen, external cardiac massage, and the Heimlich maneuver. Because teamwork is the key to success all auxiliary personnel should be involved in both the initial training and in subsequent review sessions.

As one contemplates writing a book difficult decisions regarding content. The authors feel that the material presented is the minimal prerequisite to an adequate understanding of the subject. We offer a broad base of knowledge with which we feel every dentist should be conversant.

We are, of course, indebted to a large number of individuals for having made this publication a reality. All contributors were cooperative, and expended much time and energy in an effort to insure the accuracy and relevancy of their sections.

Special thanks from both of us go to Philip Godfrey, D.M.D., M.D. and Janet Mintzer for their help in preparing the text.

Louis F. Rose/Barry H. Hendler

Table of Contents

Contributors

James T. Amsterdam, D.M.D., M.D.
Instructor of Surgery, Section of Dental Medicine, Medical College of Pennsylvania, Resident, Emergency Medicine, Medical College of Pennsylvania

Jeffrey G. Garber, D.M.D.
Assistant Professor of Anesthesia, Hospital of the University of Pennsylvania, Assistant Professor of Oral Surgery and Anesthesiology, University of Pennsylvania School of Dental Medicine

Barry H. Hendler, D.D.S., M.D.
Director Oral and Maxillofacial Surgery, Medical College of Pennsylvania, Associate Professor of Surgery, Section of Dental Medicine, Medical College of Pennsylvania, Assistant Professor of Oral Surgery and Anesthesiology, University of Pennsylvania School of Dental Medicine

Richard Lammers, M.D.
Assistant Chief of Emergency Medicine, Valley Medical Center of Fresno, Fresno, California

B. Kyle Martino, D.D.S., F.A.D.S.A.
Clinical Assistant Professor of Surgery, Section of Dental Medicine, Medical College of Pennsylvania, Clinical Assistant Professor of Oral Surgery and Anesthesiology, University of Pennsylvania School of Dental Medicine

Louis F. Rose, D.D.S., M.D.
Chief, Section of Dental Medicine, Medical College of Pennsylvania, Associate Professor of Surgery, Section of Dental Medicine, Medical College of Pennsylvania, Associate Professor of Periodontics, University of Pennsylvania School of Dental Medicine

Barbara J. Steinberg, D.D.S.
Director General Practice Dental Residency, Medical College of Pennsylvania, Assistant Professor of Surgery, Section of Dental Medicine, Medical College of Pennsylvania, Assistant Professor of Oral Medicine, University of Pennsylvania School of Dental Medicine

Scott Ulin, M.D.
Director Emergency Medicine, Hurley Medical Center, Flint, Michigan

Section I

Prevention and Evaluation

Chapter 1

Patient Evaluation

Louis F. Rose, D.D.S., M.D., Barbara J. Steinberg, D.D.S. and
Barry H. Hendler, D.D.S., M.D.

The incidence of medical emergencies is most prevelant in geriatric and medically compromised patients. This is a rapidly growing segment of the population whose physical or psychosocial problems may complicate dental treatment. It is the elderly or medically compromised patient who is frequently taking one or more medications, such as steroids, anticoagulants, cardiac drugs, and immunosuppressive agents and may therefore require special consideration before undergoing dental treatment. As ever-increasing numbers of such individuals seek dental care, it becomes the responsibility of the dentist to avoid therapeutic conflict and to deal with medical emergencies when they occur.

Many may ask why there need be such emphasis placed upon the management of what seems to be such a small group of patients. Careful study, however, has shown that the compromised patient is actually in the majority, with more than 50% of 4,365 patients recently surveyed giving history of more than one significant medical problem. By virtue of advancing medical technology, the chronically ill have taken their place amongst the general outpatient population.

Sophisticated surgical manipulation and medical intervention have made possible the ambulatory nature of people with cardiovascular, endocrine and degenerative diseases; disorders which just a few years ago would have meant confinement or death. Coupling these facts with the increasing public awareness of dental health (spurned largely by third party payment groups), one can easily explain the increase in numbers of elderly and chronically ill patients occupying the waiting rooms of America's dentists.

Considering the increasing likelihood of the occurrence of medical emergencies (as well as malpractice cases), with this compromised population, it is the responsibility of every practicing dentist and his auxiliary staff to identify any patient who may be a potential medical risk by securing a comprehensive pre-treatment physical evaluation. Physical evaluation is performed in order to determine the physical and emotional status of a patient to tolerate a specific dental procedure.

Little and King in their article on the significance of physical diagnosis, patient history, data and medical screening in the dental office, summarize the reasons for physical evaluation as follows:

1. To identify patients with undetected systemic disease that could be a serious threat to the life of the patient or that could be complicated by dental treatment.
2. To identify patients who are taking drugs or medication that could be potentiated by drugs we may prescribe, that would complicate therapy we may plan, or that may serve as a clue to an underlying systemic disease that the patient has failed to tell us about.

3. To allow the dentist to modify the treatment plan for the patient in light of any systemic disease the patient may have or drugs he may be taking.
4. To protect the patient and the dentist from commitment (or allegations thereof) of any malpractice.
5. To enable the dentist to select and communicate with a medical consultant concerning a patient's possible systemic problems.
6. To help establish a good patient doctor relationship by showing patients that we are interested in them as individuals and we are also concerned about their overall well being.

The data obtained from a comprehensive physical may prevent the occurrence of a medical emergency. A well conceived evaluation method involves the following: 1) recording a complete medical history, 2) recording of appropriate findings on physical examination and when indicated, 3) ordering and interpreting necessary laboratory studies, 4) initiating medical consultation or referral.

In addition, the medical evaluation must be periodically updated to be an effective mechanism to prevent common medical emergencies.

Medical history

History taking is a technique for eliciting subjective information. This data is organized in a logical manner so that it conveys the patient's physical and emotional status. As dentists, we are obligated to identify those problems that might compromise the patient's well-being, rather than diagnose a specific medical disorder. The medical history puts the physical examination into perspective by supplying information which should alert the examiner to areas of suspected abnormalities. The importance of an accurate medical history cannot be overly stressed. Even in a life threatening situation, once the immediate threat has been contained, a history should be obtained from the patient if possible, or from a relative or friend when the patient is unable to respond.

Two basic methods for obtaining a medical history are the questionnaire and the personal dialogue interview. At first, it might seem that a great deal of time and trouble could be saved if we were to have each patient complete a typed questionnaire and then have the answers coded. There are, however, several problems with this approach. For instance, a "no" answer may mean the patient never had the symptoms or the disease, or that the question is not understood, or felt to be irrelevant since the patient only wants to have a tooth restored or extracted.

On the other hand, a personal history elicited by dialogue allows for observation and the way he reacts to questions. This is often more important than the answer itself. The personal dialogue interview provides the practitioner with opportunity to evaluate the patient's mental status in a non-threatening atmosphere. The patient who is afraid or uninterested will respond quite differently from the one who is self confident and truly concerned about oral health.

The attitude of the clinician is not unobserved by the patient. Most patients respond well to the concerned, sympathetic and unhurried listener who regards their problems in a matter of paramount importance and with absorbing interest. Nothing can be more convincing to indicate our interest in patients than our willingness to devote time to a discussion of their concerns, and too, it has long been known that more accurate and complete histories are the products of such interactions. A questionnaire, if used, would supplant the need for this early doctor-patient contact which might serve to establish rapport. The personal history if properly taken can convey this positive attitude and therefore serve as a powerful antidote to anxiety, stress and tension. This therapeutic effect will not only facilitate subsequent dental treatment, but also may prevent the occurrence of the types of medical emergencies attributable to a psychological etiology.

The questionnaire, (Fig. 1-1) is a legitimate method of securing data if used in conjunction with the dialogue history. The questionnaire component of the combined approach may help a patient to recall frequently used medications and various symptoms which may be indicative of a medical disease. It can also assist the dentist in ascertaining which areas in the dialogue history to emphasize and further explore.

A comprehensive dialogue medical history (Fig. 1-2) helps the dentist to evaluate the present health status of a patient, past medical history, allergies, medications the patient may be taking, pertinent familial and social history, and a review of body systems. The following information may be elicited under each of the aforementioned areas of the medical history.

Present Health Status: The patient should be asked the date and results of his last complete physical examination. If the patient states, for example, that he has diabetes it is important to determine the date of the initial diagnosis, the degree of success in controlling the disease, the therapeutic regimen, as well as the date, type and results of the last complete blood count and blood glucose study. If the patient has not had a recent complete physical examination it would be advisable to make a recommendation for him to do so. The present health status gives the dental practitioner an awareness as to how the patient perceives his present general state of health. This may be an important indication of the patient's psychological makeup, how he views his oral health status and how readily he will accept the dental diagnosis and proposed treatment.

Past Medical History: The date, diagnosis, and treatment of significant hospitalizations and illnesses during childhood and adult life will help evaluate the patient's past medical history and clearly indicate whether his average state of health has been one of normal vigor or chronic illness.

Allergies: The patient should be asked if he is allergic or has reactions to any food or medications. Be sure to specifically mention aspirin, local anesthesia, and penicillin (abbreviated, ASA, LA and PCN).

Medications: In questioning about medications, it is imperative to determine the brand and/or generic name of the drug, why and by whom it was prescribed, the dosage, and the length of time the medication has been taken. It should be noted that a number of patients will not include medications used for allaying anxiety or for inducing sleep, such as tranquilizers and sedative/hypnotic drugs. An effective way of ascertaining this information is by asking patients if they ever have to take anything to help them rest, relax, or sleep. Also some women will not include oral contraceptives (abbreviated OC) and supplemental hormones, both of which may affect the oral tissues.

Review of Systems: The review of body systems (Fig. 1-3) is the main component of the interview approach to history taking. It provides additional data about each system and reveals signs and symptoms not already elicited which may be indicative of a previously treated or undiagnosed disorder. The review of systems helps to refresh the patient's memory about problems that may be indicative of a specific disorder and hopefully prevents inadvertent forgetfulness on the part of the patient.

Family History: This is taken in order to determine if there is a predisposition of the family toward inheritable diseases or diseases in which inheritance seems to be an important factor, such as diabetes. For example, a patient with a strong family his-

Dental care center
Planned care health questionnaire

Name ______________________________

Date ______________ Referred by ______________

Previous Dentist ______________________________

Address ______________________________

Physician ______________________________

Address ______________________________

Reason for appointment ______________________________

DIRECTIONS TO PATIENTS:

Answers to these questions will help the dentist decide how to best treat your dental problems. Try to check each answer "yes" or "no." If you have no idea of the answer to the question, do not check either answer.

Medical history	Yes	No
1. Have you been treated by a physician or been in the hospital in the past year?	___	___
2. Has there been any change in your general health in the past year?	___	___
3. List all the medications or drugs you are taking at the present time:		

Medications	Dosage
______________	______________
______________	______________
______________	______________
______________	______________

	Yes	No
4. Have you ever been told you had a Thyroid problem?	___	___
5. Have you ever been told you had sugar diabetes?	___	___
6. Have you taken daily cortisone medication (Prednisone) in the past year?	___	___
7. Have you ever had persistent pain or difficulty swallowing?	___	___
8. Have you ever had jaundice, hepatitis, or some other liver problem?	___	___
9. Do you get short of breath on mild exertion or when you lie down?	___	___
10. Have you ever had TB (tuberculosis) or lived with anyone who had TB?	___	___
11. Have you ever had asthma?	___	___

12. Have you ever been told you had:
    - Rheumatic fever ___ ___
    - Heart murmur ___ ___
    - Heart attack or coronary ___ ___
    - Angina ___ ___
    - Heart surgery ___ ___
    - High or low blood pressure ___ ___
13. Have you ever had prolonged bleeding (more than is normal for you) for a cut, injury, or tooth extraction? ___ ___
14. Have you ever had hemophilia or some other bleeding disorder? ___ ___
15. Have you ever had anemia, low blood or thin blood? ___ ___
16. Have you ever had gonorrhea, syphilis, bad blood, or venereal disease? ___ ___
17. Are you pregnant or think you are pregnant? ___ ___
18. Are you now taking birth control pills? ___ ___
19. Have you ever had troublesome pain in your jaw joint? ___ ___
20. Have you ever had fits, seizures, convulsions or epilepsy? ___ ___
21. Have you ever had a stroke? ___ ___
22. Have you been treated for some allergic condition? ___ ___
23. Are you allergic to penicillin? ___ ___
24. Has anyone ever told you not to take a particular drug (aspirin, novacaine, sulfa, etc.)? ___ ___
25. Are there any medications that make you sick or ill? ___ ___

Fig. 1-1 Health questionnaire.

tory of diabetes mellitus, with no apparent signs or symptoms of the disease, should be evaluated periodically since clinical manifestations may appear later in life. The dentist should inquire specifically for family history of diabetes, cancer, heart disease, high blood pressure, seizure disorders, mental disorders, etc.

Social History: The social history should not be underemphasized. It may assist in determining how well the patient responds to the demands and conflicts of modern society. In addition, it may help to explain the untoward reactions of a patient to his particular medical/dental problems and to the therapeutic recommendations. For example, the alcoholic patient may have difficulty in communicating and may be unwilling to follow recommendations (e.g., diet and oral hygiene). Also, the alcoholic is an anesthetic risk and may develop prolonged and profound hypotensive episodes secondary to various anxiety and pain control drugs. The social history should include: occupation and any associated health haz-

Name ______________________ Tel. Home ______________ Date ______________
Address ______________________ Tel. Bus. ______________ Date of Birth ______________
Referred by ____

Dental History:
Dentist ______________________ Telephone # ______________ Last Visit ______________
Chief Complaint:

History of Present Illness

Past Dental History:

Medical History:
Physician ______________________ Telephone # ______________ Last Visit ______________
Present Health Status

Hospitalizations

Illnesses
Allergies ______________________ A.S.A. ________ L.A. ________ PCN ______________
Meds. ____________________________________ O.C. ______________
Review of Systems
Skin ____
EENT ____
Respiratory ____
Cardiac ______________ RhF ______________ RhHD ______________ M ______________
Gastrointestinal ____
Genitounnary ____
Menstrual Hx. ______________ Pregnancy ______________ Children ______________
Endocrine ______________________ Diabetes ______________________
Extremities ____
Nervous ______________________ Psychiatric ______________________
Hematopoietic ____

Family History
Diabetes ______________ Hypertension ______________ Cardiac ______________
Epilepsy ______________________ Other ______________________
Social History
Occupation ____________ Smoking ____________ Alcohol ____________ Other ____________

Regional Examination
1. Face ______________ 5. Floor ______________ 9. Gingiva ______________
2. Lips ______________ 6. Plate-Hard ______________ ______________
3. Buccal Mucosa ______________ 7. Plate Soft ______________ 10. Lymph nodes ______________
4. Tongue ______________ 8. Pharynx ______________ **Vital Signs** ____ B.P. ____ P. ____________

Medical Summary:

Recommendations:

Fig. 1-2 Comprehensive dialogue medical history.

Review of systems

1. *Skin:* itching, rash, ulcers, changes in hair, hair loss.

2. *Eyes:* vision, diplopia, blurring

3. *Ears, Nose, Throat:* hearing, earache, epistaxis, sore throat, hoarseness, sinus pain.

4. *Respiratory:* cough, sputum (describe quantity, color, odor, blood) wheezing, infections, exposure to tuberculosis.

5. *Cardiac:* chest pain on exertion, palpitation, dyspnea, orthopnea, swelling of ankles. History of rheumatic fever, rheumatic heart disease, "heart attack", high blood pressure, murmur.

6. *Gastro-intestinal:* appetite, nausea, vomiting, dysphagia, heartburn, indigestion, food intolerance, abdominal pain, jaundice.

7. *Genito-urinary:* dysuria, nocturia, polyuria, hematuria, frequency, difficulty starting stream; venereal disease and treatment, kidney infection.

   For women:
   a. *Menstrual history:* last menstrual period and previous menstrual period; dysmennorrhea
   b. *Menopause:* age of occurrence, hot flushes
   c. *Obstetrical history:* pregnancies, miscarriages, living children

8. *Extremities:*
   a. Vascular: varicose veins, phlebitis
   b. Joints: pain, stiffness, swelling of joints
   c. Muscles: weakness, pain, tenderness, cramps

9. *Nervous System:* syncope, convulsions, headache, vertigo, tremor, paralysis, paresthesias, anesthesias

10. *Hematopoetic:* bleeding tendency, excessive bruising, anemia, known exposure to radiation or toxic agents.

11. *Psychiatric:* "nervousness," irritability, depressions, history of previous "nervous breakdown."

Fig. 1-3 Information that should be obtained regarding each body system.

ards, marital status, diet, use of alcohol, tobacco or other drugs.

Medical Summary and Recommendations: All positive findings should be summarized and any recommendations relating to those findings recorded. This will enable the dentist and his staff to quickly review a patient's medical status at each visit and facilitate the diagnosis and treatment of any medical emergency that may arise.
Initially, the medical history form described here may appear to be somewhat cumbersome and lengthy, and the information sought excessive, and possibly irrelevant. In actual practice, this usually is not the case, but rather represents one of the most accurate methods for determining the physical and emotional status of the patient, his tolerance for a specific procedure and the presence of any medical risk factors. In essence, this form will aid in deciding whether one can proceed with dental treatment with relative safety or whether medical consultation should be sought prior to beginning therapy.
In conclusion, the comprehensive medical history is an important procedure for dentists to adopt and routinely utilize in order to assure that their patients are receiving the optimum benefit of the many diverse health resources that are available to us today.

Physical examination

The second aspect of the medical evaluation is the physical examination. Emphasis should be placed on a regional examination of the head and neck and oral cavity (Fig. 1-4). In addition, every patient who enters the dental office should have baseline vital signs recorded. Without these parameters, the evaluation of a medical emergency would be most perplexing and the management could be inappropriate and ineffective. (Vital signs and monitoring will be considered in chapter 2.)

The examination of the head and neck and oral cavity is mainly conducted through the application of the following principles of physical examination: inspection, palpation and auscultation.

Inspection: This represents the first step of every physical examination and generally contributes more pertinent information to a diagnosis than any other physical technique. Through inspection the practitioner can obtain both quantitative data of measurement and qualitative data of description. Simply by observation the dentist may be able to help identify certain undetected illnesses, i.e., liver and heart disease by noting skin color. Inspection is an invaluable tool when examining the oral cavity. In order to perform a visual examination of this region one should have adequate lighting, a mouth mirror, 2x2 gauze, tongue depressors and disposable gloves.

Palpation: The practitioner can ascertain the size, consistency, mobility and character of structure with this technique.

Auscultation: This involves the use of a stethoscope and is dependent on the differential transmission of sounds which are provided by normal and pathologic organs. We may be able to appreciate a bruit or temporomandibular click when applying auscultation to head and neck examination. When compared to inspection and palpation, the technique of auscultation has limited value in the examination of the head and neck.
The dentist should develop an orderly and systematic method of physical examination such as the one that will be discussed.

Skull: Observation is made noting general size and contour of the skull. Palpation should be performed by placing both hands on the skull, and with even pressure, palpating for any masses, lumps or areas of tenderness. The contour and size of the skull varies considerably within normal limits and even extreme deviations from nor-

Regional examination

VITAL SIGNS B.P. ______________ P ______________ R ______________

HEAD AND NECK

Face—color, expression, lesions, eyes

Trachea—midline

Thyroid—enlarged, tender

Carotics—patent, prominence

Jugular Veins—prominence

Lymph nodes—palpable

ORAL CAVITY

Lips

Buccal mucosa

Gingiva

Floor of mouth

Tongue

Hard palate

Soft palate

Pharynx

Gag reflex

Other

Fig. 1-4 Regional examination of head and neck, and oral cavity; baseline readings of vital signs.

mal may not indicate any disturbance. However, mild degrees of altered contour and size which may be difficult to detect may result from a pathologic disturbance and should be continually observed. Observing an abnormally large head may be related to such entities as hydrocephalus, Paget's disease or acromegaly. When examining the skull it is also important to note signs of injuries and operations of the head. The scar of an operation for tic douloureux, intracranial tumor, or gunshot wound may be the basis for dysfunction of the oral structures.

Face: When examining the face, facial expression should be noted. The term, "facies" refers to the appearance of the patient's face as a whole. The appearance may be suggestive or pathognomonic of a particular disease entity. Some characteristic facies include those of: acromegaly (enlargement of both bone and soft tissues of the head, with bony prominence of the forehead, nose and lower jaw, soft tissues of the nose, lips and ears are also enlarged); myxedema (dull puffy facies, edema pronounced around the eyes which does not pit with pressure, hair and eyebrows are dry, coarse and thinned, skin is dry); Cushings Syndrome (round or "moon" face with red cheeks, excessive hair growth may be present in the mustache and sideburn areas and on the chin); Down's Syndrome (transverse groove on tongue, prominent epicanthal folds along with outer slant to the eyelids).

Normally the skull and face are fairly symmetrical; however, perfect symmetry is not usually found and the two halves of the face and skull will often differ somewhat. It is necessary that the practitioner develop an appreciation for asymmetry of the face in order to recognize skeletal defects that may have a bearing on growth and development of the maxilla and mandible, to properly evaluate past traumatic injury and to recognize the presence of disease whose beginning may present only minimal facial asymmetry. The cause of facial asymmetry may be skeletal, muscular, neurologic, glandular, occlusal or soft tissue in origin.

When examining the face, the skin should be observed noting the color, pigmentation, textures, and any lesions. The color of the skin may be a key to an underlying problem. Pallor may be observed in the patient with anemia, leukemia or a vasomotor phenomena. It may result from a decrease of hemoglobin pigment, a diminished flow of blood to the tissues, the presence of edema or a decrease in melanin pigments. An increased redness of the skin may be caused by capillary dilatation (often associated with liver disease) or associated with blushing, fever, burns, exposure to sunlight and telangiectasia resulting from X-ray therapy. Abnormal redness may infrequently be caused by polycythemia vera. Cyanosis, a bluish color of the skin, is associated with diminished oxygen-carrying capacity of the blood. It results when the absolute reduced hemoglobin in the blood reaches five grams. It may be present with cardiac or pulmonary disease. Jaundice is most commonly caused by bilirubin pigment and is associated with prehepatic, hepatic or obstructive disease of the bile duct, such as that caused by neoplasms or gallstones.

Alterations of the basic pattern of pigmentation must be noted by the dentist. Changes in the color of the skin caused by increased melanin pigmentation may be related to external causes such as sunlight, mechanical irritation, wind and heat. Increased melanin pigmentation may be noted in certain systemic diseases such as Addison's disease and may be seen in pregnant individuals with a hormone imbalance.

The texture of the skin is also noted when examining the face. As a person ages, the skin loses some of its elasticity. Some diseases also produce various changes in skin texture. In hyperthyroidism, skin feels smooth and silky and is generally moist and elastic. In hypothyroidism and myxedema, dryness and inelasticity prevail.

Eyes (Visual Acuity): For screening purposes the patient is asked to read any available print. Each eye is used separately, covering the other with an opaque card.

Visual Fields: This procedure is usually omitted in a routine examination, but should be included whenever a neurological problem is suspected. To conduct the test for visual fields, the patient should cover one eye and look at the examiner's nose directly opposite. Starting at the periphery of each quadrant of vision, the examiner moves his finger or a cotton tipped applicator in front of the patient, toward the center of vision. The patient is asked to signal as soon as he sees the finger or applicator. The test is performed for each eye. This procedure will reveal gross defects. The tests for visual fields may reveal disturbances in function along the optic pathways, including sense organs and neurons in the retina, fibers of the optic nerve and tract and abnormalities in the temporal, parietal or occipital lobes.

Position and Alignment: The eyes are surveyed for their position and alignment with each other. Exophthalmos is a protrusion of the eyeball and is a characteristic finding in hyperthyroidism.

Eyelids: The eyelids are examined noting the position of the lids in relationship to the eyeballs. Edema, color, lesions and condition and direction of the eyelashes, if present, are also noted. Ptosis is drooping of an eyelid caused by muscular weakness, interference with the oculomotor nerve which controls voluntary elevation of the eyelid and interference with the sympathetic nerves which maintain smooth muscle tone of the lid. The cause may be congenital in origin or may be caused by other conditions such as tabes dorsalis, multiple sclerosis, and neoplastic or inflammatory disease. In Bell's palsy there is inability to close the lid. Lid lag may be present in patients with hyperthyroidism and is noted when the eye is rotated downward and the lid fails to follow synchronously.

Sclera: The sclera is normally bluish-white and variation in this color should be noted. Jaundice may be seen and may be indicative of liver, gallbladder or pancreatic disease. Of dental significance is the relationship of blue scleras to osteogenesis imperfecta or odontogenesis imperfecta. Patches of melanin are commonly seen in the sclera of many persons of dark complexions, especially in blacks. This is not a pathologic finding and should not be confused with jaundice.

Conjunctiva: When examining the conjunctiva, color must be noted. Jaundice may be noted as well as pallor, which may be indicative of anemia. Petechiae if observed may be associated with subacute bacterial endocardititis and purpuras.

Pupils: Size, shape and equality of the pupils is noted. The change in the pupil most significant to the dentist is miosis associated with tabes dorsales of tertiary syphillis and the pinpoint pupil of the narcotic addict. Pupils of unequal diameter may be of congenital origin or may be related to disease of the central nervous system.

The pupillary accommodation reflex is tested by checking pupillary constriction as the patient changes his focus from a distant to a close object.

Pupillary light reflexes are evaluated by shining a light into each eye from the side. Both direct and consensual (opposite eye) reaction should be that of pupillary constriction.

Extraocular Movements: The range of ocular movements is checked by asking the patient to follow the movement of the examiner's fingers as they are moved in all six cardinal fields of gaze (Fig. 1-5). Given involvement of the oculomotor nerve, the patient will not be able to look up, down or medially with the affected eye. There will

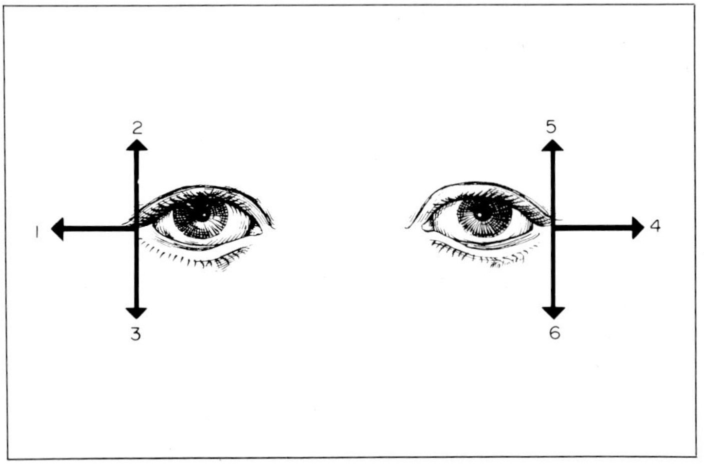

Fig. 1-5 Extraocular movements. Numbers indicate sequence of movement.

be ptosis of the lid and dilation of the pupil. If the trochlear nerve is affected, he is unable to look downward and laterally. If the abducens nerve is affected, the patient will not be able to look laterally with the involved eye. In any of these cases, the patient will complain of double vision. Either the nerves themselves or their nuclei in the midbrain and pons may be involved. During the examination of ocular movements, one should observe for nystagmus, e.g.,a rhythmic fine oscillation of the eyes. Minor grades of oscillation are often encountered under normal conditions. True nystagmus is a pathologic sign and is seen in a variety of neurological conditions.

No evaluation of the eye is totally complete without a thorough ophthalmoscopic examination. The ophthalmoscope is used to inspect the fundus of the eye, which includes the retina, choroid, fovea, macula, optic disc and retinal vessels. Many conditions and systemic diseases present with positive findings when performing this examination: most commonly optic atrophy, papilledema, hypertension and diabetes. If the medical history and brief clinical examination so indicate, the patient should be referred to an internist or an opthalmologist.

Nose and Sinuses: The contour of the nose is inspected, noting asymmetry and abnormalilties of profile. The patency of each naris is tested by closing the other with digital compression, while the patient inhales with the mouth closed. With the left thumb the soft nasal tip is pushed upward, while a lighted penlight in the other hand closes one naris so the observer, through the open naris, can view the transilluminated septum for deviations, perforations and masses. The nasal mucosa is observed, noting color, swelling, exudate and bleeding. The inferior and middle turbinates and the middle meatus between them are examined noting color, swelling, exudate and polyps.

The cheeks and supraorbital ridges are palpated for tenderness over the maxillary and frontal sinuses. Tenderness may be present in acute sinusitis.

Ears: The auricle and surrounding tissues should be inspected for deformities, lumps and skin lesions. Lymph nodes and sebaceous cysts are often found around the ears. If ear pain, discharge or inflammation is present, tenderness should be checked by moving the auricle and pressing on the tragus and mastoid process. Movement of

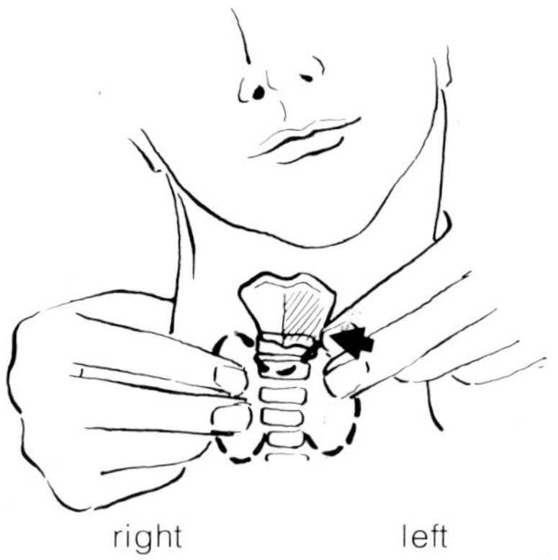

Fig. 1-6 Palpation of thyroid.

the auricle and tragus is painful in acute otitis externa but not in otitis media. Tenderness of the mastoid process suggests mastoiditis or posterior auricular lymphadenitis.

An otoscope must be used to examine the ear canal and drum. Using the largest speculum that the canal will accommodate, the canal is inspected for wax discharge, and foreign bodies, making note of any redness or swelling of the canal. Redness, scaliness, narrowing, swelling and pain are observed in acute otitis externa. The entire drum should be visualized noting color, position of the handle of the malleus and any lesions. Abnormalities of the eardrum often seen include otitis media, perforations and myringitis.

Auditory acuity can be grossly tested by moving a ticking watch away from the ear until the patient can no longer hear. Tests can also be conducted by moving the watch toward the ear. Each ear should be tested. Normal acuity must also be established.

Trachea: The trachea is palpated in the area of the supra-sternal notch noting deviation from the midline. The trachea deviates from masses in the neck, mediastinum or from pleural and pulmonary abnormalities.

Thyroid: The thyroid is palpated noting its size, shape, symmetry, tenderness and presence of nodules. The easiest method for palpation is for the examiner to stand behind the patient resting both thumbs on the nape of the patient's neck and with the index and middle fingers of both hands feeling for the thyroid isthmus and for the anterior surfaces of the lateral lobes (Fig. 1-6). The patient flexes his neck slightly forward and to the right. The thyroid cartilage is then displaced to the right with the fingers of the examiner's left hand and the palpation is performed with the right hand, placing the thumb deep to and behind the sternomastoid and the index and middle fingers in front of it. The patient then swallows at which time the thyroid should rise. The procedure is reversed for the other side. The ability to palpate the thyroid varies considerably depending on a person's stature. In a thin person, the isthmus is usually but not always palpable. It may be impossible to find in a stocky neck. Although normal lobes are sometimes palpable, they more often are not.

Both the isthmus and lateral lobes of a diffusely enlarged thyroid can usually be felt. Such enlargement may be associated with hyperthyroidism with endemic goiter and Hashimotos' thyroiditis. The presence of multiple nodules suggests a metabolic rather than a malignant process, but unusual firmness and rapid enlargement of one of the nodules must raise the suspicion of neoplasm. Although a clinically single nodule of the thyroid gland may be a cyst, a benign tumor or the presence of a malignancy must be ruled out. Rapid enlargement, induration and fixation to surrounding tissues are ominous signs.

Carotid Arteries: The carotid pulse should be palpated in a medical emergency because of its size and close proximity to the heart. The patient's head should be turned slightly toward the side being examined. One side should be palpated at a time with the examiner's index and middle fingers at the medial edge of the sternocleidomastoid, pressing gently on the carotid artery in the lower half of the neck. Rate and rhythm can be noted as well as amplitude graded on a 0 to 4+ scale. Decreased or absent carotid pulse suggests arterial narrowing or occlusion.

Jugular Veins: Venous pulsations are rarely palpable, usually absent in an upright position and are diminished by inspiration. Venous distension should be observed with the patient's head in a 30-45° position. In general, the position of the patient in the dental chair is such that congestion and pulsation of the jugular veins may sometimes be noticed in association with vascular hypertension, severe thyrotoxicosis and congestive heart failure. Engorgement of the veins of the neck is suggestive of right sided congestive heart failure or of some obstructive process that prevents venous return to the heart.

Lymph Nodes: Lymph nodes are palpated, using the pads of the index and middle fingers, moving the skin over the underlying tissues in each area rather than moving the fingers over the skin (Fig. 1-7). The patient should be relaxed, and the neck tilted slightly forward. The examiner should palpate in sequence for the following nodes:

1. pre-auricular
2. posterior auricular
3. occipital
4. tonsillar
5. submaxillary
6. submental
7. superficial cervical
8. posterior cervical
9. deep cervical
10. supraclavicular.

Size, shape, mobility, consistency and tenderness should be noted. Small mobile, discrete non-tender nodes are frequently found in normal healthy individuals. These may be residual from a previous illness. Detection of enlarged or tender nodes often suggests inflammation. Indurated and fixed nodes suggest malignancy.

Oral Cavity: As performed during routine dental examinations.

Larynx: The larynx is the entrance to the upper airway. In order to examine this structure, the examiner must use a mirror for viewing. The technique is known as indirect mirror laryngoscopy and takes a great deal of practice on the part of the practitioner. The patient is seated in a chair with a clear 150 watt electric lamp immediately behind him and to his right. This light

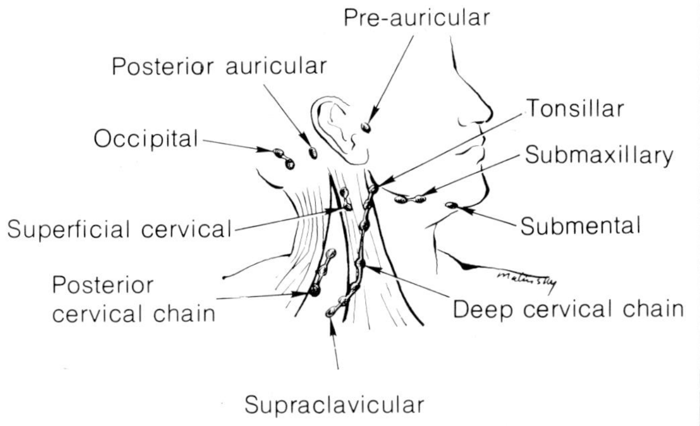

Fig. 1-7 Lymph nodes of the neck.

is reflected with a head mirror the examiner is wearing. The patient is asked to sit erect with the chin somewhat forward, both feet on the floor and the knees together. The examiner is seated in front of the patient with his knees outside the patient's. The examiner explains what he is going to do and has the patient concentrate on breathing softly and regularly through the mouth. The tongue is protruded maximally over the lower teeth while the examiner's left hand wraps a piece of gauze over the tongue and grasps the wrapped portion with thumb and middle finger while bracing the hand against the patient's teeth with the forefinger. The tongue is then gently pulled to the patient's right side. The examiner grasps a No. 5 (large) laryngeal mirror at the midpoint of its handle with the thumb and forefinger of the right hand. The mirror is heated over an alcohol flame or in warm water to avoid subsequent steaming over. The temperature is tested by touching the mirror to the back of the examiner's left wrist. The handle is held like a pencil and the mirror is inserted in the patient's mouth from the left side with the face of the mirror downward and parallel to the tongue surface (Fig. 1-8). The mirror is moved posteriorly until its back rests against the anterior surface of the uvula. The uvula and soft palate are pressed steadily upward avoiding the back of the tongue so the patient does not gag. The patient breathes steadily while the larynx is inspected. While viewing the vocal cords the patient is asked to say "e – e – e" or "he – e – e" in a highpitched voice. The structures as shown in Fig. 1-9 should be observed. The true vocal cords should be observed during quiet respiration when the rima is tent shaped and during phonation when they meet in the midline.
This method of examination is of great importance in diagnosing the following: laryngitis, laryngeal edema, nodules, ulcers, polyps and carcinoma.

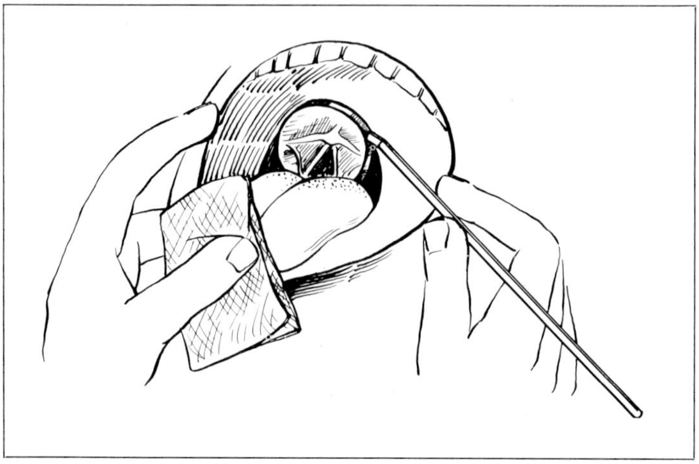

Fig. 1-8 Indirect mirror laryngoscopy.

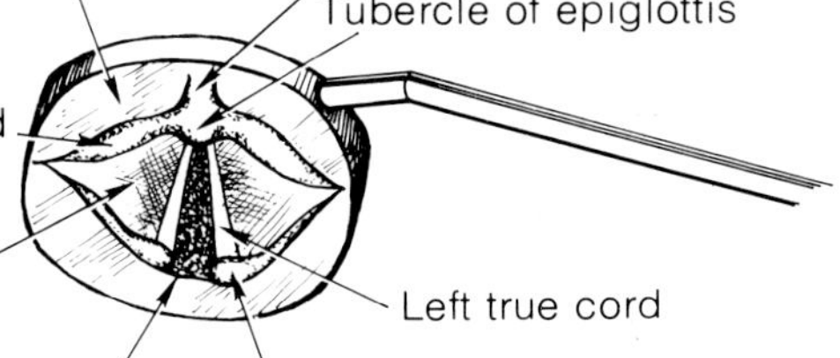

Fig. 1-9 Appearance of the larynx in the mirror.

Interpretation of clinical laboratory studies

There are certain instances when the patient's medical history and physical examination warrant the ordering of laboratory tests to confirm a diagnosis or to uncover incidental findings separate from the chief complaint. Depending on the dentist's background and experience in interpreting such tests he will either refer directly to a clinical laboratory or to a physician for appropriate examination, tests and opinion. In the first alternative the dentist assumes the responsibililty for the interpretation and then the referral to a physician for confirmation and treatment if indicated. In the second alternative the physician assumes all the responsibility for preparing the patient and evaluating the findings.
The following is a list of clinical laboratory studies, their indications and interpretations of which the dentist should have some knowledge.

Complete blood count (CBC)

The CBC will routinely include the hemoglobin (Hgb), hematocrit (Hct), red blood cell count (RBC), white blood cell count (WBC), with a differential white count and a statement on the adequacy of platelets.

Hemoglobin: It is the oxygen carrier of the blood. The hemoglobin is decreased in hemorrhage and anemias and is increased in hemoconcentration and polycythemia. The hemoglobin and red cell count do not always rise and fall equally. This is an important factor in the differention of anemias. For example, in iron deficiency anemia the hemoglobin is reduced more than the red blood cell count and in pernicious anemia the opposite is true. In males normal range is 14-18 grams per 100 ml of blood and in females 12-16 grams per 100 ml.

Hematocrit: This reflects the relative volume of cells and plasma in the blood. In anemias and after blood loss, the hematocrit is lowered. In polycythemia and dehydration it is raised. The normal hematocrit range for men is from 42-52% and for women from 37-47%.

Red Blood Cell Count: The red cells contain hemoglobin. An increase in red cells may indicate hemoconcentration or polycythemia. A decrease in the number of red cells may be indicative of blood loss or one of the anemias. The normal range is 4,000,000-6,000,000 red blood cells per cubic mm.

White Blood Cell Count: White blood cells are important in the defense of the body against invading microorganisms. An increase in the white blood count is seen in the leukemias, bacterial infections, infectious mononucleosis and in certain parasitic infections. It may also be increased after exercise and emotional upsets. A decrease in the white blood cell count is seen in aplastic anemia, lupus erythematosus, acute viral infections, and in drug and chemical toxicity. Normal white blood cell count is 5,000-10,000 per cubic mm.
There are several kinds of white blood cells that can be identified microscopically. These types of white blood cells are known as the differential. It is important to know whether the proportions of these cells have changed since they may be indicative of a particular group of diseases.
The neutrophils (54%-62%) are increased in most bacterial infections. An increase in the number of immature neutrophils is frequently found in acute infections. This is the so-called "shift to the left." The eosinophils (1%-3%) are increased in allergic conditions and parasitic infections. The basophils (0%-1%) may be increased in some blood dyscrasias. The lymphocytes (25%-33%) are noted to be increased in measles and in several bacterial or chronic infections. The monocytes (3%-7%) may be increased during recovery from severe infections and Hodgkin's disease.

Blood Glucose: This test is performed to determine glucose metabolism. Basic tests for disorders of blood glucose are the Fasting Blood Sugar (FBS), the Two-Hour Post-Prandial Blood Sugar, the Glucose Tolerance Test, and the Random Blood Sugar. An increase in blood glucose will be seen in diabetes mellitus, liver disease, and in overactivity of several endocrine glands. A decrease in blood glucose is seen in hypofunctioning of several endocrine glands, adenoma of the islet cells in the pancreas, glycogen storage disease and overtreatment with insulin. The normal range is 80 to 120 mg blood glucose per 100 ml of serum or 70 to 105 mg of blood glucose per 100 ml of whole blood.

Blood Urea Nitrogen (BUN): This test is used as a screening test for kidney function; however, it is not specific. An increased value will be seen in extensive kidney disease, congestive heart failure and dehydration. Protein intake may also directly affect the BUN. If renal disease is suspected a more reliable assessment is the serum creatinine test. The ratio of BUN to creatinine is usually 10 to 1. Normal range for BUN is 10-20 mg per 100 ml of blood.

Serology: There are several varieties of serological tests screening for syphilis. All are nonspecific tests for syphilis and may give both false-positive and false-negative results. They may occur with lupus erythematosus, infectious mononucleosis, smallpox, malaria, measles and all spirochetal diseases. Interpretation of these serological tests requires correlation with the patient's history and clinical findings. Normally these tests are negative; if positive, confirm with fluorescent treponemal antibody—absorption test (FTA—abs).

Screening tests for hemorrhagic disorders

Bleeding Time: It is the time required for hemostasis to occur in a standard wound of the capillary bed. Bleeding time varies with vascular and platelet abnormalities. Bleeding time is prolonged in thrombocytopenia purpuras and in Von Willebrand's disease, liver cirrhosis, and acute leukemia. Normal range is: 1-6 minutes.

Platelet Count: Platelets are decreased in thrombocytopenia purpura. In myeloproliferative diseases, platelets are increased. Normal platelet count is 250,000-500,000 per cubic mm.

Prothrombin Time (PT): This is an indirect test of the clotting ability of the blood. Prothrombin is converted to thrombin in the clotting process. When the prothrombin level of the blood is lower than normal, it is believed that the clotting tendency of the blood within the blood vessels is diminished. This test is extremely significant in discovering abnormalities in the clotting mechanism involving Factors V, VII, X, prothrombin and fibrinogen. It is used to establish and control the level of anticoagulant therapy of the coumarin drugs (Dicumarol) or similar drugs. These substances are given to reduce the clotting tendency of the blood and thus avoid thromboembolic phenomena. This test gives an indication of prothrombin deficiency arising from liver disease, fibrinogen deficiency, and lack of or inability of the body to utilize vitamin K. Normal range: between 11 and 18 seconds, depending on type of thromboplastin used, is considered 100 per cent of normal. In treatment with coumadin the physician tries to keep the prothrombin time at 2-2.5 times normal.

Partial Thromboplastin Time (PTT): This is a test to recognize mild to moderate deficiencies of the intrinsic clotting factor since the prothrombin time bypasses the intrinsic clotting system. Another use for the PTT is to demonstrate a circulating anticoagulant in plasma. The normal PTT is 45 seconds or less, however, since variations in technique are widespread the normal range for the PTT varies somewhat between laboratories.

Urinalysis (UA)

Volume: Increased urine output is observed in diabetes insipidus, diabetes mellitus and in chronic nephritis. Decreased urine output is observed in dehydration, toxic and metabolic diseases of the kidney and obstructive lesions of the bladder and urethra. Normal volume: 1000-1500 ml per 24 hours.

pH: This is a measure of the degree of acidity or alkalinity of the urine. The kidney maintains the blood at the correct pH by excreting into the urine any excess ions which might alter the pH of the blood. The urinary pH varies widely and changes do not indicate abnormality. However, in certain situations it is advisable to have an acid or alkaline urine and the pH measurement is important. pH may be increased with frequent vomiting and anemia while the pH may be decreased in acidosis and with fever. Normal range: pH 4.8-8.0.

Specific Gravity: This is a measurement of the ability of the kidney to reabsorb water.

Increased specific gravity occurs in diabetes mellitus and in dehydration. Decreased specific gravity occurs in chronic nephritis and diabetes insipidus. Specific gravity varies from 1.003-1.026.

Gross Appearance: Red urine may be indicative of hematuria or congenital porphyria. Green urine is characteristic of pseudomonas infection. Brown urine is associated with glomerulonephritis and obstructive jaundice. The urine that turns black on standing is found in alkaptonuria. Normal appearance is amber color.

Glucose: In some disorders glucose is found in the urine. This is most commonly observed in primary diabetes mellitus, acute disorders of the CNS (meningitis, cerebrovascular accidents) and in Cushing's syndrome. Normal range: no sugar in the urine.

Albumin: Ordinarily the albumin in the blood does not pass through the glomerular wall into the urine. However, in several conditions such as nephritis from inflammatory and degenerative changes, chronic heart disease or drug toxicity, albumin appears in the urine. Therefore, the test is not specific but indicates that more precise tests are needed. Normal range: in 5% to 15% of normal individuals small amounts of albumin are sometimes found in the urine with no disease present. This is known as orthostatic or postural albuminuria.

Acetone: This test is important in the diagnosis of ketosis, a type of acidosis produced by faulty metabolism. When available glycogen is decreased, there is an increase in oxidation of fatty acids giving rise to acetone bodies which are then excreted by the kidneys. Acetone in the urine indicates a severe disorder of metabolism. Diabetes mellitus and starvation may account for acetone in the urine. Normally there is no acetone in the urine.

Microscopic Tests: Red Blood Cells—Blood in the urine may appear as intact red blood cells (hematuria) or dissolved hemoglobin derived from destroyed red blood cells (hemoglobinuria). Hematuria comes from bleeding somewhere along the urinary tract from the glomerulus to the urethra. The site of bleeding and its cause are determined by more precise testing methods. Hemoglobinuria usually arises from conditions outside the urinary tract. The reticuloendothelial system is unable to metabolize hemoglobin resulting from increased destruction of red blood cells, and therefore it is excreted by the kidney. This is seen in extensive burns and hemolytic anemia. Normal range: a few red blood cells may be seen per high power field. In the female, blood due to menstrual flow may be found. A catheterized specimen may contain blood because of urethral bleeding from the trauma of inserting the catheter.

White Blood Cells: White blood cells when found in males or in catheterized specimens from females suggest infection in the urinary tract. Normal range: very few if any white blood cells in the urine of males, although substantial quantities may be found in the urine of females.

Casts: Large numbers of casts in the urine may appear after exercise, glomerulonephritis, various collagen diseases, and in acute tubular necrosis. Normal range: a few casts may be present.

Medical consultation

The dentist has a responsibility to his patients to consult with a physician prior to beginning therapy when there may be a medical risk involved. The decision to consult is based upon the information secured in taking the patient's medical history, findings in the physical examination and results obtained from clinical laboratory studies.

Consultation with the physician is not only

Medical Evaluation

CC and HPI: A 61-year-old woman visited this office with the chief complaint of gingival bleeding and mobile teeth. She gave a history of generalized body aches for three days. She has been diagnosed with diabetes mellitus for five to six years and has taken 45 units of U-80 Lente insulin/day. On the day of admission, she began to notice aching in her joints and extremities. On the previous day, she ran out of her insulin and stopped taking it. She reports polydipsia with a dry mouth and blurring of vision.

PMH: Jaundice as child/History of hypertension

ROS: Occasional swelling of ankles

PE: BP 130/90; P 80; R 20; T 98.8

Impression: Diabetes mellitus/Periodontal disease/Hypertension

Plan: Physician evaluation/Dental treatment/Physician evaluation

Dental Evaluation

CC and HPI: This patient reports that her gums have been bleeding on eating for three months. She states that at times she cannot eat because of this. She also experiences general pain in all of her remaining teeth. She states that several weeks ago she had an "abscess" of one of her teeth drain, and she noticed a small lump under her left mandible.

Head and neck examination: Obesity making palpation of structures difficult.
Left submandibular lymph node (diameter, 0.5 cm) which is freely movable and not tender.

Oral examination: Gingiva exhibits generalized severe inflammation with spontaneous bleeding and sulcular exudates. All remaining teeth are very mobile and carious and exhibit tenderness to percussion.

Formulation: This patient has a very severe case of generalized periodontal disease that affects all of her remaining teeth. Radiologic examination shows almost total bone loss surrounding her remaining teeth, and several teeth show evidence of abscess formation. The tentative treatment is for full-mouth extraction of remaining teeth followed by maxillary and mandibular denture construction. These extractions would be done on an outpatient basis with the use of Xylocaine and epinephrine (1:1,000,000) local anesthetic. This patient should be evaluated as to the status of her diabetes mellitus and hypertension. If the diabetes mellitus cannot be controlled, the current dental infection probably is a contributing factor, and should be coordinated with changes in insulin therapy. Antibiotics would be used after the extractions.

Impression: Severe generalized periodontal disease.

Plan: Extraction of all remaining teeth.
Maxillary and mandibular full denture construction.

Fig. 1-10 Example of data base for medical-dental consultation.

in the patient's best interest, but is educational for both practitioners. The consultation enhances the dentist's knowledge of medical disorders and how they may affect the treatment and management of the dental patient. On the other hand, the physician gains knowledge about the particular dental problem or oral disease. Both practitioners gain a clearer understanding that a patient's general health is important to dental health.

An effective means of communication has to be established between the physician and dentist to insure good patient management. A brief phone call or short note will often not suffice. Because of this, a systematic consultation format should be used which will include all pertinent patient data (Fig. 1-10). This is, in effect, an organized approach for gathering patient information and offering a subsequent diagnosis and treatment.

The medical evaluation portion of the consultation is that information elicited by the dentist when taking the patient's medical history. The physician, upon consultation by the dentist, will provide additional information, especially in the areas of physical examination and results of laboratory studies. It must be understood that the preliminary impression of the diagnosis and plan for treatment included in the medical evaluation is subject to alteration after the physician's evaluation.

The dental evaluation portion of the consultation includes the chief complaint, history of the present illness, a complete head and neck and oral examination. The formulation is a narrative that summarizes pertinent findings as well as the dentist's opinion as to the problem, the differential diagnosis, studies required or therapy indicated. This is where the dentist has an opportunity to educate the physician or vice versa. Last is the impression and plan, which is a list of the problems identified and how the dentist plans to rule out and treat each problem. After reading this, the consulting physician can more readily make recommendations to the dentist regarding the proposed dental therapy. In conclusion, use of the consultation format certainly improves upon communication between physician and dentist and provides better holistic patient care.

References

1. Bates, Barbara. *A Guide to Physical Examination.* Philadelphia: Lippincott, 1974.
2. Brasher, W.J., Rees, T.D. "The Medical Consultation: Its Role in Dentistry." *JADA* 95:961-964.
3. Cottone, J.A., Kafrawy, A.H. "Medications and Health Histories: A Survey of 4,365 Dental Patients." *JADA* 98:713-718.
4. DeGowin, E.L., DeGowin, R.L. *Bedside Diagnostic Examination,* second edition. London: Macmillan Company, 1969.
5. Hendler, B.H., Rose, L.F. "Common Medical Emergencies: A Dilemma in Dental Education." *JADA* 91:575-582.
6. Hooley, James R. *Hospital Dentistry.* Philadelphia: Lea and Febiger, 1970.
7. Kerr, D.A., Ash, M.M., Millard, D.H. *Oral Diagnosis,* Third edition. St. Louis: Mosby, 1970.
8. Little, J.W., King, O.R. "The Significance of Physical Diagnosis, Patient History, Data, and Medical Screening in the Dental Office." *Annals of Dentistry* 3:31, 42-55.
9. McCarthy, F.M. *Emergencies in Dental Practice,* Second edition. Philadelphia: Saunders, 1972.
10. Redding, S.W., Rose, L.F. "The Consultation: A Means of Communication between Dentists and Physicians." *General Dentistry* Sept./Oct. 1979:54-57.
11. Rose, L.F. "Medical History is a Dental Procedure." *Dental Dimensions* January-March 1977:13-18.
12. Rose, L.F. *Diagnosis and Management of Medical Emergencies in the Dental Office.* Senior editor—D. Walter Cohen, D.D.S. University of Pa. School of Dental Medicine, vol. 1, no. 3, 1977.
13. Rose, L.F. "Hospital Dental Practice." *Dental Clinics of North America. Vol. 19, no. 4, October 1975.* Philadelphia: Saunders.
14. Sonis, S.T., Jandinski, J.J. "Physical and Laboratory Diagnosis." *Dental Clinics of North America* vol. 18, no. 1, January 1974. Philadelphia: Saunders.
15. Vazuka, F.A. *Essentials of the Neurological Examination.* Philadelphia: Smith, Kline and French Laboratories, 1968.
16. Wasserman, B.S. "Teaching Physical Evaluation and Physical Diagnosis in a Hospital Setting." *JADA* 95:103-105.
17. Zambito, R.F. *Hospital Dental Practice, A Manual.* New York: Medical Examination Publishing, 1978.

Chapter 2

Vital Signs and Monitoring

James T. Amsterdam, D.M.D., M.D.

Introduction

Whether one is performing a physical evaluation or a complete physical examination, the procedure of taking and recording vital signs is always completed first. The definition of vital signs includes an overall impression of the patient's appearance (inspection) and report of the patient's height and weight, temperature, pulse, blood pressure and respiratory rate. The weight should be converted to kilograms for calculation of drug dosage and recorded in a prominent place on the patient's chart. When obtaining the above information, any change in the patient's weight should be noted and correlated with both the patient's appearance and other aspects of the history and physical examination.

In medical practice, body temperature is usually recorded. This is probably unnecessary under normal circumstances in dental practice with the exception of patients who are present with infection, lymphadenopathy or history and physical consistent with a possible malignancy. As a routine procedure for an initial visit, the patient's pulse, blood pressure and respiratory rate must be recorded. This information should be updated every six months during standard dental care, but may be repeated more frequently according to clinical situations such as patients undergoing sedation (I.V. and/or inhalation) or known hypertensives who are difficult to control or unreliable.

Appearance

It is most helpful to observe a patient walk into a consultation room or operatory rather than seeing a patient for the first time fully draped. Is the patient neat and clean or unkempt? The latter may be secondary to organic disease, e.g., organic brain syndrome, ethanol or other drug addiction, or parietal lobe lesions with characteristic inattention to one side of the body. An unkempt appearance may also be functional, e.g., severe depression. Is the patient's dress appropriate? Heavy clothing in a rather warm atmosphere might suggest hypothyroidism, while light clothing in the winter might suggest hyperthyroidism.

Height and weight

Any disparity in a patient's reported height and weight can be evaluated by checking these values on various published tables (Fig 2-1). For pediatric patients, height and weight can be plotted on growth curves so that significant deviations can be noted (Fig. 2-2). Any unexplained gain or loss in weight should be elaborated upon by additional questioning concerning dietary habits and appetite and investigated further.

Vital signs: *Temperature*

Normal body temperature orally ranges from 97°F to 99°F. Rectal temperatures

Height (in shoes)	Weight in pounds (in indoor clothing)		
	Small frame	Medium frame	Large frame
5′ 2″	112-120	118-129	126-141
3″	115-123	121-133	129-144
4″	118-126	124-136	132-148
5″	121-129	127-139	135-152
6″	124-133	130-143	138-156
7″	128-137	134-147	142-161
8″	132-141	138-152	147-166
9″	136-145	142-156	151-170
10″	140-150	146-160	155-174
11″	144-154	150-165	159-179
6′ 0″	148-158	154-170	164-184
1″	152-162	158-175	168-189
2″	156-167	162-180	173-194
3″	160-171	167-185	178-199
4″	164-175	172-190	182-204

Fig. 2-1 Desirable weights for men according to height and frame: Age 25 and over.

which are more accurate are usually one degree higher than adequate oral temperatures. Axillary temperature might also be used and is a convenient method for approximating body temperature during an office procedure. Since oral temperatures will most often be used in an office setting, several minor precautions are advised. The patients should abstain from hot or cold beverages for ten minutes and they should be able to keep their mouths closed while the temperature is recording (for a minimum of two minutes). Excessively high or low temperatures which are inappropriate for the patient's clinical state should be reperformed under constant supervision in case the patient is meandering. Specific emergencies resulting from extreme changes in body temperature are:

Hypothermia: Most likely encountered during long anesthetic procedures especially with pediatric patients. This situation is usually preventable and treated by use of a controlled thermal blanket beneath the patient, blankets on the patient and an environment in the operatory that is not excessively cold.

Hyperthermia: Best avoided by careful medical history including family history of difficulties with general anesthetic procedures. This entity is preventable by careful monitoring of the patient's temperature during anesthetic procedures with rapid institution of measures to prevent and treat hyperthermia if it occurs: 1) cooling the patient, e.g., alcohol rub, ice blanket, 2) reversing hypoxia and acid-base disturbance by increasing 0_2 concentration (100%) and hyperventilation to eliminate CO_2 generated by the acidosis, 3) pharmacologic therapy, e.g., chlorpromazine, sodium bicarbonate, dantrolene sodium, 4)

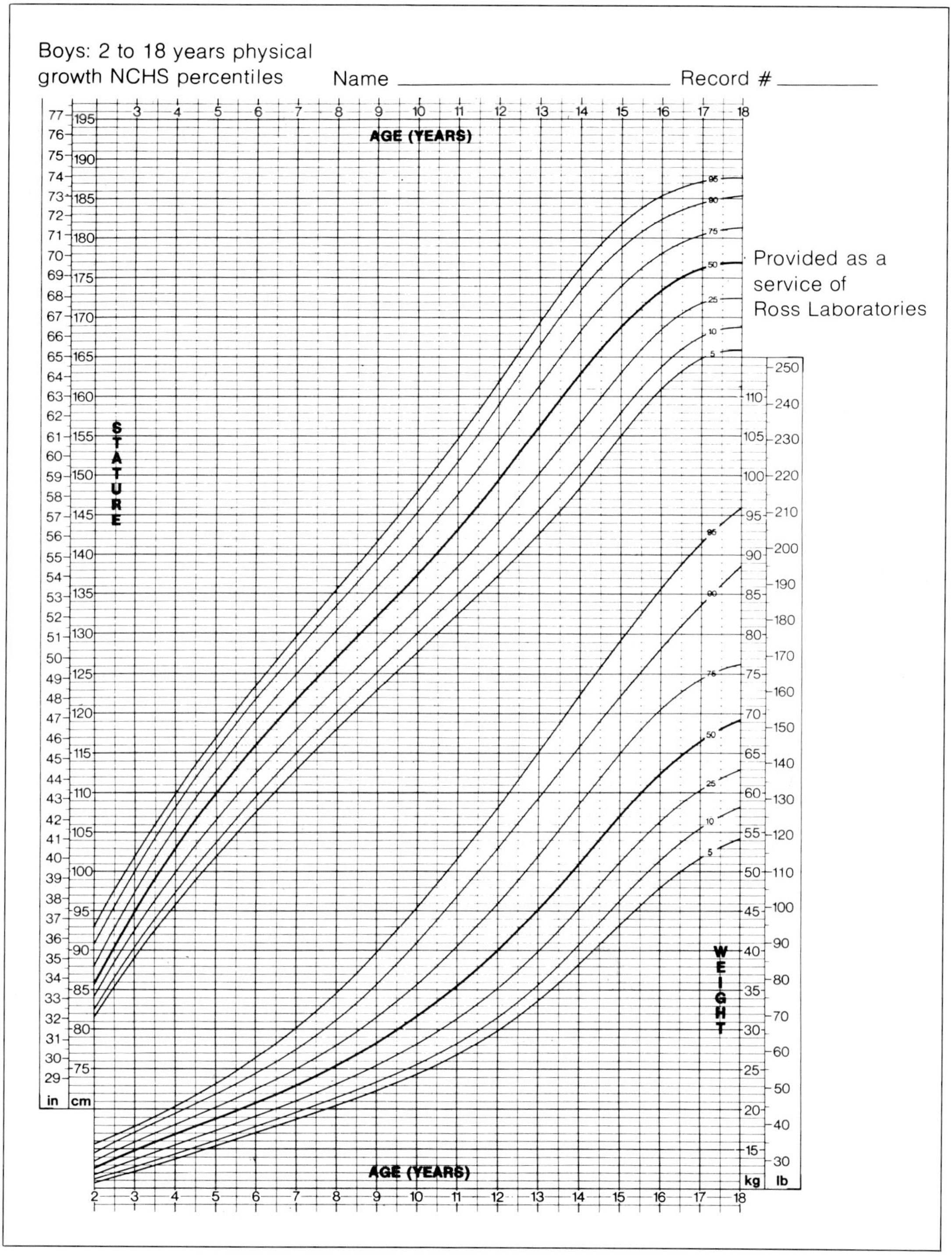

Fig. 2-2 Pediatric growth chart.

volume replacement to correct hypotension secondary to hyperthermia and dehydration, and 5) steroids. Hyperthermia is one of the most dreaded anesthetic emergencies and its prognosis extremely poor, especially in a non-hospital environment.

Vital signs: *Respiration*

The patient's respiratory rate is routinely recorded after a sufficient rest interval. Normal respiratory rate ranges from 14-20 breaths per minute in the adult and is usually slightly higher in children. It is important to note the character of the respirations: shallow, deep, stridorous, or labored. Shallow and slow respiratory rate should raise suspicion of respiratory depression secondary to sedative drugs. Rapid respiratory rate is usually secondary to a combination of anxiety and/or pain; a suspicion of the hyperventilation syndrome is easily confirmed by inspection of the patient and verbal confirmation of lightheadedness, circumoral and distal extremity paresthesis (especially the fingers). Respiratory depression is treated by drug reversal or assisted ventilation and hyperventilation by verbal reassurance and/or rebreathing through a bag as discussed in more detail later in this text.

Vital signs: *Pulse*

Perhaps the most classic of all the recorded vital signs is the arterial pulse. Information determined from an arterial pulse contributes to an understanding of the character of the circulation; the arterial blood pressure measures the quality and effectiveness of the circulation (cardiac output). For routine pulse determination the *radial* pulse is adequate; this pulse is best detected by depression of the radial artery of the wrist with the pads of the index and middle fingers. However, in an emergency situation, especially involving shock and/or impending cardiopulmonary arrest, the dental team should be familiar with other pulse locations which are easier to locate and more accurate:

1. *Carotid Artery:* Only one carotid artery should be examined at a time. The artery must be examined with gentle pressure, since active stimulation of the carotid sinus under emergency conditions can result in decrease in pulse and blood pressure perhaps compounding existing hypotension and/or arrhythmias. This pulse gives the most accurate information regarding the nature of the cardiac output. Locate the carotid by placing the index and middle fingers on the trachea, sliding them laterally until locating the medial aspect of the sternocloidomastoid muscle and applying gentle pressure (Fig. 2-3).
2. *Brachial Artery:* The brachial artery is located by palpation of the medial aspect of the antecubital fossa (routinely done during determination of the arterial blood pressure) (Fig. 2-4).
3. *Femoral Artery:* This is the artery most frequently palpated during CPR to determine effectiveness of chest compressions, since the artery is easily found, very accessible during CPR, and may be continuously palpated with any degree of pressure, and may be palpated simultaneously with no danger to the patient. Locate the femoral artery by palpating the anterior superior iliac crest (point a), the pubic symphysis on the same side (point b), and palpating in the center of the line connecting points a and b, to locate the pulse (Fig. 2-5).

Once the arterial pulse has been located the following information should be noted:

1. Rate and Rhythm
   —Normal Rate 60-100 per minute
   —Slow Rate (Bradycardia) less than 60
   —Fast Rate (Tachycardia) 100-160

Is the pulse regular (a constant or rela-

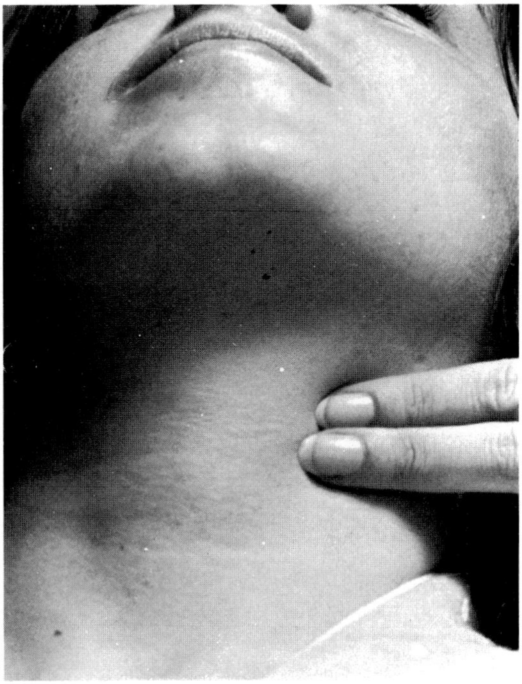

Fig. 2-3 Carotid pulse—in locating the carotid pulse, the thyroid cartilage is first palpated; the fingers are then brought laterally to the medial aspect of the sternocloidomastoid muscle; gentle pressure is applied.

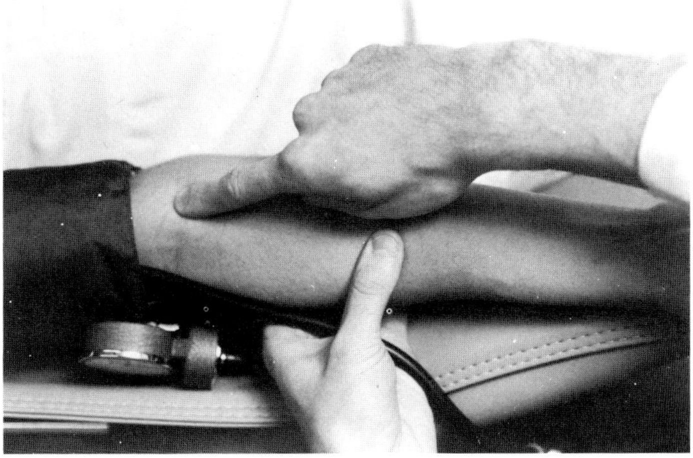

Fig. 2-4 Brachial pulse.

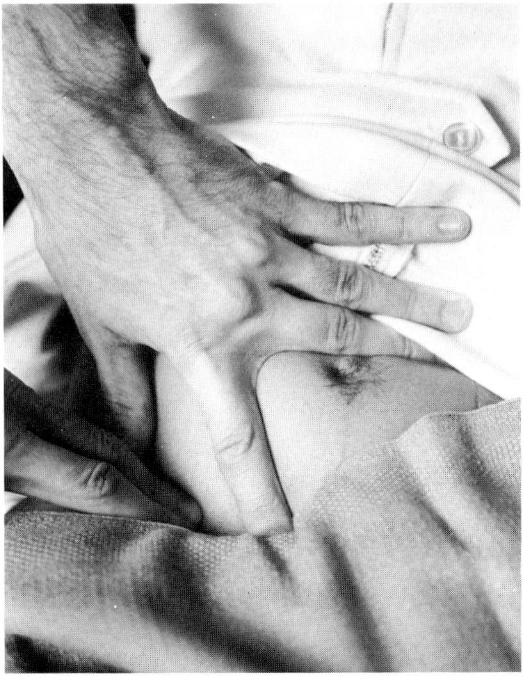

Fig. 2-5 Femoral pulse—the forefinger palpates the pubic symphysis while the thumb palpates the anterior superior iliac crest. The pulse is located at the midpoint of the line connecting these two points.

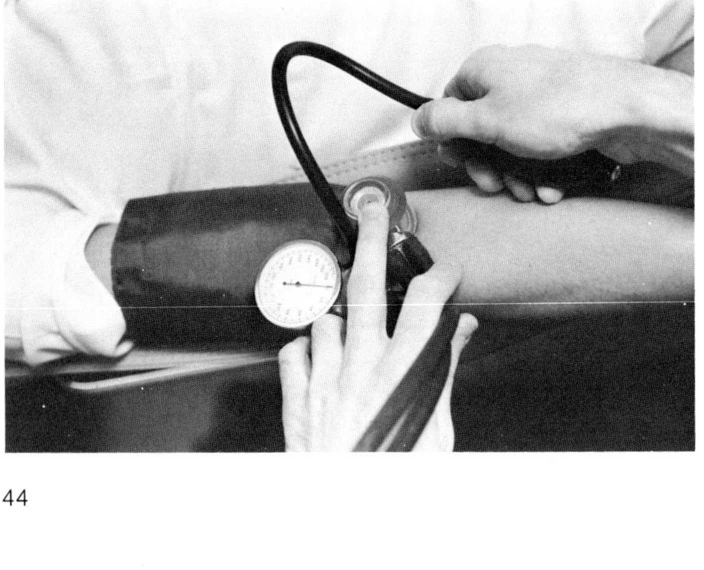

Fig. 2-6 Blood pressure measurement (See text).

tively constant time interval between pulsations) or irregular? If irregular, is the pulse predictably irregular, e.g., two normal beats then a delay, (regularly irregular) or is the pulse totally and unpredictably irregular with no consistent pattern (irregular-irregular) such as occurs in atrial fibrillation (see arrythmias section below). Irregularities in pulse warrant auscultation of the heart and a rhythm strip from a cardiac monitor, if available.

2. Amplitude and contour (speed of upstroke, peak duration, and nature of collapse)
   a) Large and Bounding
      —High Output States (consider anxiety, pain, exertion, fever, anemia, and hyperthyroidism)
      —Aortic Regurgitation (due to rapid runoff of blood) this results in so called "pistol-shot" pulse and may result in actual head bobbing by the patient).
   b) Slow Upstroke (aortic stenosis)

3. Alteration in amplitude with beats
   —Pulsus Alternans (pulse alternates from high and low amplitude from beat to beat and is found in left sided heart failure).

While considering arterial pulse, mention should be made of venous pulse. Neck veins are routinely examined during physical examination. Distention of the internal jugular veins, with the patient seated at 45° and pulsation of this vessel independent of the carotid pulse, is highly suspicious of increased right sided filling pressure of the heart secondary to congestive heart failure or compression of the vena cava. (See physical examination.)

Vital signs: *Blood Pressure*

Blood pressure is measured routinely using a sphygmomanometer which is available in two different types: aneroid or mercury. Both types give accurate recordings and should be calibrated on a periodic basis (yearly). In order to obtain an accurate and reproducible pressure the proper size cuff for the limb to be used (usually upper arm) must be selected. The guidelines are that the cuff should be 20 per cent wider than the diameter of the limb and should be able to fully encircle the limb. Inflated cuffs should not unravel.

Technique: The patient should be sitting and comfortable; the arm should be free of constrictive clothing. (Note: patients should be requested not to wear constrictive clothing to any appointment, especially for sedation procedures, since this makes access for monitoring difficult). Prior to recording blood pressure patients should have sufficient time to relax. Abnormal vital signs recorded by an auxiliary should always be reconfirmed by the dentist.

The arm should be gently flexed and maintained (antecubital fossa) at heart level. The appropriately sized cuff is centered above the brachial artery 2.5-3 cm above the antecubital fossa and wrapped and secured around the arm. The cuff is inflated 30-40 mm Hg above the point at which the palpable radial pulse disappears; while continuing to palpate the pulse the cuff is deflated and the point at which the pulse is felt is the palpable systolic pressure. This procedure avoids the mistake of beginning to listen for a systolic pressure during an auscultatory gap (see below).

The stethoscope is now placed gently at the point of maximal pulsation of the brachial artery, touching nothing by skin. The cuff is then reinflated 30-40 mm Hg above the palpable systolic pressure. The cuff is slowly deflated approximately 3 mm Hg/sec; the point at which the first beat (first Korotkoff sound) is heard is the systolic pressure. These sounds will continue to become louder from turbulent flow and then become muffled. The point of muffled sound is the diastolic pressure; some also record a further point at which all sounds

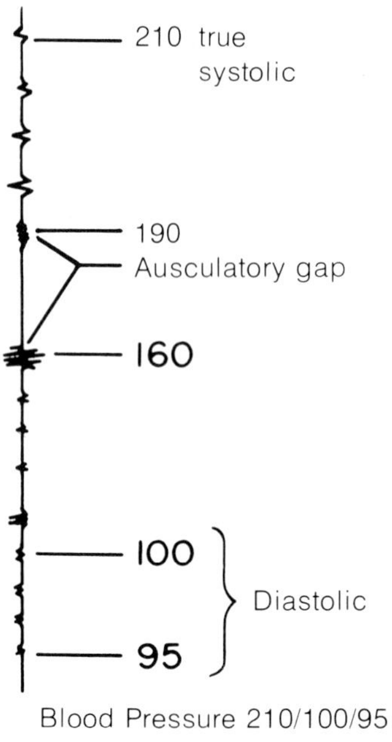

Fig. 2-7 The ausculatory gap: in the region of 190 to 160 no pulse can be ausculated; failure to initially pump the cuff to a pressure beyond the beginning of the gap will result in the recording of falsely low pressures.

disappear. Therefore, a patient's blood pressure might be recorded as 135/70 or 135/70/65 (Fig. 2-6).

Special considerations

Several errors in the recording of blood pressure are common:

1. *Inaccurate Calibration:* Use of equipment that is not properly calibrated results in erroneous readings (high or low).
2. *Improper Cuff Application:* Loose cuffs result in high readings. It should be possible to place two fingers under a properly placed cuff.
3. *Improper Cuff Size:* This is a frequent problem since most offices do not have multiple cuff sizes. Too small a cuff results in erroneously high blood pressure recording. Standard armamentarium should include an average pediatric, average adult and obesity (thigh) cuff.
4. *The Auscultatory Gap:* Many patients, especially hypertensive patients, have a pronounced auscultatory gap. This gap is defined by a loss of Korotkoff sounds between systolic and diastolic pressure which reappear prior to diastole (Fig. 2-7). The problem here is clear. If one failed to estimate the palpable systolic pressure in a patient, for example 200 mm Hg, who had an auscultatory gap in the range of 190-170, arbitrary inflation of the cuff to 180 would result in hearing the first sound around 170 mm Hg. Therefore, 170 mm Hg would be recorded as the systolic pressure which in reality was 200 mm Hg. This problem becomes more significant as pressures go higher, and the consequences of this error become potentially more serious accordingly. The

simple procedure of determining a palpable pressure and then reinflating the cuff 30-40 mm above this level prior to listening avoids this problem.

5. *Diagnosis:* No patient is judged as a hypertensive patient based on one blood pressure recording. It is true that anxiety and pain may elevate pressure and a general rule allows for a 20-30 mm Hg rise in systolic and 5-10 mm Hg in diastolic to be attributed to this cause. Abnormal recording should be confirmed with the patient's physician. For example, a pressure of 170/100 may be high for a patient, but consultation with the physician may reveal that this is the best level the patient has ever reached under antihypertensive therapy. Known hypertensives in addition to bringing a current list of all medications with them for a dental visit, should also present their last blood pressure recording at the physician's office if possible. This is a good reference source for comparison of the value obtained in the dental office at the present appointment.

Monitoring

With advancing modern technology the list of electronic monitoring equipment is endless. However, due to cost, the most sophisticated equipment is usually found in the hospital setting. Therefore, if a patient requires very sophisticated monitoring equipment for safe dental treatment, then treatment in the hospital is desirable. The following is a presentation of practical monitoring equipment for the dental office or hospital dental center. Examples of equipment are illustrative only. One should always compare competitive items and choose the unit which is the best for the price both in terms of quality and ease of operation.

Central nervous system

Monitoring of the central nervous system is based on observation. From initial physical evaluation the dentist should have a record of the patient's cranial nerve function with special attention to the size, equality and reactivity of the pupils and extraocular muscle function. This system is easily monitored during anesthesia or CPR by observation of the pupils and their reactivity to a light. Under conditions of depolarizing and non-depolarizing muscle blockers some find the use of electronic muscle stimulators to be helpful in determining degree of blockade; however, most anesthesiologists find these units useful only on occasion.

Temperature: It can be monitored by use of the glass thermometer or portable electronic thermometer with disposable sheaths (which cover removable leads for oral or rectal use). Both of these thermometers are cumbersome during anesthetic procedures and an electronic unit is available for continuous temperature monitoring via leads placed rectally, nasally, esophageally and now in some cases via a tympanic membrane electrode (Fig 2-8). Many now find a disposable thermosensor strip taped to the forehead to be useful for routine temperature monitoring (Fig. 2-9).

Cardiopulmonary system

Heart and Breath Sounds: One of the least expensive yet most valuable monitoring devices is the precordial or esophageal stethoscope with a single custom-fitted earmold. The precordial stethoscope when placed above the left nipple or the esophogeal attachment (used only in the anesthetized patient) enables the anesthetist to hear both heart and breath sounds simultaneously; the esophogeal component has the advantage of transmitting early sounds reflecting swallowing activity which is especially useful when neuromuscular block-

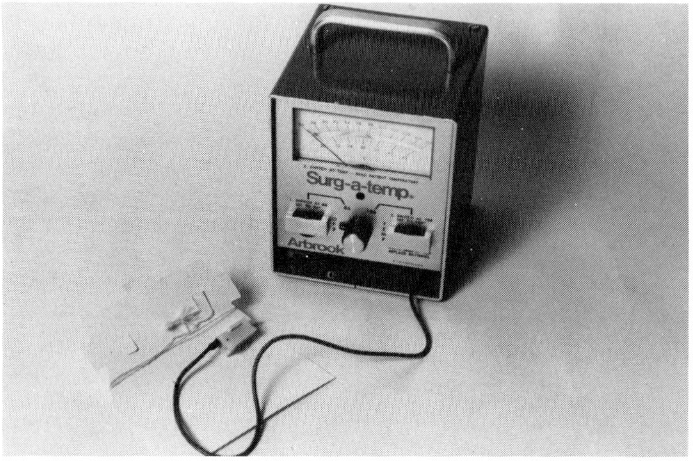

Fig. 2-8 Electronic thermometer: tympanic membrane probe is attached.

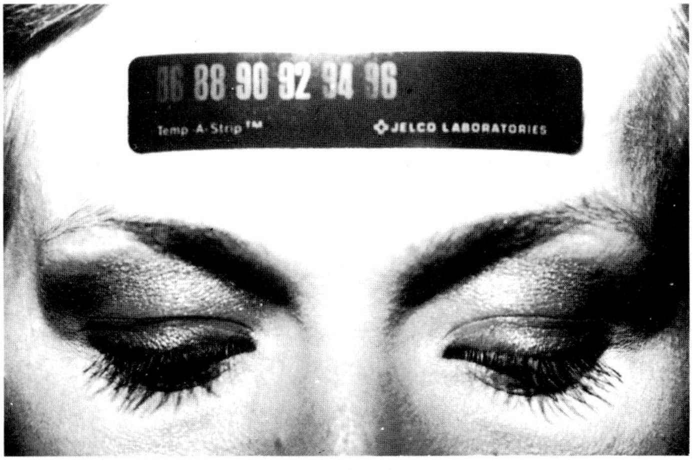

Fig. 2-9 Thermosensor strip.

ers are employed (Fig. 2-10 and 2-11). Even in the presence of a cardiac monitor beeping loudly with a normal rhythm pattern, one must still listen for heart sounds. A condition of electromechanical dissocation is possible in which there is conduction of the electronic impulse within the heart but no corresponding myocardial contraction and zero cardiac output. Under conditions of endotracheal intubation and/or when the patient is covered with drapes, inspection of chest movement is difficult; therefore, it is best to hear breath sounds. The monaural feature of this stethoscope is both comfortable to wear for long periods of time and allows the wearer to hear other activity occuring in the operatory.

Arterial blood gas

The quality of the cardiopulmonary system's capacity to carry and deliver oxygen to the tissues and to eliminate CO_2, is best monitored by an arterial blood gas. This test determines pH, O_2 saturation, Hemoglobin level, pO_2, pCO_2, HCO_3 and base deficit or excess. This equipment is found only in the hospital environment. It should be added that management of an acid/

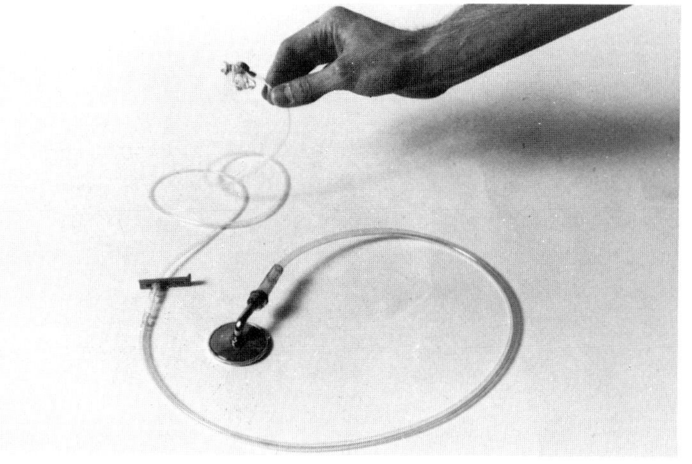

Fig. 2-10 Monaural pre-cordial stethoscope.

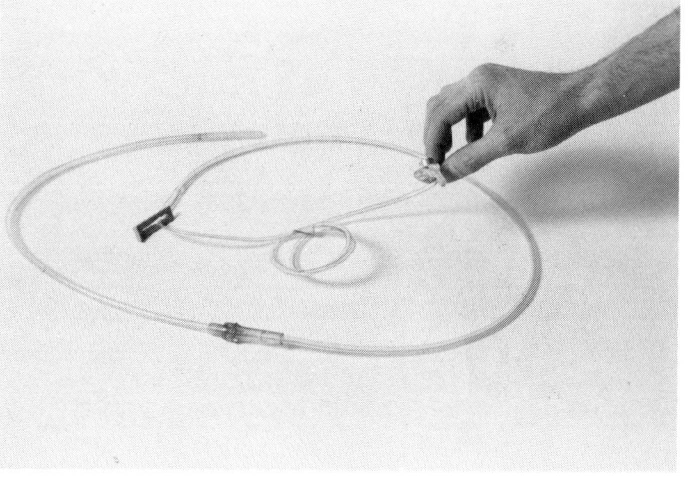

Fig. 2-11 Esophageal stethoscope with monaural earpiece (unconscious patients only).

base disturbance such as the patient with hyperthermia or one undergoing advanced cardiac life support (CPR) can only be accomplished with the information obtained from this study.

Pulse

Pulse can be monitored manually in the manner described above or with an electronic pulse meter. Pulse meters work by an electric eye principle. The pulsation of arterial blood interrupts the beam, creating a beep and rate is registered on a meter.

This unit has two disadvantages. First, the audible tone is frequently masked by high speed handpieces and suction. In addition, under conditions of hypotension and shock, the peripheral circulation may shut down making the device of little help.

Blood pressure

Blood pressure can be manually recorded in the manner described above. A convenient technique for serial monitoring used in the operating room is to tape the dia-

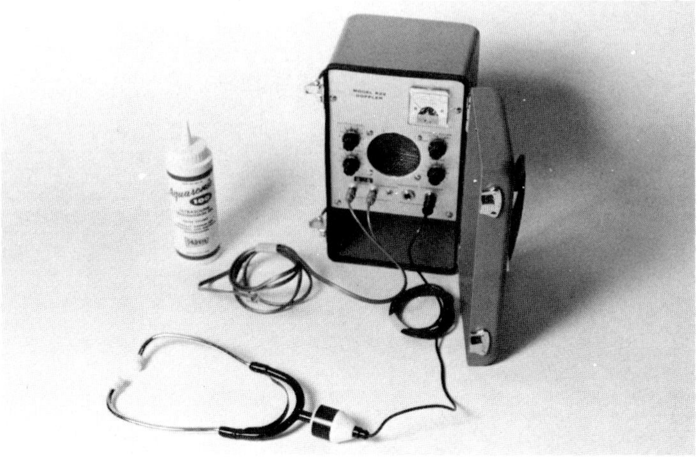

Fig. 2-12 Electronic doppler stethoscope.

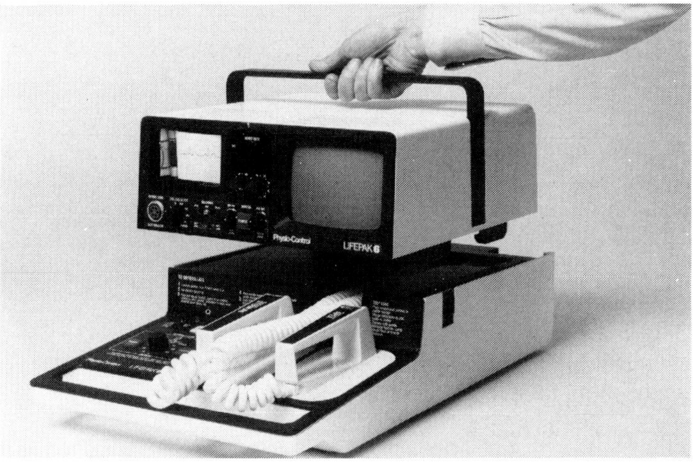

Fig. 2-13 Monitor—DC defibrillator. The monitor is detachable from the defibrillator. The defibrillator is equipped with "quick-look" paddles so that the EKG can be read from the paddles themselves.
Courtesy of Physio-Control Corp., Redmont, WA 98052

phragm of an extra long stethoscope in place over the brachial artery; this eliminates fishing under drapes during a procedure. It is also possible to connect the B.P. stethoscope to the precordial tubing by means of a three-way stop-cock. The stopcock is manually turned to hear either the Korotkoff sounds or heart and breath sounds. A more elaborate system is available utilizing the Ploss automatic switch valve. In this system, the valve automatically switches to the blood pressure when the cuff is inflated and returns to the precordial component when the cuff is fully deflated.

A variety of electronic devices are available which automatically inflate the blood pressure cuff and record both systolic and diastolic pressures; some work on a time setting so that the frequency for recording can be preset. Perhaps a more useful system for the dental office is a manually controlled device with blinking light and/or beep tone which signals each Korotkoff sound. These systems are valuable in the dental setting where Korotkoff sounds normally heard by the human ear are difficult to appreciate due to the extraneous noise of a handpiece or suction.

With the improvement in ultrasound tech-

nology, Doppler devices are available for the recording of blood pressures. These are especially useful for very young patients, older patients or diabetic patients with advanced atherosclerotic disease in whom reliable Korotkoff sounds are difficult if not impossible to hear (Fig. 2-12).
Any of the electronic sphygmomanometers require meticulous placement of a microphone over the brachial artery for accurate determination. These instruments (other than the Doppler) should have their readings confirmed by conventional techniques. Under emergency conditions, conventional techniques are best.

Cardiac monitors

Patients undergoing sedation or general anesthetic procedures, whether in-patient or out-patient, should be monitored routinely on an electrocardioscope. Patients with a past history of heart disease (coronary artery disease) or history of arrhythmias might also be monitored during routine dental care.
Electrocardiography in the dental office is becoming more practical, since recording units are more compact, simple to use, and well shielded against electronic interferences. For Advanced Cardiac Life Support, monitor-defibrillator combinations are also available. The most desirable system consists of a monitor-defibrillator system, with an EKG recording strip built into the unit, and with a quick-look feature so that an EKG can be read through the defibrillator paddles. The monitor can be detached from the defibrillator and used independently (Fig. 2-13). It should be noted that monitors are used for the detection and treatment of arrhythmias not for the diagnosis of infarction or ischemia; therefore, 12-lead EKG capability is not essential.

Dysrhythmia recognition

A complete discussion of electrocardiography and the arrhythmias is beyond the scope of this book. This material should be reviewed in a standard textbook on the subject. The reader is advised to participate in an Advanced Cardiac Life Support (ACLS) course to gain skills in interpretation of arrhythmias. As a quick reference, the ACLS section on electrocardiography and dysrhythmia recognition will now be reviewed.

Electrocardiogram

Normal conduction in the heart is initiated in the sinoatrial (SA) node in the right atrium and spreads through the atria; the depolarization of the atria results in a P wave on the EKG. The impulse proceeds to the atrioventricular node (AV) where conduction is slowed, subsequently entering the bundle of His. Here the impulse is directed down the right bundle branch through the right ventricle in the Purkinje system. The left bundle branch divides into anterior and posterior branches for activation of the left ventricle. Polarization of the ventricles results in the QRS complex and their repolarization is the T wave. A U wave after the T wave is possible usually under circumstances of digitalis toxicity, electrolyte imbalance, and premature ventricular contractions (Fig. 2-14).
The normal PR interval should not be greater than .21 seconds (measured from the beginning of the P to the beginning of the Q), just greater than five smal! squares on the EKG graph paper (one square = .04 sec.). A normal QRS complex is no greater than .10 seconds. Abnormalities in the SA node, ectopic atrial pacemaker AV node disturbances, and intraventricular conduction abnormalities, including ectopic ventricular pacemakers, all result in a variety of important arrhythmias.
These arrhythmias are frequently lethal especially in the presence of myocardial infarction.
By convention, conduction traveling toward a positive electrode results in upward deflection on the EKG. There are four con-

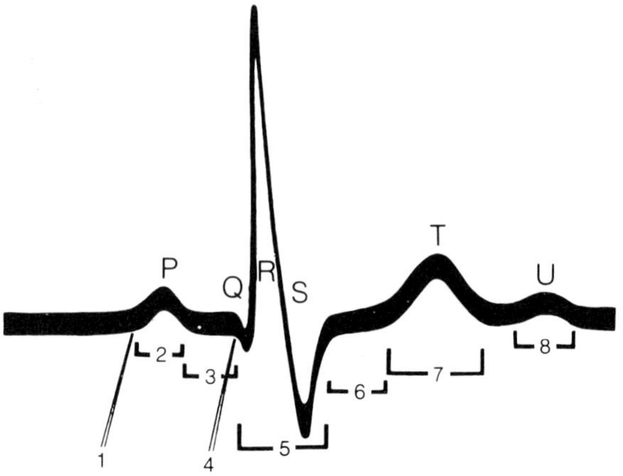

Sequential Electrical Events of the Cardiac Cycle	Electrocardiographic Representation
1. Impulse from the sinus node	Not visible
2. Depolarization of the atria	P wave
3. Depolarization of the A-V node	Isolectric
4. Repolarization of the atria	Usually obscured by the QRS complex
5. Depolarization of the ventricles	QRS complex
a. intraventricular septum	a. initial portion
b. right and left ventricles	b. central and terminal portions
6. Activated state of the ventricles immediately after depolarization	ST segment: isoelectric
7. Repolarization of the ventricles	T wave
8. After-potentials following repolarization of the ventricles	U wave

Fig. 2-14 The EKG. (Figs. 2-14—2-28 are courtesy of Phillips and Feeney, The Cardiac Rhythms)

venient leads for monitoring. *Lead 1* (positive below left clavicle and negative below the right), *Lead 2* (positive below the left nipple and negative below right clavicle, *Lead 3* (positive below left nipple and negative below left clavicle), and *MCL$_1$* (positive in the right fourth interspace next to the sternum and the negative near the left shoulder). In all cases, the *ground lead* may be placed below the right pectoral muscle. A good criterion for lead-selection is one which shows distinct P and clear QRS waves. The reader should be able to recognize the following rhythms. The management of arrhythmias will be discussed in the section on cardiovascular emergencies.

Normal Sinus Rhythm (Fig. 2-15)
Rate: 60-100
Rhythm: Regular

Sinus Tachycardia (Fig. 2-16)
Rate: 60-100
Rhythm: Regular
P waves: Precede each QRS complex (may become focal or multifocal)

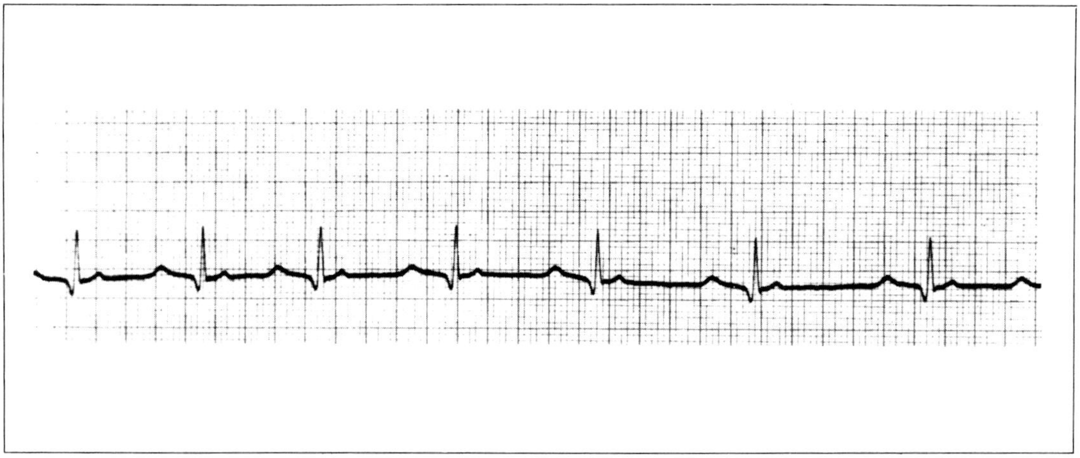

Fig. 2-15 Normal sinus rhythm.

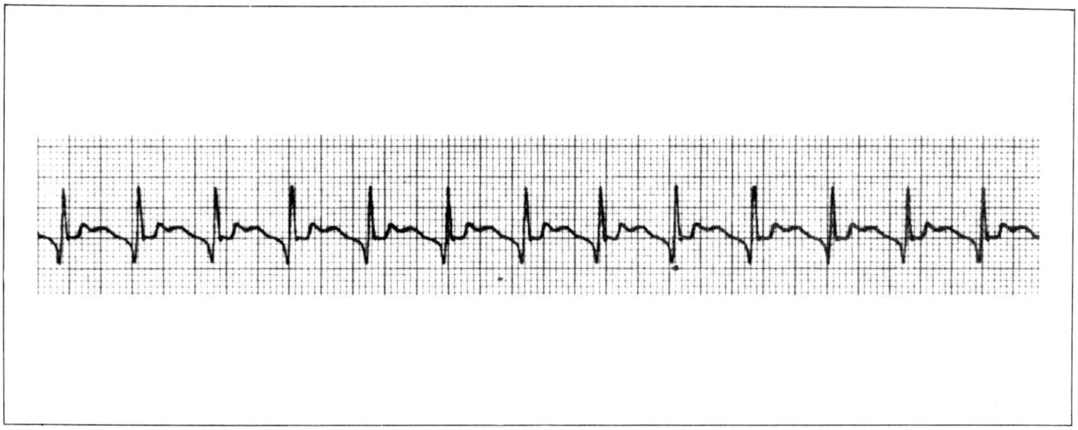

Fig. 2-16 Sinus tachycardia.

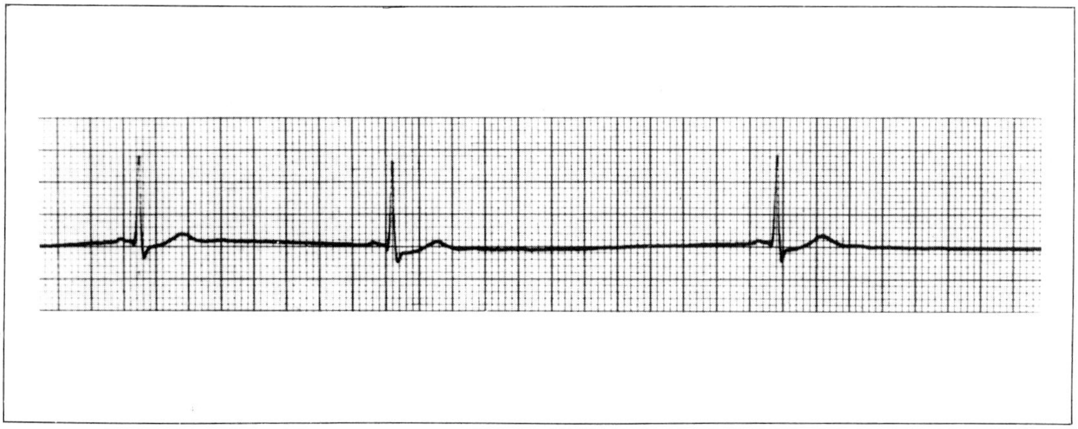

Fig. 2-17 Sinus bradycardia.

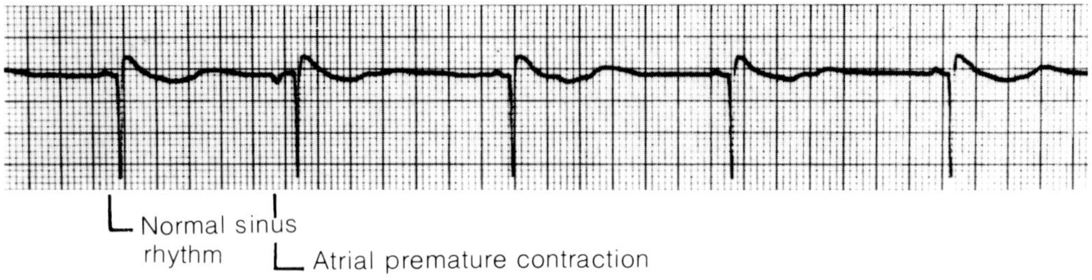

Fig. 2-18 Premature atrial contraction.

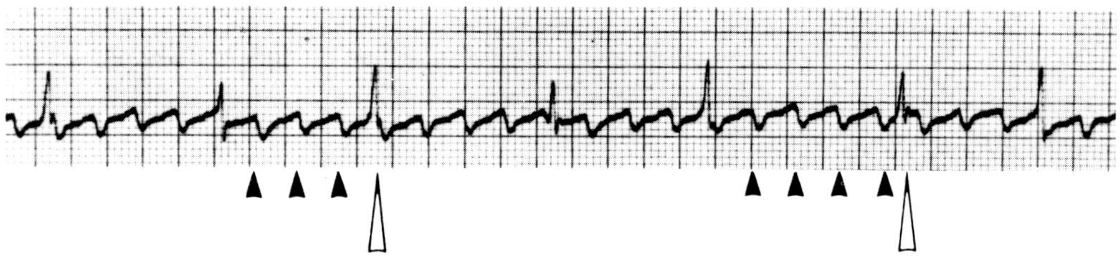

Fig. 2-19 Atrial flutter.

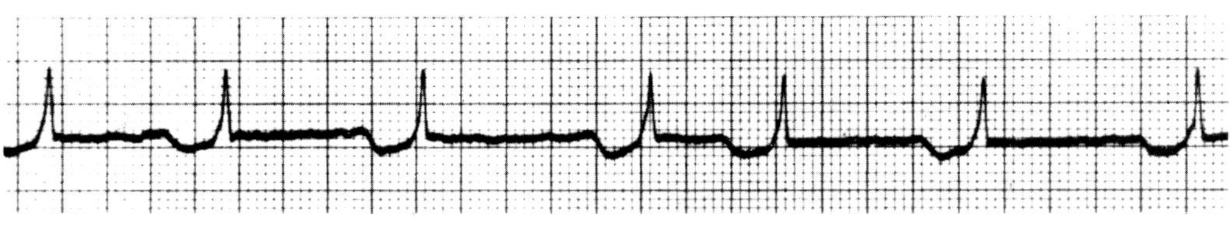

Fig. 2-20 Atrial fibrillation.

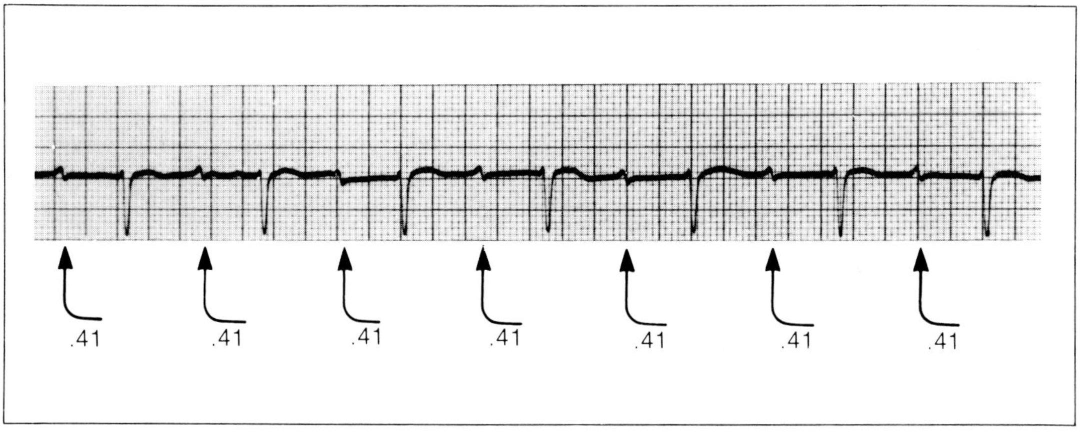

Fig. 2-21 First degree AV block.

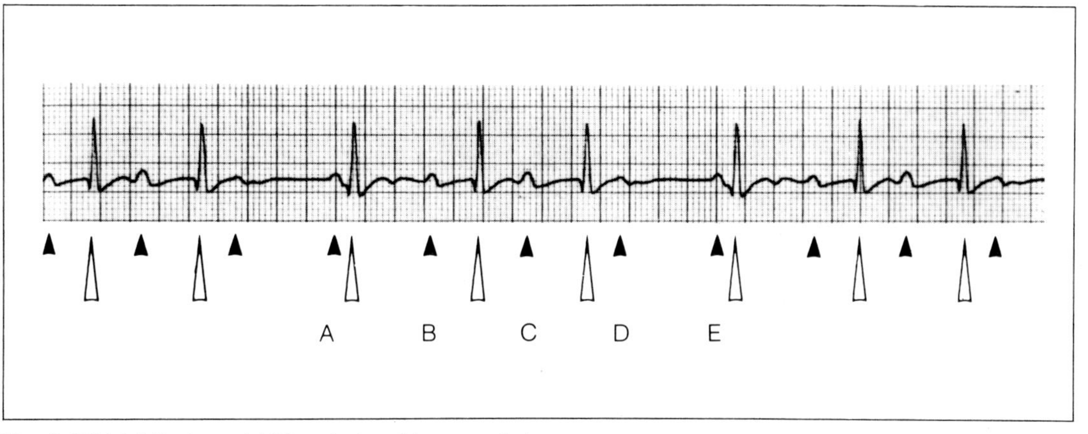

Fig. 2-22 Mobitz type I (Wenckebach) second degree AV block.

Sinus Bradycardia (Fig. 2-17)
Rate: less than 60
Rhythm: Regular

Premature Atrial Contraction (PAC) (Fig. 2-18)
Rate: Depends on number of PAC's
Rhythm: Irregular
P Wave: PAC has different P wave which may be distorted if it crowds the T wave

Atrial Flutter (Fig. 2-19)
Rate: Atrial 240-360
Rhythm: Atrial regular: ventricular response may be regular depending on degree of AV block (eg 2:1 AV conduction) but might also be irregular with 3:1 or 4:1 Av block
P Waves: "Sawtooth" pattern
PR interval: Cannot measure

Atrial Fibrillation (Fig. 2-20)
Rate: Atrial 350-600
Ventricular 100-160
Rhythm: Irregular. Highly irritable atrial focus results in fibrillatory f waves not P waves
PR interval: Not measurable

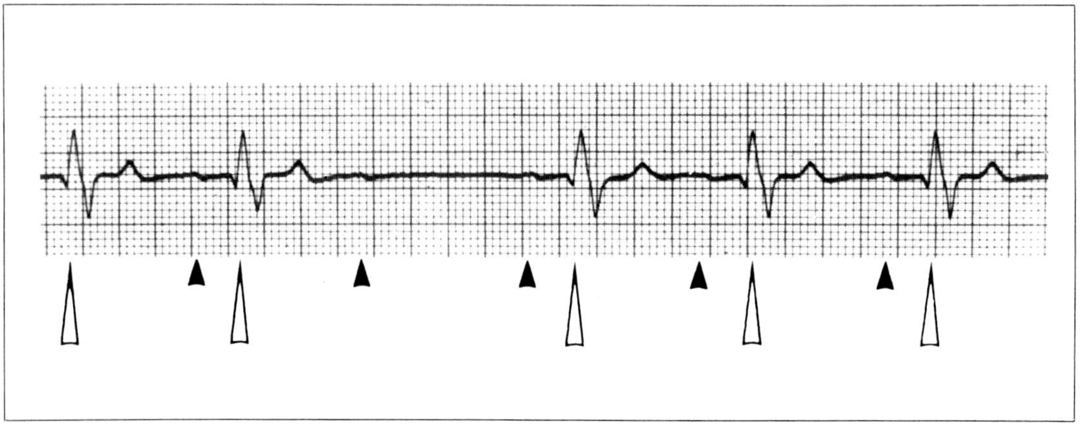

Fig. 2-23 Mobitz type II, second degree AV block.

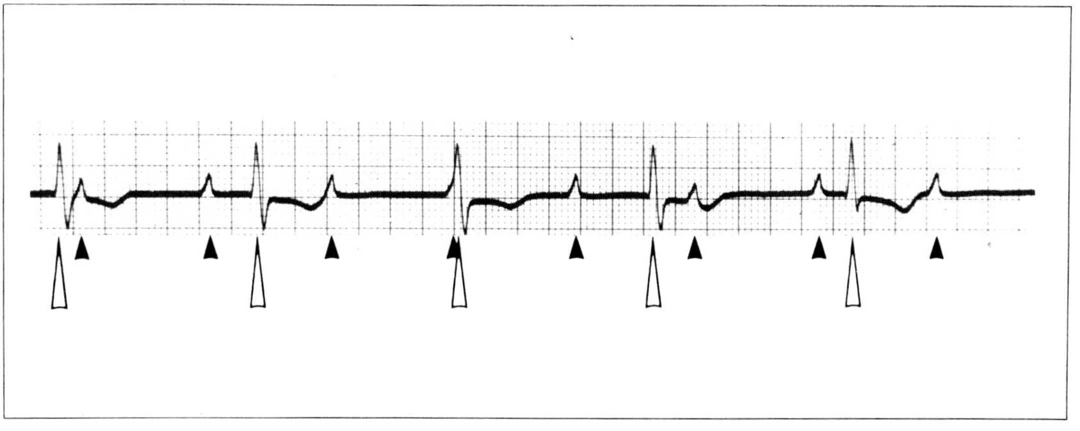

Fig. 2-24 Third degree (complete) AV block.

First Degree AV Block (Fig. 2-21)
Rate: Normal
Rhythm: Regular
P Waves QRS interval: Normal
PR interval: Greater than .21 seconds (but constant). AV Block may be occurring in the atria, AV node, His bundle or bundle branches; the seriousness increases in this same order.

Second-Degree AV Block
Mobitz Type I (Wenckebach) AV Block (Fig. 2-22)
Rate: Atrial—normal
Ventricular—depends on degree of block
Rhythm: Atrial—regular
Ventricular—Variable
P Waves: More than QRS waves
PR Interval: Progressive increase in the PR interval with each complex until a P wave is *not* followed by a QRS

Mobitz Type II AV Block (Fig. 2-23)
Rate: Atrial—Normal
Ventricular—depends on degree of block
Rhythm: Atrial—regular
Ventricular—variable

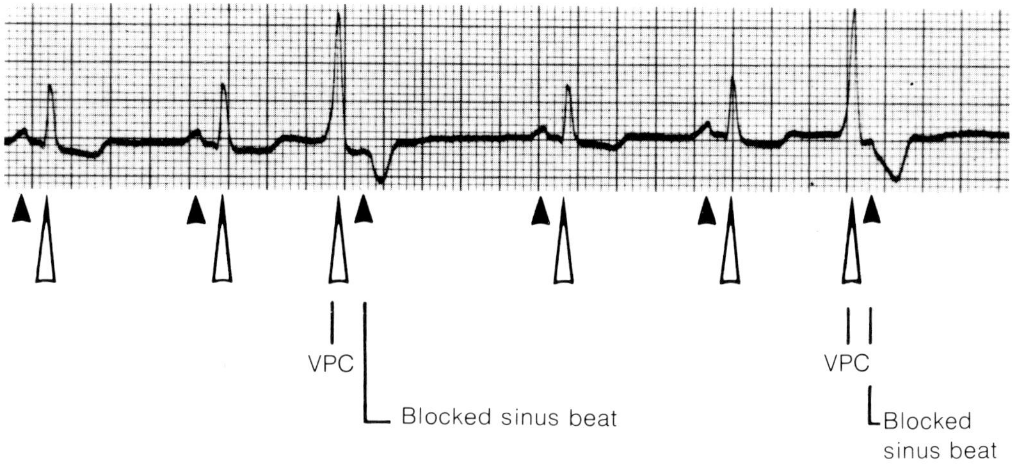

Fig. 2-25 Premature ventricular contraction.

P Waves: More numerous than QRS complexes

PR Interval: (Conducted beats have constant PR interval (which may be prolonged or normal) until a P wave occurs without a QRS. A fixed pattern may occur such as 2:1 or 3:1 etc. of atrial beats and corresponding ventricular response.

Significance: Serious arrhythmia, frequently precedes complete AV Block

Third-Degree (Complete) AV Block (Fig. 2-24)

No atrial impulses reach the ventricles and the two beat independently. This may or may not be symptomatic but is an extremely serious arrhythmia.

Rate: Atrial—normal
Ventricular—30-40

Rhythm: Atrial and ventricular regular but independent of each other

QRS: Normal configuration if ventricular pacemaker is above the bundle of His but will be widened if it occurs from below this bundle.

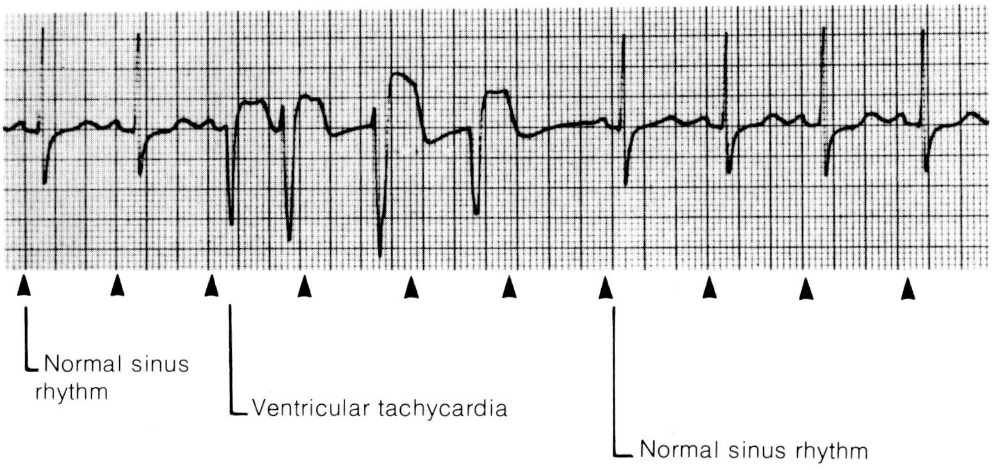

Episode of ventricular tachycardia recorded from a monitoring lead in a patient with suspected acute myocardial infarction.

Fig. 2-26 Ventricular tachycardia.

Premature Ventricular Contractions (Fig. 2-25)

These occur from an ectopic ventricular focus and are frequently followed by a compensatory pause. They may be unifocal or multifocal in nature. Three or more PVC's together constitute a "run" and may dispose to a ventricular tachycardia. PVC's falling on a T wave (R on T) may result in ventricular fibrillation.

Ventricular Tachycardia (Fig. 2-26)

Rate: 100-250
Rhythm: Regular (usually)
P Waves: Obscured
PR Interval: Not measurable
QRS Interval: Greater than .12
Significance: Cardiac output is usually poor if this persists, and usually precedes ventricular fibrillation

Ventricular Fibrillation (Fig. 2-27)

Ventricles quivering with disorganized activity result in no cardiac output, resulting in a lethal state if not corrected.
Rate: Rapid and Bizarre
Rhythm: Irregular
P Waves: Absent
QRS Interval: Oscillating

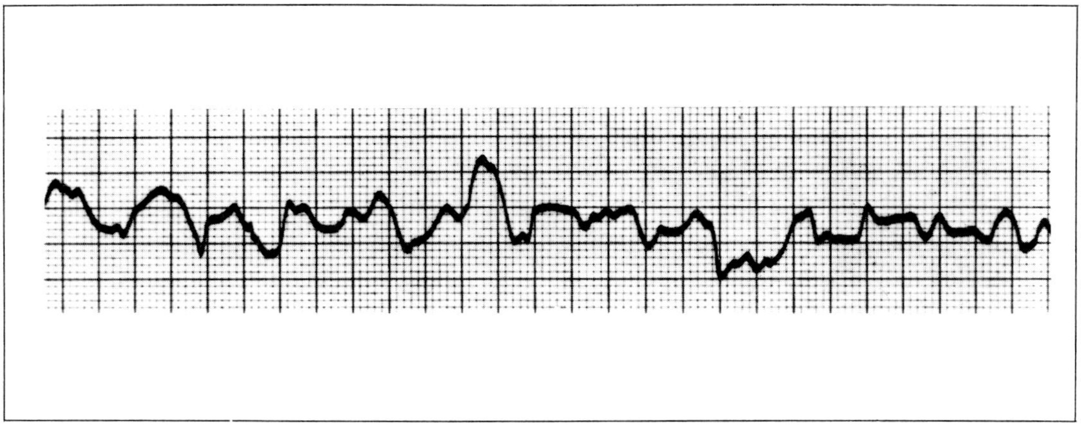

Fig. 2-27 Ventricular fibrillation.

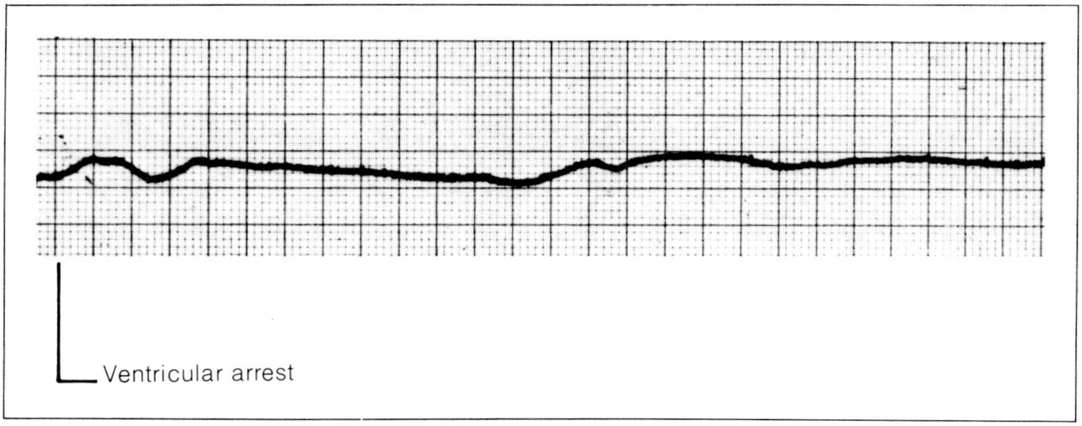

Fig. 2-28 Agonal rhythm and cardiac standstill.

Agonal Rhythm and Cardiac Standstill (Fig. 2-28)

A terminal rhythm resulting in absence of electrical activity in the heart.

Summary

Vital signs are routinely recorded on all patients on their first visit and should be updated. Medically compromised patients may require more frequent vital sign determinations, and patients during sedation or general anesthetic procedures require serial monitoring. There are a vast number of electronic devices available for the recording and serial monitoring of vital signs. An *anesthesia record* is a convenient way to record a patient's history, drug dosage, serial vital signs and the type of monitoring employed (Fig. 2-29).

EKG rhythm strips and other figures in "The Electrocardiogram" section (Fig. 2-14-28) are from the pages indicated in Phillips, Raymond and Feeney, Mary: *The Cardiac Rhythms,* Phila., W. B. Saunders, 1973 by permission of the publisher and author. Photographic reproductions of this material by Mr. David Sullivan, University of Pennsylvania School of Dental Medicine.

MEDICAL COLLEGE OF PENNSYLVANIA
ANESTHESIA RECORD

PRE OPERATIVE DIAGNOSIS

OPERATION PROPOSED

PRE-OPERATIVE SUMMARY

T.	P.	R.	B.P.	AGE	M F	WT.	DENTURES

HGB	HCT.	PRE OP DRUGS	CONSENT	PHYSICAL STATUS	LAST ORAL INTAKE

PREVIOUS ANESTHETICS

TYPE OF ANESTHESIA DISCUSSED WITH PATIENT

PERTINENT PRE OPERATIVE DATA

PREMEDICATION (DRUG, DOSE, TIME)	EFFECT	ALLERGIES

TIME — TOTALS

AGENTS

OTHER

FLUIDS

	°C				
AIRWAY	40°c	200	200	B.P. ∨ ∧
	38	180	180	
TUBE SIZE	36	160	160	PULSE •
MACHINE	34	140	140	START ANES. x
	32	120	120	START OP. ○
MONITOR	30	100	100	END ANES. ⊗
	28	80	80	
VENTILATOR	26	60	60	TEMP. △
	24	40	40	C.V.P. □
RESPIRATION S.C.A		20	20	RESP. —
POSITION OF PATIENT		0	0	

SYMBOLS

IMMEDIATE PRE-ANESTHETIC CHECK LIST COMPLETED ☐
REMARKS:

BEGAN TO WORK WITH PATIENT AT ____________

LEFT PATIENT IN CARE OF RECOVERY ROOM NURSE AT ____________

FLUID SUMMARY

BLOOD LOSS: MEASURED ____________
ESTIMATED ____________
TOTAL ____________
ADMINISTERED: BLOOD ____________
OTHER

OPERATION PERFORMED	POST OPERATIVE DIAGNOSIS

SURGEON	ANESTHESIOLOGIST	DATE OF SURGERY

CHART COPY

Fig. 2-29 The anesthesia record.

References

1. American Heart Association. *Advanced Cardiac Life Support Manual.* 1975.
2. Bates, Barbara, M.D. *A Guide to Physical Examination.* Philadelphia: Lippincott, 1974.
3. Harvey, A., et al. *Principles and Practice of Medicine,* 19th Ed. New York: Appleton-Century—Crofts, 1976.
4. Malamed, S. *Manual of Medical Emergencies in the Dental Office.* St. Louis: Mosby, 1977.
5. McCarthy, F. *Emergencies in Dental Practice.* Philadelphia: Saunders, 1979.
6. Phillips, Raymond E. and Feeney, Mary K. *The Cardiac Rhythms.* Philadelphia: Saunders, 1973.
7. Warner, Howard. ''Therapy of Common Arrhythmias.'' *Medical Clinics of North America* Vol. 58, No. 5, Sept. 1974.

Chapter 3

Basic Methodology of Cardiovascular-Respiratory Support

Jeffrey G. Garber, D.D.S.

Introduction

Life threatening emergencies can and do occur in dental offices. The ability to provide supportive care during these periods of crisis is essential. Over the past several years, organized dentistry has recognized this need and encouraged its membership, under the auspices of the American Heart Association, to attain certification in Basic Life Support as a method of learning to provide emergency cardio-pulmonary care.

Emergency cardio-pulmonary care at a supportive level requires: 1) recognition of an emergency state, 2) assessment of ventilation, 3) establishment of ventilation when necessary, 4) assessment of cardiac function, and 5) establishment of supportive artificial circulation when necessary. From the above sequence, it is obvious that an understanding of both pulmonary and cardiac function is necessary if the technical applications of airway management and circulatory support are to be truly appreciated. It is the aim of this chapter to provide the reader with the physiologic basis of ventilation and cardiac perfusion as it is applied to emergency cardio-pulmonary supportive care. In order to achieve this aim the subjects of ventilation and cardiac perfusion will be subdivided as follows:

Ventilation:

1. Basic considerations of breathing,
2. Pathophysiology of respiratory arrest or insufficiency,
3. Airway management and
4. Adjuncts to airway management.

Cardiac perfusion:

1. Physiology of cardiac compression and
2. Adjuncts for artificial circulation.

Ventilation

Fundamental Considerations of Breathing: Ventilation or respiration may be defined as the process by which oxygen and carbon dioxide are transported in the airways, blood and tissues. Changes in this process are recognized by changes in the rate and depth (volume) of breathing. Control of these changes is dependent on the respiratory center of the medulla; the pH sensitive receptors of the central nervous system which are bathed by the cerebrospinal fluid, whose pH varies in relation to arterial carbon dioxide tension; and the oxygen-sensitive receptors located in the carotid and aortic bodies, that respond to varying levels of arterial oxygen tension. These receptors which control respiration play dominant and lesser roles depending on the homeostasis of the individual. Thus a patient who is narcotized may have a depressed medullary respiratory drive as well as a decreased response to arterial CO_2 changes (pH changes of C.S.F.). Another example is the patient with chronic

obstructive lung disease (C.O.P.D.) whose primary breathing drive is a response to low arterial oxygen tensions, known as the hypoxic drive to breathe.
Respiration may be regarded as having three phases: 1) the gas phase, 2) the blood phase, and 3) the tissue (gas transfer) phase. For each of these phases a variety of factors must be considered if the process is to function normally. Changes in any of these factors will lead to abnormalities in ventilation.

The gas phase:

1. The airways must remain unobstructed and offer low resistance to gas flow.
2. Inspired air should contain an adequate partial pressure of oxygen.
3. The lungs, essentially reservoirs, should have a normal volume, a normal capacity, and normal compliance (flexibility).
4. Alveolar ventilation at the terminal gas exchange unit should maintain arterial Co_2 tension in the normal range. It should be evenly distributed to permit matching with capillary perfusion at the terminal alveoli.

Let us consider as a model the situation of a patient who is semiconscious or unconscious. As consciousness diminishes the possibility of airway obstruction occurs. This obstruction prevents passage of gas exchange from the external source to the internal source (alveoli of the lungs). If this flow of gas (air) is sufficiently obstructed, less and less of the lung gets filled and therefore an increasing area of lung tissue becomes nonfunctional. As less functioning lung is available, less gas is exchanged into the blood phase, hence oxygenation and the removal of CO_2 becomes inadequate.

The blood phase:

1. The arterial oxygen tension must have a concentration of oxygen sufficient to utilize fully the oxygen-carrying capacity of the blood.
2. The hemoglobin level (oxygen-carrying capacity) must be within normal limits.
3. The cardiac output must be normal and appropriately distributed through the lungs.
4. The pulmonary circulation must have a normal volume and distribution in order to permit proper matching of alveolar ventilation with pulmonary capillary perfusion at the terminal alveoli.
5. The chemical environment must be such that the blood has a normal pH, temperature and buffer and electrolyte content.

The tissue phase:

This phase has one basic requirement.

1. The capillaries and tissues must have normal membrane permeability and tissue metabolism for respiratory transfer to occur.

As a part of understanding the respiratory process, it is important to be aware of those factors that are pertinent to the relationship between ventilation and perfusion in the lungs. The lungs in normal function serve as a reservoir area for gas exchange. In other words, the entire gas exchange area of the lungs is not in constant use (i.e., all parts of the lungs are not always ventilated and perfused). The extent to which the lung is used is influenced by the amount of physical activity and by position. Increases in the level of physical activity increase areas of lung both effectively ventilated and perfused. Also effecting ventilation and pulmonary blood flow is position. Dependent portions of the lung receive the greater amount of flow and ventilation during rest, leaving the less dependent areas in reserve.
Since the relationship between ventilation and pulmonary blood flow is so important to normal respiratory function, a basic respiratory exchange unit can be defined as a terminal alveolus and its capillary blood supply. One can then further define a series of normal and abnormal gas exchange units which may exist: 1) The nor-

mal gas exchange units consist of a ventilated alveolus and a perfused capillary supply; 2) A "dead space" exchange unit consisting of a ventilated alveolus but an unperfused capillary supply; 3) A "shunt" exchange unit as a nonventilated alveolus and a perfused capillary supply; and 4) A "silent" exchange unit with a nonventilated alveolus and nonperfused capillary supply (Table 3-1).

With this basic understanding of the respiratory process, some of the factors which occur with respiratory insufficiency or arrest can be examined. Respiration has been defined as the transport of oxygen and carbon dioxide and can therefore define those processes which interfere with this transport as being causative of respiratory insufficiency. These disturbances include: 1) An increase in shunting, 2) An increase in dead space, 3) An increase in the work of breathing, and 4) A decreased oxygen transport in blood.

To understand the above physiological disturbances, it is important to discuss in detail oxygenation, ventilation, and the relationship between ventilation and perfusion. Oxygenation, which involves the transport of oxygen, depends on many factors, such as: 1) inspired oxygen concentration, 2) alveolar ventilation, 3) gaseous diffusion, 4) distribution of ventilation and perfusion, 5) hemoglobin content, and 6) cardiac output—its volume and distribution.

1. Inspired Oxygen Concentration: This is concentration of oxygen which the patient is breathing. In the assesssment of oxygenation, knowledge of this value is imperative. For example: If the arterial oxygen tension is measured at 100 torr, the patient's ability to oxygenate will be normal if room air is the oxygen source and very abnormal if the source is 100% oxygen.
2. Alveolar Ventilation: This is a measure of the amount a patient is breathing and is reported as liters/minute. It is a measure of the tidal volumes and the rate of breathing over a given period of time.

Table 3-1 Normal and abnormal gas exchange units

	Ventilation	Perfusion
1. Normal	Yes	Yes
2. Dead Space	Yes	No
3. Shunt	No	Yes
4. Silent	No	No

3. Gaseous Diffusion: This term relates to the ability of oxygen and carbon dioxide to pass across the membrane of the alveoli into the pulmonary circulation. Any change in the ability to diffuse across this membrane will effect oxygenation.
4. Distribution of Ventilation and Perfusion: To insure adequate matching, the flow of gas and blood must reach the same parts of the lungs.
5. Hemoglobin Content: The amount of hemoglobin in blood. There must be an adequate amount to carry the available oxygen. Very little oxygen is dissolved in blood and therefore hemoglobin is the tool for oxygen transport.
6. Cardiac Output: The heart's output must be sufficient to have an adequate circulating volume in those areas of ventilated lungs for oxygenation to occur.

To assess these factors, a knowledge of arterial oxygen tension (concentration), arterial oxygen content (arterial oxygen tension and oxygen-carrying capacity) and oxygen transport (cardiac output) must be known. Normal values of arterial oxygen tension on room air (O_2 = 21%) are 80-100 mm Hg, while on 100% O_2 they are 610-670 mm Hg.

Arterial oxygen content is usually measured indirectly by measuring the arterial oxygen tension (values previously given) and the hemoglobin content (oxygen-carrying capacity). Normal values for hemoglobin content are: Males 14-18 gm/100ml, Females 12-17 gm/100ml. Oxygen transport is a measure of cardiac output which has a normal value of 5-6 liters/min. Since this is somewhat difficult to measure, the cardiac output is usually assessed as a function of heartrate, arterial blood pressure, urine output, and arterial pH.

Ventilation is defined as the amount (volume) of breathing necessary to maintain a normal arterial carbon dioxide tension (normal Pa_{CO_2} 34-44 mmHg). By measuring the volume of ventilation and the arterial Co_2 tension and comparing these values to predicted values, an assessment of the respiratory state can be obtained.

To properly assess ventilation, both the value of arterial carbon dioxide tension and the value for the minute ventilation must be known. The minute ventilation is derived by measuring tidal volumes and counting breaths for one minute and then multiplying the results. Normally a person will need to ventilate approximately 90 ml/Kg of weight/minute to maintain the arterial carbon dioxide tension within the normal range. Therefore a 70 Kg person will have a 6.3 liter/min minute ventilation. To accomplish this the person will breathe between ten and twenty times per minute. If the same 70 Kg person needs to breathe, for example, two or three times the expected value of his minute ventilation to maintain a normal arterial carbon dioxide tension, then we can say that for some reason ventilation is impaired.

We can also define two ventilatory states:

1. Hyperventilation—overventilation. When the arterial carbon dioxide tension is less than 34 torr.
2. Hypoventilation—underventilation. When the arterial carbon dioxide tension is greater than 44 torr.

The relationship between ventilation and perfusion can be assessed through estimations of the pulmonary shunt and the pulmonary dead space. These aspects are beyond the scope of this text. But it is not hard to understand that as alveolar dead space increases it significantly contributes to pulmonary ventilation-perfusion abnormalities. These abnormalities lead to a decrease in oxygenation and effective ventilation.

Using our understanding of the physiologic aspects of respiration, we can now understand the importance of ventilation and oxygenation during cardio-pulmonary emergency situations.

Since the ability to oxygenate and ventilate requires maintenance of an open airway in the emergency patient, we will proceed with a discussion of airway management.

Airway management

The patient with a cardio-pulmonary problem must be evaluated for adequacy of ventilation. The initial assessment involves determining if spontaneous breathing is present or if it is absent. If breathing is present, then determining whether the breathing is occurring with free exchange or whether the breathing is being attempted through a partially or completely obstructed airway must be ascertained. If the latter is the case, corrective means must be undertaken by readjusting head and jaw position and/or the use of adjunctive measures (to be discussed later). The use of supplemental O_2 is advised in all cardio-pulmonary emergencies.

When spontaneous ventilation is not present, then artificial ventilation must be quickly instituted to overcome the adverse physiological changes previously discussed. Artificial ventilation may be instituted as mouth-to-mouth ventilation or with one of the adjunctive measures to be discussed.

Airway management during an emergency necessitates being able to position the head and jaw of the victim in such a way that a clear breathing passage is maintained. By tilting the head back and extend-

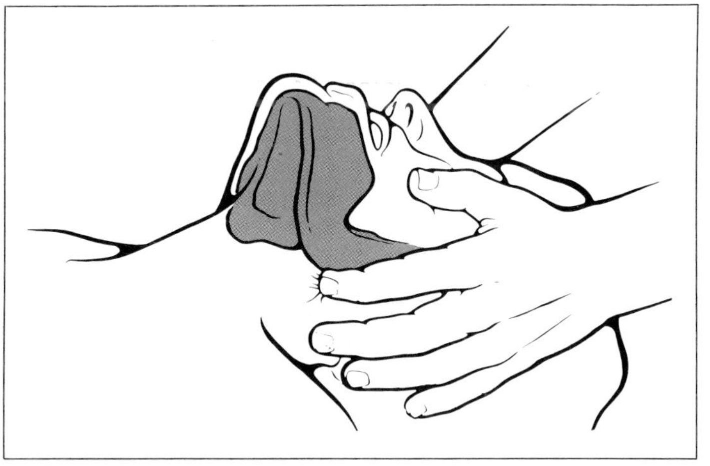

Fig. 3-1 Forward thrust of the mandible.

ing the mandible (lower jaw) forward, such a position can be achieved (Fig. 3-1). The forward thrust of the mandible serves to pull the tongue forward away from the posterior wall of the pharynx thus clearing the airway. The most common cause of airway obstruction in the unconscious or semiconscious victim is a relaxed tongue falling backward against the pharyngeal wall. The lower jaw can be thrust forward by using the index fingers placed under the mandibular angles and pushing forward. Another method is to grasp the anterior segment of the mandible with the thumb and index finger and pull forward, thus pulling the tongue forward.

When spontaneous ventilation is greatly depressed or absent, artificial ventilation must be instituted. Evaluation of effective ventilation under these circumstances may simply be the visible observation of the expansion of the chest. With positive pressure ventilation an elastic feel of an unobstructed airway is also indicative of successful ventilatory effort. Under emergency circumstances, hyperventilation tends not to be a problem although with overly vigorous ventilatory efforts, gastric distention may become troublesome.

Physiologically, a rescuer's exhaled ventilation contains an oxygen concentration of approximately 15%. This compares with the 21% present in room air. For this reason, the use of supplemental oxygen with adjunctive airway measures is recommended at the earliest possible moment. The need to increase the inspired oxygen concentration in order to improve oxygenation has been discussed previously. Certainly in the emergency or suspected emergency this need is of the utmost importance.

Adjuncts for the airway and respiration

Probably of greatest importance as an adjunct to cardio-respiratory support is the use of oxygen therapy. During any cardiopulmonary emergency, hypoxia is likely to be the result of a decreased cardiac output with resultant decreased oxygen tension in arterial blood. Associated with and complicating the emergency are: 1) Airway obstruction, along with, 2) Alveolar hypoventilation, which may lead to, 3) Increased physiological shunting. This shunting may result from abnormal anatomical shunt, diffusion block, abnormal relation of perfusion to ventilation, or atelectasis (collapsed alveoli), all of which are usually factors during a cardio-pulmonary emergency. The decreased cardiac output usually results from multiple factors such as: 1) Myocardial depression, 2) Decreased coronary perfusion, 3) Increased peripheral vascular resistance, 4) Increased pulmonary vascular resistance, 5) Cardiac arrhythmias, and 6) Decreased circulating blood volume.

The physiological basis of oxygen therapy is to ensure adequate tissue oxygenation, particularly of the heart and brain, and to prevent compensatory responses which may stress an already maximally stressed system. These responses include, increased cardiac output, peripheral sympathetic overactivity and hyperventilation. Pharmacologically these responses represent an increased stimulatory effect of the adrenergic sympathetic nervous system.

Clinical indications for adjunctive oxygen therapy other than in cardio-pulmonary arrest include: 1) Angina, 2) Acute hypotension, 3) Tachypnea—rapid breathing as an indication of alveolar hypoventilation or hyperventilation, and 4) Cyanosis—this often being a very late sign of hypoxia.

Adjunctive oxygen therapy can be delivered via the following equipment: 1) Nasal cannulas, 2) Plastic face masks, 3) Venturi masks, 4) Oxygen reservoir masks, 5) Pocket masks, 6) Bag-valve and mask devices, and 7) Oxygen-powered breathing devices.

Proper choice of the above equipment will be dependent upon the physiological state of the patient. Patients who are conscious and spontaneously breathing will need a different method of oxygen delivery from the patient who is unconscious and unable to support his own airway. The emergency patient unable to maintain and protect the airway, and who requires positive pressure ventilation may need adjunctive aid for airway support such as a nasopharyngeal airway, oropharyngeal airway, esophageal obturator airway, or tracheal intubation (Figs. 3-2 through 3-7).

The above aids to airway maintenance vary in their usefulness and the need of the rescuer to be skilled in their placement. Both the nasopharyngeal and oropharyngeal airways are relatively simply to place, and function to provide a space between the tongue and the posterior wall of the pharynx so that a free passage of air can move to the lower airway. The advantage of the nasopharyngeal airway over the oropharyngeal airway is that it is less reactive in a responsive patient who is experiencing upper airway obstruction. The oral airway is more likely to cause gagging and vomiting.

Placement of an esophageal obturator airway and endotracheal intubation require considerably more clinical skill and should not be attempted unless the rescuer has developed that skill previously. Although the former does not require the use of a laryngoscope and is designed for ease of placement, both devices allow a method of delivery of positive pressure ventilation and protection of the trachea from gastric aspiration.

The choice of delivering supplemental oxygen, as previously mentioned, will depend on the patient's needs and the availability of adjunctive equipment. The following is a list of these oxygen delivery devices and their capabilities (Figs. 3-8 through 3-12).

1. Nasal cannulas—spontaneously breathing patient
   flow rate 6 1/min
   O_2 concentration 30%
2. Plastic face masks—spontaneously breathing patient
   flow rate up to 10 1/min
   O_2 concentration up to 50%
3. Venturi mask—a mask designed to deliver variable O_2 concentrations—particularly useful in the patient with chronic lung disease
   O_2 concentrations of 24, 28, 35 and 40%
4. Oxygen reservoir mask—spontaneously breathing patient
   has O_2 storage
   high flow rate of 10–12 1/min
   can get O_2 concentrations up to 90%

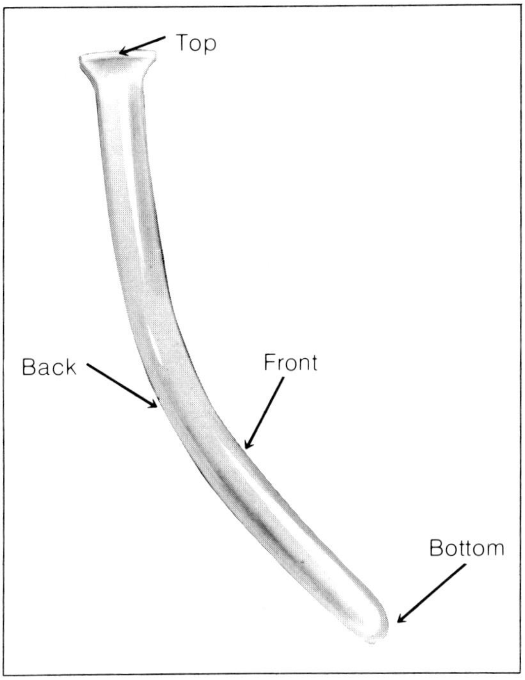

Fig. 3–2 Nasopharyngeal airway.

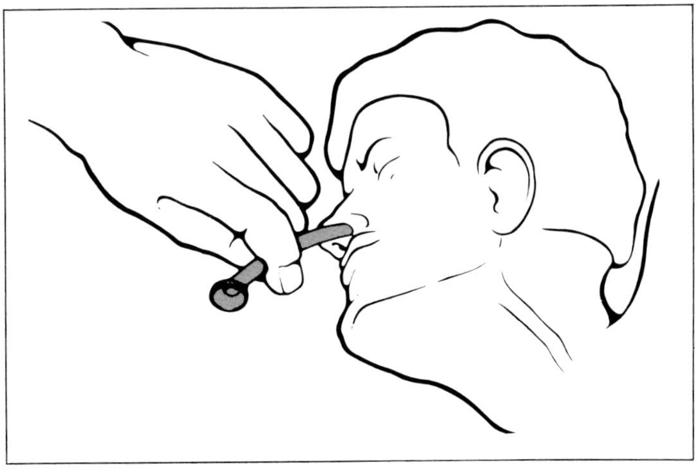

Fig. 3–3 Placement of naso-pharyngeal airway.

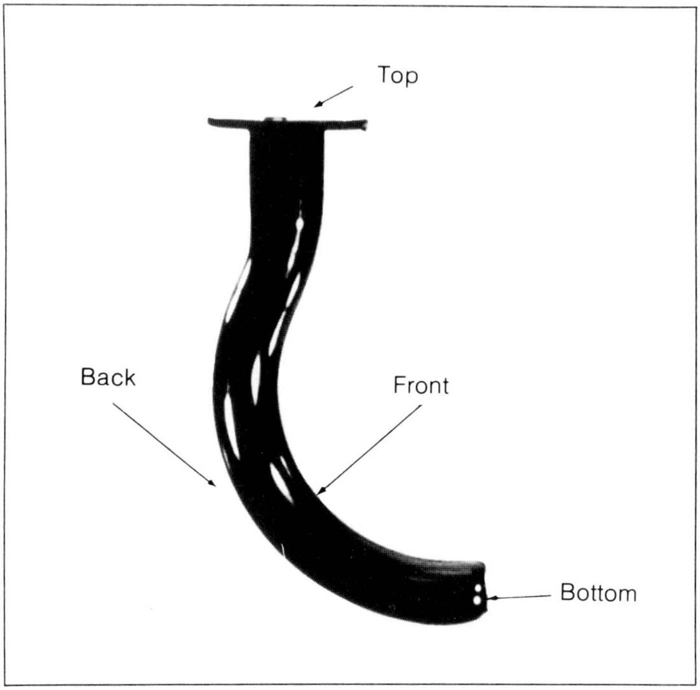

Fig. 3-4 Oropharyngeal airway.

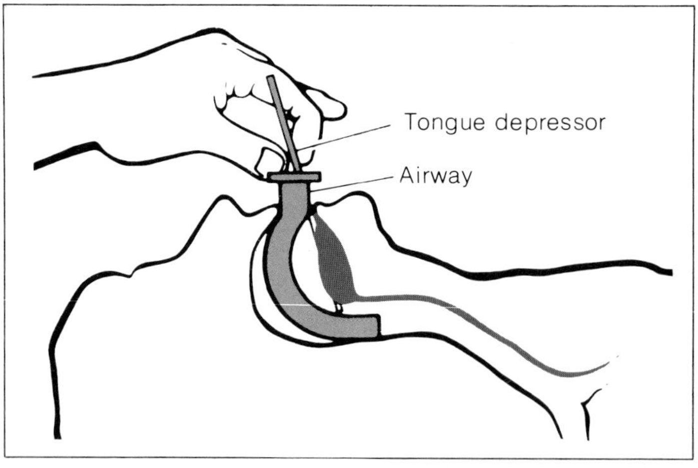

Fig. 3-5 Placement of oropharyngeal airway.

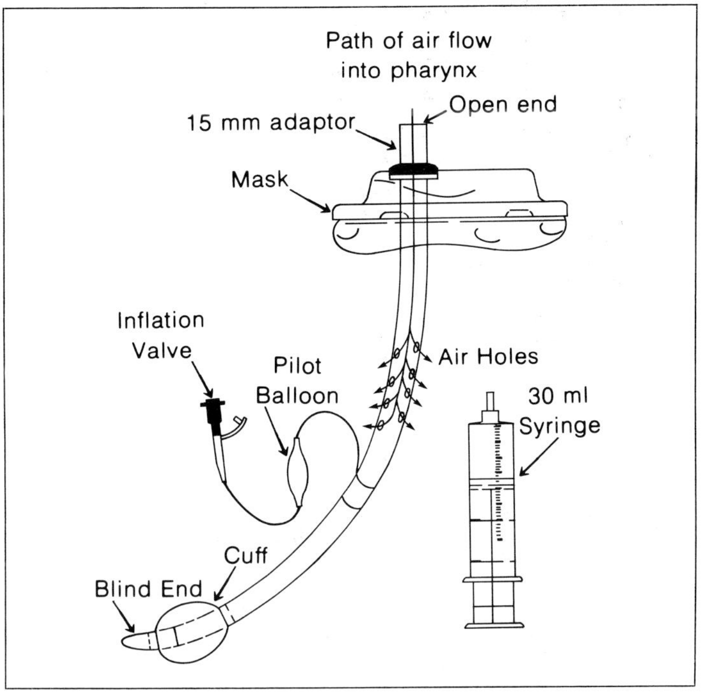

Fig. 3-6 Esophageal obturator airway.

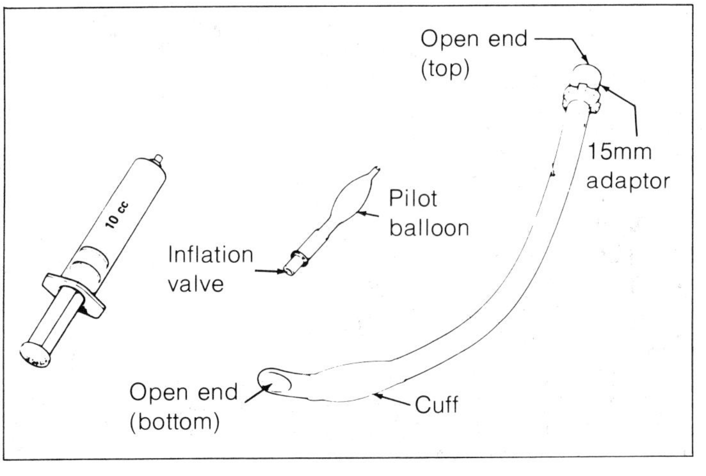

Fig. 3-7 Endotracheal tube.

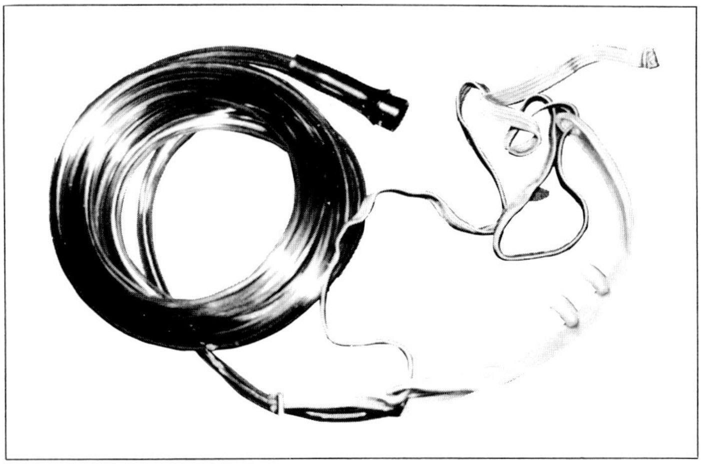

Fig. 3-8 Nasal cannula (See chapter 4).

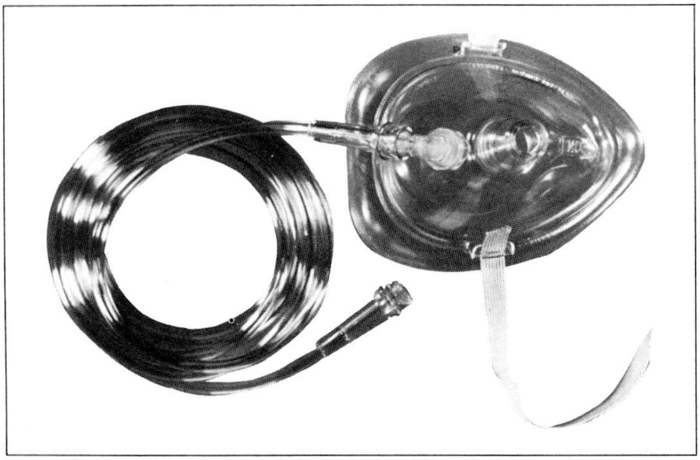

Fig. 3-9 Plastic oxygen face mask.

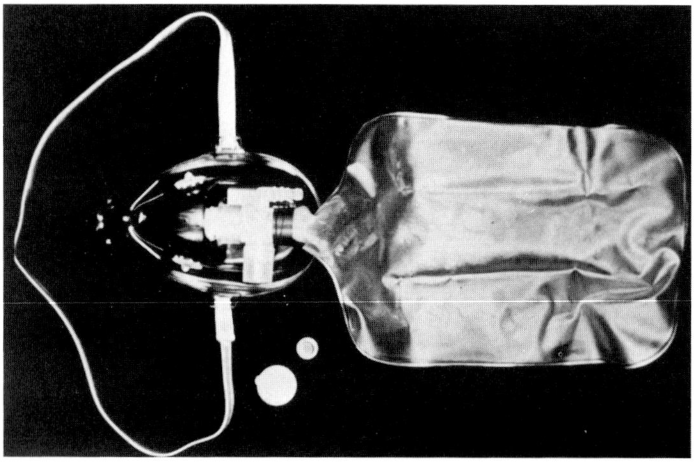

Fig. 3-10 Oxygen reservoir mask.

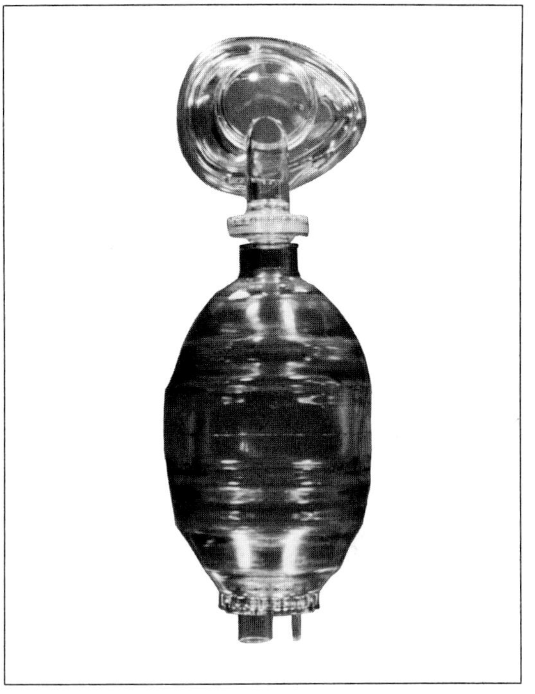

Fig. 3-11 Bag-valve mask devices.

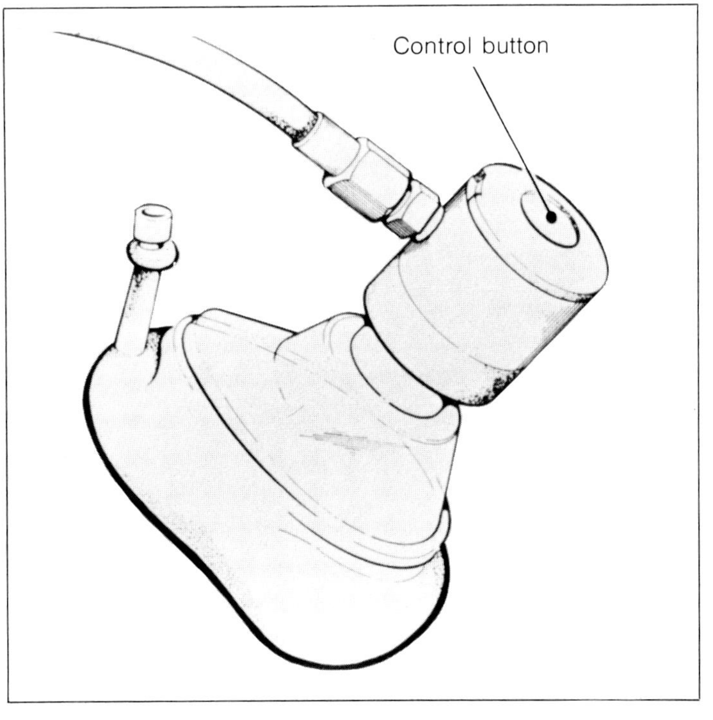

Fig. 3-12 Oxygen powered breathing device.

5. Pocket mask—patient requires positive pressure ventilation
   allows rescuer a method of delivering mouth-to-mouth resuscitation without touching patient's mouth
   supplemental O_2 can be attached.
6. Bag-valve mask devices—Patient who needs positive pressure ventilation. Resuscitation bags that are self-inflating and can deliver room air or be attached to a supplemental oxygen source to allow inspired concentrations of oxygen of greater than 90%. This device can also be used with a spontaneously breathing patient.
7. Oxygen-powered breathing devices—Manually triggered devices that delivery oxygen at a flow rate of at least 100 1/min. It is necessary to observe the chest rise and fall to assure proper ventilation.

Patients sustaining a cardiopulmonary emergency need immediate basic life support in ascertaining both respiratory and cardiac function. We have discussed in some detail those factors effecting pulmonary physiology and will now direct our attention to those factors effecting cardiac function and those methods of external circulatory support.

When cardiopulmonary emergencies are the result of a myocardial infarction, it is now believed that if arrest occurs, it is likely to be from a fatal dysrhythmia such as ventricular fibrillation. It is also felt that ventricular fibrillation is usually preceded by a more benign cardiac dysrhythmia such as a sinus bradycardia, possibly with premature ventricular contractions. It is during this in-between-time when supportive care and monitoring can play a preventive role.

For the dentist confronted with a cardiopulmonary emergency, the supportive care provided may mean the difference between life and death. Depending on the dentist's training and skill, supportive care may encompass only administration of oxygen or include monitoring and treatment of cardiac dysrhythmias. Certainly basic life support (i.e., mouth-to-mouth resuscitation and external cardiac compression) is a necessary holding action that should be within the capability of every dentist.

Once a cardio-pulmonary event has reached the stage where the heart can no longer sustain an adequate cardiac output, the need to restore at least a life-sustaining circulation is of the utmost importance. The ability to perform and sustain perfusion of the vital organs by the use of external cardiac compression requires detailed attention to the mechanical principles so as to effect the maximum cardiac output. Anything less than near perfect external cardiac compression will result in an inadequate cardiac output necessary to sustain biologic function. With more advanced training, monitoring of cardiac dysrhythmias and electrode defibrillation of ventricular fibrillation has improved the chances of survival of the patient in cardio-pulmonary arrest.

Knowledge of the electrophysiology of the heart is a necessary tool if an understanding of dysrhythmia initiation is to be achieved. Heart muscle is able to contract innately because of specialized tissue which has the ability to depolarize spontaneously. This tissue, having the property of automaticity, enables the heart to contract by sending out a wave of electrical activity. The sino-atrial node (S.A. node) is the heart's primary pacemaker. This pacemaker located in the right atrium sends out an electrical impulse which spreads through both atria and reaches the atrioventricular node (A.V. node). This node is located near the interventricular septum. From here the impulse spread through the bundle of His to the right and left bundle branches on either side of the ventricular septum. The final spread of the impulse is through the ventricular walls via the Purkinje fibers. It should be noted that any portion of the conducting system has the ability to fire automatically, and should impulses fail to arrive along the normal pathways, spontaneous discharge may occur along any point (Fig. 3–13). It is the possibility of

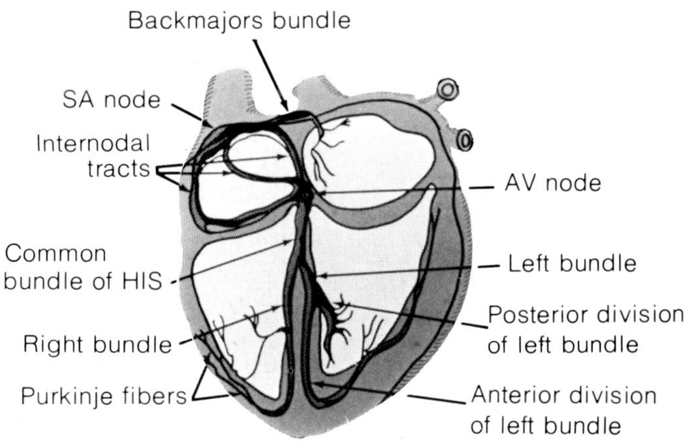

Fig. 3-13 Conduction system of the heart.

such ectopic beats which may initiate fatal dysrhythmias.

Electrophysiologically, this electrical impulse formation or action potential that is propagated, is associated with ion changes across cell membranes. These ions include Na^+, K^+, and Ca^{++}. As the waves of electrical depolarization spread through the heart muscle, they cause its contraction (Fig. 3-14).

When the electrical activity of the heart ceases to cause a productive contraction of the myocardium such as occurs during ventricular fibrillation, the need to institute artificial circulation is urgent. Palpation of the carotid artery pulse informs the rescuer of an adequate central circulation. Absence or questionable presence of the pulse is the indication for starting artificial circulation. Note that peripheral pulses are not useful in evaluating central circulation. Peripheral vasoconstruction is usually present during cardio-pulmonary emergencies.

External cardiac compression consists of the rhythmic application of pressure over the lower one-half of the sternum. Intermittent pressure applied to the sternum compresses the heart and produces a pulsatile artificial circulation. Properly performed cardiac compressions can produce systolic blood pressure of approximately 100 mmHg. The mean pressure achieved is rarely above 40 mmHg. These compressions produce a cardiac output of only 25-33% of a normal output. This output is just sufficient to maintain profusion in the vital organs (heart, brain, lungs). Ventilation provides the necessary supply of oxygen to keep the machine running. Circulation of unoxygenated blood is a useless exercise. Optimally, cardiac compressions should not be interrupted because with each stoppage the blood pressure drops to zero and effective blood flow ceases.

Adjuncts for artificial circulation include manual and gas-powered chest compressors (Figs. 3-15 and 3-16). The major advantages of these mechanical devices are that they require less effort to use and can provide prolonged, effective cardiac compression. Like any mechanical device, they are only as effective as the ability of the people applying them. Other mechanical aids for artificial circulation include bed boards and other devices to make it possible to compress a patient's sternum against a firm surface. A custom-made board to fit the narrow dental chair is usually necessary. Compression of the pa-

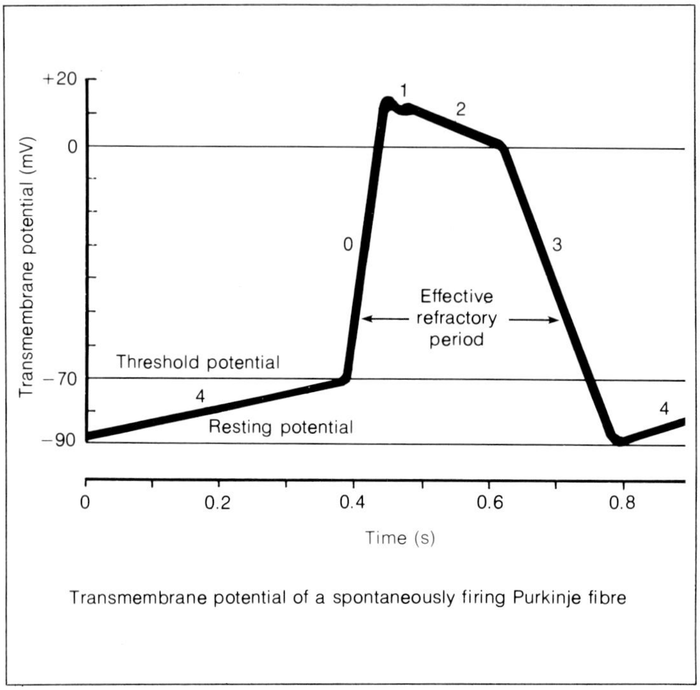

Fig. 3-14 Myocardial action potential.

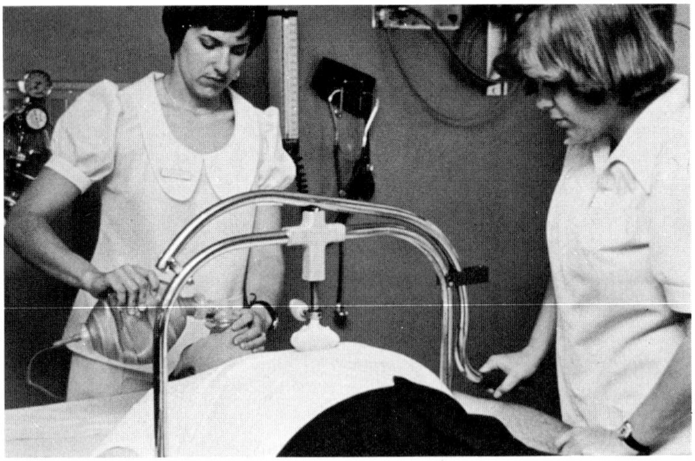

Fig. 3-15 Cardiac compression bedboard.

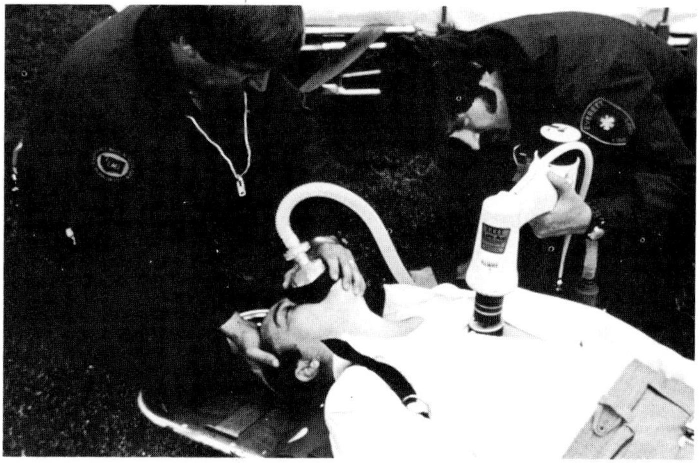

Fig. 3-16 Gas powered cardiac compressor.

tient's chest against a giving surface will result in an inadequate compressive force. It cannot be overemphasized that near perfect technical compressions are necessary to give the patient any chance of survival. This chapter has attempted to provide an overview of the physiological aspects of respiration and cardiac function as they apply to the technical skills of basic and advanced cardiac life support.

References

1. Bendixen, Egbert, Hedley-Whyte, Laver and Pontoppidon. *Respiratory Care.* St. Louis: Mosby, 1965.
2. Dripps, Eckenhoff and Vandam. *Introduction to Anesthesia.* Philadelphia: Saunders, 1977.
3. Goldber, Alan H. *Advanced Cardiac Life Support—Adjuncts for Airway and Breathing.* American Heart Assoc., 1975.
4. Guildner, C.W. *Advanced Cardiac Life Support—Adjuncts for Artificial Circulation.* American Heart Assoc., 1975.

Chapter 4

Pharmacologic Aspects of Emergency Drugs in Dental Practice

Jeffrey G. Garber, D.D.S.

Introduction

Successful use of drug therapy during emergency situations requires a knowledge and understanding of 1) a drug's major pharmacologic actions, 2) its clinical indications, 3) the correct dosages, 4) the necessary precautions and 5) the available clinical forms in which the drug is provided.

Effective drug therapy, as with any therapeutic mode, requires practice and a "feel" for what a given drug will do. Since emergencies requiring drug intervention are rare in dental practice, most clinicians find themselves last having used many of these agents during their school or residency years. With this in mind, the chapter is so designed as to limit the number of drugs with which the clinician must keep abreast and yet enable treatment of emergencies that do arise.

Emergencies that may necessitate drug therapy in the dental office include:

1. Cardiovascular emergencies
   a) cardiac arrest
   b) myocardial infarction
   c) disturbances of heart rhythm and conduction
   d) angina
2. Allergic reactions
   a) anaphylactic reactions
   b) edematous type reactions
   c) urticarial type reactions
3. Convulsive disorder emergencies
   a) epileptic seizures
   b) drug induced seizures
4. Respiratory emergencies
   a) asthmatic reactions

These and other medical emergencies are detailed in greater depth in other parts of this text. In order to compose a drug inventory, a core of drugs must be identified that are useful in treating emergencies in each of the four groups presented. Many of the groups will present overlapping drug management. Those drugs selected are, in the author's opinion, the simplest and most effective way of achieving the desired effect. They are by no means the only therapeutic choices.

Drugs in cardiovascular emergencies

The most frightening thought for any dentist is that of a patient experiencing a cardiovascular problem while in the office. Yet the likelihood of just such emergencies occurring seems greater because of the increasing number of patients being seen in dental offices with medically and surgically compensated cardiovascular disease.

The drug armamentarium for cardiovascular emergencies in a dental office includes the following: 1) Oxygen, 2) Epinephrine, 3) Sodium Bicarbonate, 4) Atropine, 5) Lidocaine (Table 4-1).

It must be remembered that emergency care in the dental office is meant to be supportive rather than diagnostic and corrective. The goal is to help a patient through

Table 4-1 Drugs for cardiovascular emergencies

a. Oxygen
b. Epinephrine
c. Sodium Bicarbonate
d. Atropine
e. Lidocaine

an emergency period until more advanced care can be obtained.

Cardiovascular emergencies usually present one or more of the following problems which may require drug intervention. 1) The heart is unable to develop an adequate perfusion pressure. 2) Hypoxia occurs as the result of inadequate transport of oxygen by the circulation. 3) Hypoxia-induced anaerobic metabolism results in the development of metabolic acidosis and 4) The heart develops dysfunctional rhythms which causes it to become an ineffective pump.

With these problems in mind the pharmacology of each drug will be evaluated and related to clinical practice.

Oxygen (See Table 4-2)

Oxygen represents one of the basic essentials for life. As a pharmacological agent oxygen is a significant therapeutic tool in disease states that interfere with normal oxygenation of the blood and body tissues. As a therapeutic agent it is unusual in that it is delivered as a gaseous agent. Unfortunately, because of this it is often not conceptualized as a drug.

Most cardiovascular emergencies result in an inadequate transport of oxygen by the circulation. This interference in the transport of oxygen may be localized to one organ such as the heart and express itself as anginal pain, or it may be widespread and effect all organ systems as occurs during cardiac arrest. Hypoxia as a result of cardiovascular impairment is a medical emergency requiring active support. Most dentists are not prepared to treat the basic defect causing the emergency, but they should be able to administer oxygen. The administration of oxygen will usually not correct the defect, but acts as a stopgap measure until more definitive therapy can be undertaken. As a stopgap measure, the administration of oxygen can be lifesaving. In fact, the astute clinician can often anticipate a crisis, administer oxygen, and avert disaster.

Oxygen is carried in the blood mainly as oxyhemoglobin, with a small amount of the gas present in physical solution. The normal oxygen tension (concentration) in arterial blood is about 90 torr when breathing air which contains about 21% oxygen. This is significant if we look at the oxygen hemoglobin dissociation curve, which indicates that on the steep (vertical) portion of the curve, small changes in the arterial oxygen tension substantially increase hemoglobin saturation (i.e., oxyhemoglobin) and thus increase arterial oxygen content. (Fig. 4-1). This is pharmacologically significant for the patient with circulatory insufficiency who has localized or generalized tissue hypoxia because the increased arterial oxygen concentration and content and the additional oxygen carried in physical solution may aid in the delivery of oxygen to hypoxic areas. This improved tissue oxygenation may improve myocardial oxygenation with a resultant relief of pain and restlessness; more effective circulation and the relief of cyanosis. For this reason, oxygen should always be given in the presence of suspected cardiovascular difficulty (i.e., chest pain, abnormal rhythms) and certainly in all cases of cardiopulmonary arrest.

Oxygen preparations are marketed as a compressed gas in steel cylinders fitted with reducing valves for delivery of the gas. These tanks come in various sizes, E

Table 4-2 Clinical pharmacology of oxygen

Pharmocologic Action	↑Arterial oxygen content and concentration ↑Hemoglobin saturation
Clinical Indications	Suspected respiratory or cardiovascular insufficiency
Dosage	100%—During emergency situations
Precautions	Support ventilation in patients with known chronic respiratory disease
Clinical Preparation	Gaseous agent

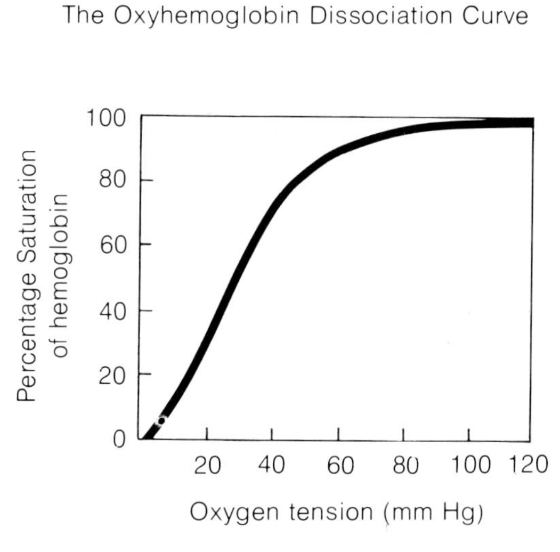

Fig. 4-1 Oxyhemoglobin curve: Arterial oxygen tension vs. hemoglobin saturation.

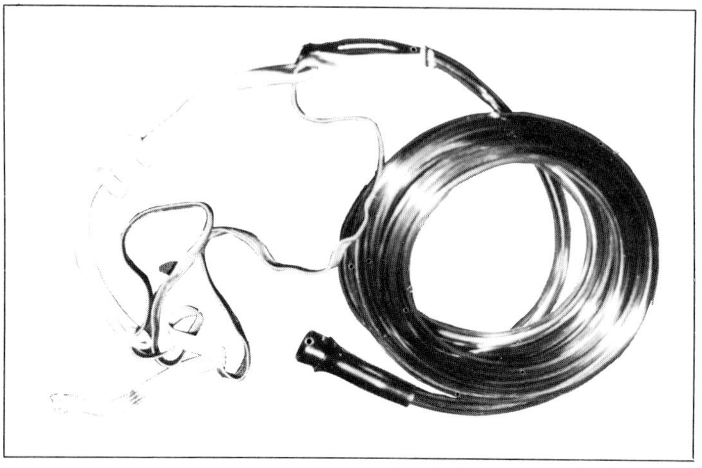

Fig. 4–2a Nasal cannula.

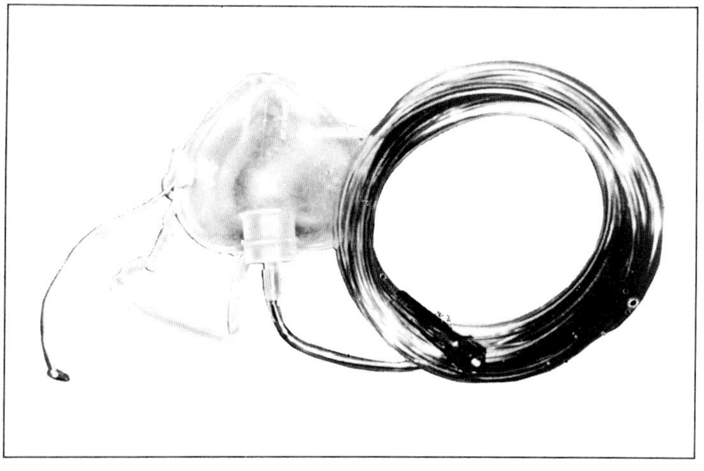

Fig. 4–2b Oxygen face mask.

and H cylinders are the ones most commonly found in dental offices. The E cylinders are the small portable tanks while the H cylinders are the large-sized central system tanks. These tanks are routinely colored green and their connections are pin indexed so as to avoid inadvertent wrong connections with other gaseous agents.

Oxygen administration is most commonly accomplished through nasal cannulas and masks both nasal and full face type (Figs. 4-2a and 4-2b). Nasal cannulas permit the delivery of oxygen at a flow rate of 4-6 liters/min. allowing the inspired oxygen concentration to be in the 30-50% ranges. More effective administration of oxygen can be achieved with face masks where it is possible to deliver a concentration of nearly 100%.

The use of high concentrations of oxygen during emergency situations presents no particular hazard and therefore should never be withheld. If there is ever any doubt as to the nature of the emergency, oxygen therapy should not be postponed if its need is suspected. In patients with chronic pulmonary disease, respiration may have to be assisted if oxygen therapy abolishes their hypoxic drive to breathe, but under no circumstances does this warrant withholding oxygen therapy when indicated.

Epinephrine (See Table 4-3)

A problem most often associated with cardiovascular emergencies is the heart's inability to pump effectively. This can and often does necessitate the need for a vasoactive drug effective in supporting the circulation. Epinephrine is one of the most potent vasopressor drugs known. The premise of this chapter is that the use of drug therapy should be undertaken only when other supportive measures have failed, or when hemo-dynamic changes incompatible with life (i.e., blood pressure, pulse and respiration) occur. It is only at these times that the use of a drug such as epinephrine, which has been found to be clinically effective in emergency situations, appears to be justified.

The pharmacology of epinephrine is complex; its many effects are often dose related with accompanying reflex changes. Nonetheless, certain cardiopharmacologic responses can be understood and expected when used in doses recommended for emergency administration.

Epinephrine is an endogeneous catechloamine having effects which simulate the stimulation of the adrenergic nervous system. Upon this system epinephrine stimulates both alpha and beta type receptors. Of interest to us is the prominent pharmacologic effect on the actions of the heart, the vascular system and on other smooth muscle.

Specifically, epinephrine: 1) increases heart rate, 2) increases the strength of myocardial contraction, 3) increases systemic vasoconstriction, 4) increases the automaticity of the heart's conduction system, 5) increases systemic arterial blood pressure and 6) increases the heart's need to consume oxygen.

Epinephrine's effect in increasing blood pressure can be viewed as a trifold response occuring because of 1) its direct stimulation of the myocardium thus increasing contractile force, 2) the direct increase on the heart's rate and 3) the vasoconstriction of many vascular beds, particularly precapillary resistance vessels as well as many venous beds.

Because of epinephrine's complex actions and the reflex changes associated with these actions, the effects described above are not as clearcut as they may seem and are dose dependent as well as being dependent on the rate and site of administration. In spite of this an increased perfusion pressure, improved myocardial contractility and the stimulation of spontaneous myocardial contractions are observed directly. The latter being very helpful when ventricular standstill has occurred.

Specifically, epinephrine's cardiac effects can be attributed to the direct stimulation of the β receptors of the myocardium and the cells of the pacemaker and conducting tissues. Although these direct cardiac effects achieve many desired results during emergency usage, it should be noted that a physiological price is paid. Cardiac efficiency is decreased while output is being increased. This can be viewed as the cardiac work performed relative to the amount of oxygen (the fuel) that is necessary to drive the machine. As epinephrine drives the heart harder, more oxygen is demanded by the cells doing the work. Supplemental oxygen to improve myocardial oxygenation in situations where epinephrine is required can now be understood.

It is also important to note that the action of epinephrine is impaired when tissue acidosis has occurred. This will be discussed in greater detail later in this chapter.

Epinephrine's other major pharmacological effect is on smooth muscle. In a later section of this chapter we will discuss its effects on the smooth muscle of the respiratory tract. The constrictive effect seen on the smooth muscle of the vascular system is the result of direct stimulation of adrenergic receptors. This effect can be principally seen on the smaller arterioles and

Table 4-3 Clinical pharmacology of epinephrine

Pharmacologic Action	Adrenergic stimulation of both α and β receptor sites
Clinical Indications	Cardiac arrest Life threatening hypotension Life threatening bronchoconstriction
Dosage	0.1 mg—0.5 mg, Depending on route of administration and emergency status
Precautions	Potent vasoactive drug Greatly increases myocardial O_2 consumption
Clinical Preparation	Prefilled syringes with 0.1 mg/ml of epinephrine

Table 4-4 Clinical pharmacology of sodium bicarbonate

Pharmacological Action	Combine with hydrogenion (H+) to correct acidosis
Clinical Indications	Following cardiac arrest or for correction of known metabolic acidosis
Dosage	1 mEq/Kg initial dose
Precautions	Metabolic alkalosis combining with other drugs such as epinephrine

precapillary sphinctors. As with its direct cardiac effects, epinephrine's effect on vascular smooth muscle can be dose dependent and biphasic with adrenergic receptor stimulation.

The dose of epinephrine during emergency situations such as cardiac arrest, or hypotension incompatible with life is 0.5 mg given intravenously. This dose should be repeated at five minute intervals if a physiologic response such as an adequate measured blood pressure or palpable central pulse is not obtainable. Two other routes of administration that may be useful in situations where an intravenous site cannot be established are 1) into the sublingual plexus of vessels and 2) if the patient is intubated, directly into the tracheobronchial tree. A third method, the intracardiac route, is certainly least desirable because it requires the greatest skill and has a high incidence of complications.

Epinephrine is available for emergency usage in prefilled syringes containing 10 ml of 1 mg of epinephrine in a 1:10,000 dilution. That is, each ml contains 0.1 mg of epinephrine. Epinephrine is also available in ampules which contain 1 ml having 1 mg of epinephrine in a dilution of 1:1,000. Use of ampules requires that the drug be drawn up during the emergency. In this case, 0.5 ml of a 1:1,000 solution of epinephrine would contain the necessary 0.5 mg of drug recommended (Table 4-3).

Sodium bicarbonate ($NaHCO_3$) (See Table 4-4)

Using a drug effective in reversing the acidotic effects of hypoxia-induced anaerobic metabolism during cardiopulmonary arrest is essential if more than basic life support (ventilation and cardiac compression) is to become part of the dentist's ability to successfully treat cardiovascular emergencies.

With cardiopulmonary arrest there is a cessation of both effective ventilation and cardiac output. This leads to an acidotic state having a metabolic and respiratory component. The metabolic component is the accumulation of organic acids, such as lactic acid, from anaerobic cellular metabolism. The respiratory component resulting from the retention of CO_2 (hypercarbia) is due to inadequate ventilation. Both forms of acidemia must be treated effectively if cardiac arrest is to be successfully reversed. Effective ventilation as a form of basic life support will be a significant factor in managing the acidemia of cardiac arrest, including the presence of a significant metabolic component.

Since it is predictable that metabolic acidosis will occur shortly after cardiopulmonary arrest, the use of sodium bicarbonate to manage this metabolic component is indicated. With management of the metabolic and respiratory components of acidosis the effectiveness of other vasoactive drugs is greatly enhanced.

Pharmacologically the bicarbonate ion of sodium bicarbonate combines with the hydrogen ions (H^+) produced by the organic acids in the following reaction:

$$HCO_3^- + H^+ = H_2CO_3 = CO_2 + H_2O$$

This reaction as it proceeds toward the right 1) removes H^+ ions from the blood, thus decreasing the hydrogen ion concentration and thereby increasing the pH and 2) produces CO_2 as an end product. The importance of adequate alveolar ventilation can be understood from this reaction. It is necessary to remove the CO_2 so the reaction will not be driven back to the left, again increasing the hydrogen ion concentration.

Reversal of acidosis which can cause a decrease in ventricular contractile force and decrease the effectiveness of catecholamines is apparent if the likelihood of resuscitation is to be increased.

When cardiopulmonary arrest occurs in the office, the procedures for basic life support should be instituted as rapidly as possible. If an intravenous route has been established and the steps of basic life support have not produced spontaneous effective ventilation and effective cardiac output, then a decision to proceed with drug therapy may be made. The initial dose of sodium bicarbonate is 1 mEq/Kg in the adult. This will translate to 50 mg of an 8.4% solution (50 mEq) or 50 ml of a 7.5% solution (44.6 mEq). It is possible that only a single dose will be necessary since transportation from the dental office to an advanced medical facility should be undertaken as soon as possible. One half the initial dose can be given at 10 minute intervals if necessary, although it is preferable to monitor arterial pH to guide administration (Table 4-4). In an arrest situation, it is unlikely that an I.V. trial dose of sodium bicarbonate will be anything but helpful.

The major precaution to be considered in administering this drug in an office setting is that no other drug should be mixed with the bicarbonate containing solution. Sodium bicarbonate will inactivate epinephrine if the two drugs mix in the intravenous tubing. Therefore it is a good idea to inject all of the bicarbonate solution and then flush the I.V. line prior to injection of other drugs.

Emergency sodium bicarbonate is best kept in the office in a prefilled 50 ml syringe, containing either the 8.4% solution

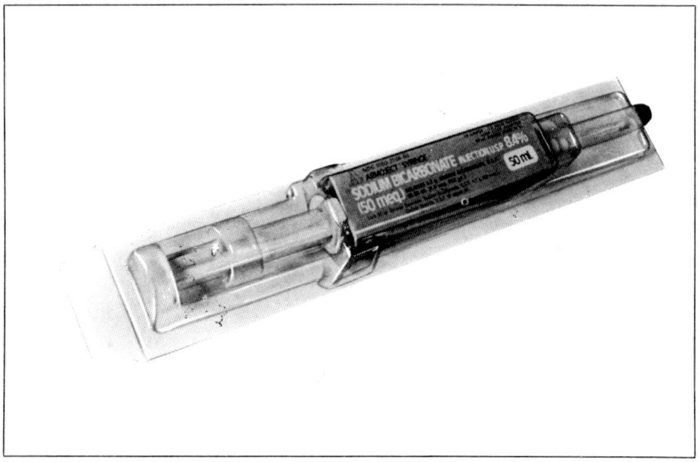

Fig. 4-3 Sodium bicarbonate prefilled syringe.

with (50 mEq) or the 7.5% solution with (44.6 mEq) (Fig. 4-3).

Atropine (See Table 4-5)

Acute myocardial infarction is one cardiovascular emergency that occasionally is followed by a severe bradycardia (heart rate 60). Atropine may be the drug of choice when attempting to treat a severe bradycardia that is accompanied by symptomatic hypotension with loss of consciousness. The important indication for atropine's use as an emergency drug is: significant bradycardia accompanied by significant hypotension. Significant bradycardia indicates a slow heart rate, well below a patient's normal resting pulse. Significant hypotension indicates a blood pressure low enough that cerebral perfusion is decreased sufficiently to cause a loss of consciousness.

Pharmacologically, atropine is a parasympatholytic drug which by its cardiac vagolytic action reduces vagal tone and thereby accelerates the rise of discharge of the SA (Sino-Atrial) node. Hence, one sees an increase in the heart's rate. This same vagolytic action seems capable of improving atrio-ventricular conduction. This may be quite useful in the treatment of certain types of heart block.

The intravenous route is the perferred route of administration. The usual emergency dose is 0.5 mg, which can be repeated at five minute intervals up to a maximum dose of approximately 2.0 mg. An acceptable heart rate can usually be established with doses less than 2.0 mg. Doses above 2.0 may lead to an increased appearance of central nervous system (CNS) symptoms such as sedation and generalized CNS depression. It should be noted that atropine crosses the blood-brain barrier.

Since atropine causes acceleration of the cardiac rate with an associated increase in myocardial oxygen consumption, many patients having ischemic heart disease; patients in the process of an acute myocardial infarction may exhibit further ischemic changes. Therefore, use of oxygen for treatment of bradycardia should be restricted to situations in which there is severe hypotension, with loss of consciousness or frequent ventricular ectopic beats. In those cases where bradycardia is severe enough to require drug therapy, atropine should be tried before resorting to

Table 4-5 Clinical pharmacology of atropine

Pharmacologic Action	Increase the rate of discharge of the S.A. node
Clinical Indications	Severe bradycardia with accompanying hypotension
Dosage	0.5 mg I.V. up to 2.0 mg
Precautions	Cause increase in myocardial oxygen consumption
Clinical Preparation	Prefilled syringes with atropine 0.1 mg/ml

Table 4-6 Clinical pharmacology of lidocaine

Pharmacologic Action	Inhibit the rate of Phase 4 depolarization
Clinical Indications	Acute myocardial infarction Ventricular prematuer contractions Ventricular tachycardia Ventricular fibrillation
Dosage	50—100 mg I.V. bolus
Precautions	Patient with known advanced heart block
Clinical Preparation	Prefilled syringes containing 10 mg/ml of lidocaine either in a 1% or 2% solution

the more potent vasopressor epinephrine (Table 4-5). As with the other emergency drugs recommended, atropine is available in prefilled syringes containing a 10 ml, 1.0 mg/ml (0.1 mg/ml) or a 5 ml, 0.5 mg/5 ml (0.1 mg/ml) solution.

Lidocaine (See Table 4-6)

Lidocaine, most familiar to dentists for its role as a local anesthetic, is also a useful drug in the emergency treatment of cardiac dysrhythmias (Table 4-6). The drug is particularly helpful in the treatment of ventricular dysrhythmias which may commonly occur after acute myocardial infarction. The drug may be used in the treatment of: 1) ventricular premature contractions, 2) ventricular tachycardia and 3) ventricular fibrillation. Recognition of these dysrythmias requires electrocardiographic monitoring although premature ventricular contractions may be determined by careful palpation of the pulse. In the patient suspected of having an acute myocardial infarction, the prophylactic use of lidocaine may be helpful in preventing fatal dysrythmias. Lidocaine, when used as will be recommended, has no significant effect on

Table 4-7 Drugs for hypersensitivity/allergic reaction

a. Diphenhydramine (Benadryl)
b. Epinephrine

myocardial contractility or arterial blood pressure and therefore has a low risk, high benefit aspect for use in emergency situations.

Pharmacologically, we know that lidocaine as a local anesthetic interrupts nerve conduction by blocking action potentials. Similarly, lidocaine is effective in blocking electrical conduction from ectopic foci of the ventricles. Specifically, by inhibiting the rate of spontaneous phase 4 depolarization it reduces automaticity of these ectopic sites. Automaticity is a response through which cells of the heart slowly depolarize without a stimulus until a critical threshold potential is reached, and then develop a maximal action potential causing a wave of action potentials to be produced. This results in the muscle's contraction.

For office emergency a single intravenous bolus of 50-100 mg may be administered. If needed, this dose can be repeated at 5 minute intervals. The total dosage given should not exceed 300 mg. Blood levels decline rapidly after an intravenous bolus of lidocaine because the drug is rapidly redistributed. In the 70 kg man toxic levels of lidocaine are usually reached when doses of 400-600 mg are administered over a short period of time.

It should be noted that lidocaine undergoes hepatic degradation, therefore when it is known or suspected that hepatic function is impaired, the dose of lidocaine should be reduced.

Lidocaine toxicity can usually be seen as effects relating to the central nervous system. These CNS effects may range from slight agitation to grand mal seizures with loss of consciousness. Other findings may include drowsiness, parathesias, muscle twitching, decreased hearing and disorientation.

Again, a most useful way of keeping lidocaine for emergency use is in prefilled syringes. These are available as 5 ml, 50 mg/ml (1%); 10 ml 100 mg/10 ml (1%) or a 5 ml 100 mg/5 ml (2%) syringes. Note that lidocaine in dental carpules contains preservatives and often has a vasoconstrictor such as epinephrine added and therefore is not recommended for use in the treatment of cardiac dysrythmias.

Drugs in the treatment of allergic reactions (See Table 4-7)

Hypersensitivity or allergic reactions can result in minor manifestations such as urticaria, itching, edema formation or in a more severe form known as anaphylaxis where vasomotor collapse with hypotension and bronchospasm may result (Table 4-7). It is likely that the urgency of the latter condition may require a drug that is both powerful and rapid and capable of reversing the broncho-constriction and hypotension seen. Epinephrine is such a drug, and although already discussed, its specific pharmacology related to allergic manifestations will be discussed in this section (Table 4-3).

Minor allergic reactions such as urticaria and edema may also require drug intervention. These reactions may cause considerable patient discomfort and may even be life-threatening if the edematous response causes airway obstruction from swelling in the floor of the mouth or laryngeal edema. For the treatment of minor allergic reactions the pharmacology of diphenhydramine (Benadryl) will be reviewed (Table 4-8).

Selection of both epinephrine and diphenhydramine represents, in this author's view, the simplest and most efficient means of dealing with the spectrum of allergenically manifested emergencies.

Table 4-8 Clinical pharmacology of diphenhydramine (benadryl)

Pharmacologic Action	Antagonist to H_1 receptor sites
Clinical Indications	Minor allergic manifestations such as urticaria, itch and edema
Dosage	25—50 mg either I.V. or orally
Precautions	Drowsiness
Clinical Preparation	Ampules of Benadryl 25 mg/cc

The therapeutic objective of this drug treatment of the hypersensitivity or allergic response is to be able to block the effects of the substances that are released or produced during these reactions. These substances called autacoids play both a direct and intermediary role in anaphylaxic and other allergic responses. Histamine is the substance primarily associated with the allergic phenomena and has been studied extensively leading to the development of drugs which antagonize the endogenous release of this substance.

The antagonism of the effects of histamine on smooth muscle, e.g. vascular and bronchial smooth muscle or capillary permeability characterizes a drug such as diphenhydramine. This histamine blocking effect is directed at specific histamine receptors called H_1 receptors.

Histamine or H_1 antagonists such as diphenhydramine (Benadryl) afford their protection in hypersensitivity reactions by blocking the effects of histamine. They are only as effective as the degree to which the response is caused by histamine release. In man, histamine release serves an intermediary function so that the H_1 blocking drugs seem most efficacious in treating those allergic responses seen in skin and mucous membranes. Therefore one finds diphenhydramine effective in the treatment of urticaria, itch and edema. On the other hand, its effects on bronchoconstriction and hypotension are limited. This may be due to the fact that histamine is not the primary substance involved in these responses.

Pharmacologically, diphenhydramine in therapeutic doses causes central nervous system depression causing the patient to feel sleepy. This may be of some significance if the drug is administered on an outpatient basis. Degradation of dephenhydramine occurs principally in the liver. Excretion is via the kidney.

Diphenhydramine (Benadryl) comes as both an oral preparation and as an injectable. The usual adult dose is 25-50 mg. This may be given during acute allergic manifestations through an intravenous infusion for rapid response. If given via the oral route the duration of action is in the range of 4-6 hours.

For the more life-threatening emergency situations where severe hypotension and bronchoconstriction has occurred, the use of epinephrine is recommended. Epinephrine has a powerful bronchodilator action, particularly when bronchial muscle is contracted, such as may occur during an anaphylactic reaction. Its cardiovascular effects in reversing hypotention have been discussed previously.

For severe allergic responses, epinephrine can be given by either the subcutaneous or intravenous routes. The route of administration will be dictated by the clinician's

Table 4-9 Drugs for convulsive emergencies

a. Oxygen
b. Diazepam (Valium)

skill and the severity of the emergency state. The use of the prefilled syringes is recommended with an initial dose range of 0.1 mg to 0.5 mg being selected.

Drugs in convulsive disorder emergencies (See Table 4-9)

Patients who develop convulsions frequently present the clinician with a difficult management problem. The most common causes of convulsions are 1) uncontrolled epileptics having seizures and 2) drug-induced seizures such as might occur with a toxic dose of local anesthetic. Whatever the underlying cause of the seizure, the greatest danger to the patient is the loss of a patent airway. Therefore, before drug therapy is considered, support of the airway should be uppermost in the clinician's list of priorities. In many instances no other treatment is necessary as the seizure is self-limiting and the patient needs only to be protected from himself.

In those instances where the seizure is prolonged or airway management compromised, drug therapy may be necessary to break the seizure and overcome its adverse effects. The two drugs selected for the emergency treatment of seizures are 1) oxygen and 2) diazepam. The pharmacological importance of oxygen has previously been discussed and its use during and after seizure activity is recommended particularly with the increased oxygen consumption seen during seizure activity compounded by the possibility of airway obstruction. Diazepam, the most common of the class of drugs known as the benzodiazepines, is the agent of choice for the treatment of status epilepticus. The drug is commonly used for its sedative-antianxiety properties. Its anticonvulsant properties are most likely the result of its suppression of neuonal activity in the reticular activating system. It may accomplish this by mimicking inhibitory neurotransmitters.

Central nervous system effects occur rapidly after intravenous administration of diazepam and the drug is then redistributed to other tissues. The drug is broken down by hepatic microsomal enzymes, one of the products being an active metabolite (N–demethy/derivative). The drug is excreted for the most part in the urine. It is interesting to note that the half-life of the parent compound and its active metabolites is in the 24-48 hour range. This is probably of more significance when chronic oral doses accumulate, although it is possible that impaired psychomotor function may persist after single intravenous boluses are used for sedation or anticonvulsant treatment.

Diazepam is a central depressant and its respiratory and cardiovascular effects may be additive when used with other depressants. As with the administration of any centrally depressant drug, the ability to maintain an airway and support ventilation is an absolute necessity.

When administered intravenously for control of seizure activity, the usual dose in adults and older children is 5-10 mg. Diazepam is available in prefilled syringes containing 10 mg in 2 ml (5 mg/cc) as well as in 2 ml ampules (5 mg/ml) and as oral medication 2, 5 and 10 mg tablets (See Table 4-10).

Drugs useful in respiratory emergencies (See Table 4-11)

Respiratory distress associated with acute bronchial asthma can pose an office emergency requiring therapeutic intervention. Again, the use of two drugs already discussed is recommended. These drugs are

Table 4-10 Clinical pharmacology of diazepam (valium)

Pharmacologic Action	Supression of neuronal activity reticular activating system of the brain
Clinical Indications	Nonself-limiting seizure activity
Dosage	5—10 mg I.V.
Precautions	Central depressant—respiratory and cardiovascular collapse
Clinical Preparations	2 ml prefilled syringes 5 mg/ml or 2 ml ampules 5 mg/ml

oxygen and epinephrine. In the selection of any therapeutic mode, simplicity and effectiveness of use must be considered. Both oxygen and epinephrine meet these criteria. The use of these drugs (particularly epinephrine) is indicated only when a truly life-threatening emergency exists. Often lessor therapeutic measures will be effective. These may include the use of antihistamines, inhalors, and specific remedies with which the patient is familiar. Epinephrine is effective in the symptomatic relief of acute bronchial asthma. Its effectiveness may be the result of relaxing bronchial smooth muscle, a β_2 receptor action and also an α receptor action which constricts bronchial vessels thereby reducing congestion and edema formation.

Treatment of an acute bronchial asthmatic attack where respiration is severely compromised is instituted by administering 0.2 — 0.5 mg of epinephrine subcutaneously. Relief of symptoms usually occurs within 5 minutes. It is also recommended that supplemental oxygen be given by mask during this period. Both the pharmacological effects of oxygen and epinephrine have been discussed previously. The reader is referred to those sections.

It must be stressed that drug therapy need not be instituted unless the severity of the respiratory distress is such that the value of transporting the patient to an emergency care facility would be lessened unless such therapy were instituted initially.

Table 4-11 Drugs for respiratory emergencies

a. Oxygen

b. Epinephrine

This chapter has attempted to provide a pharmacological approach to the treatment of emergency situations which occur in dental practice. The number of drugs discussed have been limited with the understanding that a greater knowledge of a few drugs makes for a more effective clinician. An office drug armamentarium of oxygen, epinephrine, sodium bicarbonate, atropine, lidocaine, diphenhydramine and diazepam has been selected and the appropriate pharmacological considerations for their use in the treatment of cardiovascular, allergic/anaphylactic, convulsive and respiratory emergencies, have been presented.

References

1. Goodman and Gillman. *The Pharmacological Basis of Therapeutics,* 5th Ed. New York: MacMillan Pub. Co., Inc., 1975.
2. McIntyre, Kevin M.. *Advanced Cardiac Life Support—Use of Drugs.* American Heart Assoc., 1975.
3. White, Rogers. *Advanced Cardiac Life Support—Essential Drugs in Emergency Care.* American Heart Assoc., 1975.

Section II

Management

Chapter 5

Conditions of Altered Consciousness

Louis F. Rose, D.D.S., M.D. and Barry H. Hendler, D.D.S., M.D.

Syncope

Syncope is the abrupt and transient loss of consciousness. Although the term is usually applied to unconsciousness caused by temporary decrease in cerebral blood flow, in this discussion a broader definition is employed that includes the brief disturbances in consciousness caused by changes in the chemical composition of the blood as in hyperventilation or hyperglycemia. Syncope has been found to occur in as many as 25-30% of young, healthy adult males. It should be carefully differentiated from such disorders as epilepsy, vertigo, cataplexy and strokes, all of which may produce transient disturbances in consciousness, generalized weakness, or inability to stand erect. The loss of consciousness in syncope may not be complete, but may consist of varying degrees of sensorial impairment, with transient blurring of vision, weakness and loss of postural tone. Such attacks may be described by the patient as dizziness, faintness, lightheadedness, or a "drunk feeling." These partial manifestations have the rapid onset, brief duration, and complete recovery characteristic of the fully developed faint.

Syncope is most frequently caused by reduction in cerebral blood flow below a critical level and is usually associated with a sharp fall in blood pressure. This, in turn, is the result of either a loss of peripheral resistance, as seen in vasodepressor faint and in orthostatic hypotension, or a decrease in cardiac output as in Adams-Stokes attacks. In many patients, however, loss of consciousness is not caused by a reduction of blood pressure but by a decrease in such essential blood components as glucose, carbon dioxide, or oxygen. In other instances, such as that of cough syncope, the faint seems to result from cerebral ischemia caused by extra cardiac disturbances.

There are several features common to almost all types of syncope. Electroencephlographic changes usually appear, and consist of high voltage, 2-4 cycle per second slow waves that promptly return to normal after consciousness is regained. Brief convulsive movements, such as tonic or clonic contractions of the arms and turning of the head, can occur in all types of fainting, depending on the degree and duration of the cerebral ischemia. Fully developed seizures with tongue biting and urinary incontinence, however, are unusual. Recovery is usually hastened by assumption of the recumbent posture, which helps to restore the normal cerebral circulation. The critical level of cerebral blood flow necessary to maintain consciousness has been estimated to be about 30 ml per 100 grams of brain per minute (normal value is 50-55 ml). The duration of asystole or the degree of hypotension necessary to produce critical levels of cerebral ischemia varies, depending upon the posture of the patient, the ability of the cerebral vessels to dilate, and other factors. In normal, erect subjects, a mean arterial blood pressure as low as 20-30 ml of mercury or an asystole of 4 or 5 seconds duration can produce syncope. In the recumbent position, longer periods of asystole may occur before loss of consciousness develops.

Vasodepressor syncope (common faint)

Vasodepressor syncope is by far the most frequent cause of transient unconsciousness. The condition is characterized by a fall in blood pressure associated with the development of a variety of autonomic manifestations. In the early presyncopal period, there may be pallor, nausea, and sweating; in later stages pupillary dilatation, yawning, hyperpnea, and bradycardia appear. When the mean arterial pressure falls below critical levels, loss of consciousness and characteristic electroencephalographic changes occur. Bradycardia is often severe at the onset of unconsciousness, and pulse rates of 50-60 per minute may be observed even after recovery. The duration of syncope is brief, ranging from a few seconds to several minutes. In the postsyncopal period the patient may complain of headaches, weakness, nervousness and slight confusion. Vasodepressor faint is most often evoked by sudden emotional stress associated with fear, anxiety or pain. Injections, trauma, minor surgery and the sight or withdrawal of blood are common precipitating events. Attacks usually occur in the standing or upright posture, and consciousness returns quickly once the patient is recumbent.

The initial event in this complex, vascular and neurogenic reaction is dilitation of the vascular bed throughout the body, particularly in peripheral muscles. Vasodilatation in the limb muscles is a normal response to emotional stimuli and is thought to represent preparation for "fight or flight." The fall in peripheral resistance attendant upon muscular vasodilatation is unaccompanied by compensatory increase in cardiac output, and as a result, leads to a reduction in cerebral blood flow.

Diagnosis

The diagnosis of syncope depends almost entirely upon a careful history of the attack and the setting in which it occurs. Differentiation of vasodepressor syncope from an akinetic epileptic seizure, such as petit mal or psychomotor attack, may be difficult. Careful evaluation of the electroencephalographic findings, the onset and duration of the attack and the post-syncopal manifestations can usually distinguish these conditions. These factors are also helpful in differentiating the various types of syncope. In vasodepressor faint, the patient usually has prodromal manifestations of autonomic hyperactivity such as pallor, sweating, salivation, and bradycardia. In cardiac arrest, orthostatic hypotension, and carotid sinus syncope, loss of consciousness occurs abruptly and prodromal symptoms are not usually present. Post syncopal confusion, headache and weakness often follow vasodepressor faint and the hyperventilation syndrome. In chronic orthostatic hypotension recovery of consciousness is rapid and complete without post-syncopal symptoms. Most types of fainting occur in the erect or upright position, but in cardiac arrest, syncope may occur while the patient is recumbent. The duration of syncope is brief in postural hypotension but prolonged in hyperventilation. Most of these differentiating manifestations can be determined by eliciting a careful medical history.

Treatment

As soon as the signs and symptoms of a vasodepressor episode are noted, the patient should be placed in a supine position with the legs elevated slightly (Trendelenburg position, Fig. 5-1). Manipulation and movement of the extremities frequently will increase the return of blood from the periphery. An upright position in the chair may cause prolonged cerebral anoxia, which can precipitate convulsions, nausea,

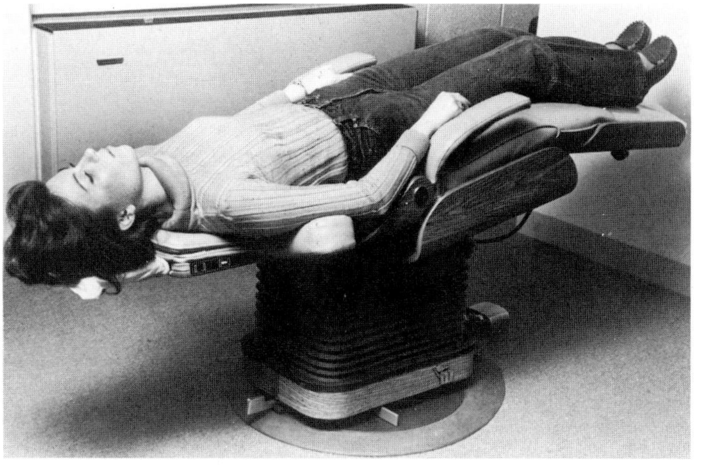

Fig. 5-1 Trendelenburg position.

etc. The proper positioning is the most important aspect of treatment since the majority of clinical manifestations in this emergency are due to inadequate flow of cerebral blood.

The establishment of a patent airway is the next step in treatment. Frequently the head-tilt position will be sufficient to develop a patent airway, stimulating spontaneous respiration. Occasionally it will be necessary to administer oxygen when the head tilt is not successful. The patient should immediately regain consciousness once the appropriate position of the patient is instituted and the airway is patent.

If the patient is not responding rapidly to the above, a respiratory stimulant, such as aromatic spirits of ammonia, should be crushed and placed under the patient's nose in order for him to inhale the spirits. This acts as a chemical stimulant to breathing. In addition, it is helpful to loosen the patient's tight clothing, such as belt, necktie, etc. Placing a cold towel on the patient's forehead may be soothing and may assist the patient in feeling comfortable.

During the episode, vital signs must be monitored, including blood pressure, pulse and respiration. They must be evaluated against the patient's baseline values in order to determine the severity and progression of the emergency. In addition, the dentist and his staff should remain calm and display a feeling of confidence and reassurance to the patient.

Once the patient has regained consciousness he should remain seated until vital signs are stable and all discomfort and anxiety have passed. The patient should not be allowed to stand quickly or walk unattended. Dental treatment should be discontinued and the practitioner should attempt to discover the syncopal precipitant so that future therapy may be modified to prevent recurrence.

Postural hypotension and syncope

Postural hypotension may occur when the patient assumes the upright position. The autonomic factors compensating for the upright posture, such as reflex arteriolar and venous constriction or increase in heart rate to compensate for pooling of vascular volume in the lower extremities, either are inadequate or fail. There is a fall in systolic and diastolic blood pressure and a variable heart rate response. The patient may develop weakness, dizziness, or syncope on sitting or standing. This may be a manifestation of various disease states, such as diseases with autonomic nervous system involvement, i.e., diabetic neuropathy, amyloidosis, or subacute combined sclerosis. It also may be a result of intravascular volume depletion, as in severe gastrointestional hemorrhage, marked dehydration or massive diuresis. Postural hypotension is commonly associated with prolonged bed rest and represents an imbalance between the hemodynamic and neurologic response to changes in position. It may occur on standing when no other abnormality is present in older people who are relatively inactive and who have poor muscle tone and peripheral venous insufficiency.

A patient who has a history of postural hypotension should be repositioned in an upright position slowly, at the conclusion of dental treatment. The patient should be instructed not to shift positions from a lying to a sitting position very rapidly. Assistance may be required. In addition to the precautions mentioned above, the same steps taken to treat vasodepressor syncope should be utilized when treating postural hypotension, i.e., position and airway maintenance.

Cough syncope

Fainting may occur during a paroxysm of vigorous coughing. It is most frequently observed in individuals with chronic bronchitis or chronic obstructive pulmonary disease. The duration of faint is brief and there are usually no serious sequelae on regaining consciousness. Vigorous coughing and an increase in intra-abdominal pressure cause a sudden sharp rise in the cerebro-spinal pressure, which may squeeze blood from the intracranial vessels. Other theories that have been expressed to explain this form of syncope include a proposed decrease in cardiac output, which results from diminished venous return to the right heart subsequent to the concussive effect of the cough. The concern is not necessarily with the episode itself, since it is self limiting, but rather with its cause. A history of chronic bronchitis or chronic obstructive pulmonary disease should be taken into consideration when formulating the dental management of these patients.

Syncope in the hyperventilation syndrome

Hyperventilation (See chapter 6) may produce a clinical syndrome in which the patient experiences numbness and tingling of the hands, feet and face; varying degrees of reduction in the level of consciousness commonly described as dizziness, lightheadedness, giddiness, or fainting; blurring of vision; drying of the mouth; stiffness of the muscles and tetany. The overbreathing which results in hypocapnia in respiratory alkolosis may represent an acute or chronic state and may have an organic or functional basis. It is seen as a manifestation of anoxia, encephalopathy, and salicylate toxicity. Most commonly, however, it is psychogenic in etiology. It is observed much more frequently in adolescent girls and in women than in men.

The symptoms may be focused in one or more systems and may suggest organic diseases. Breathlessness is common. The patient complains of shortness of breath on performing minor tasks and sensation of choking or gasping and feeling of smothering, sighing, excessive yawning, or tightness in the chest. Frequently the complaint is that the patient cannot get enough air and feels as if he is going to die. The patient may be hyperventilating while he gives his story and be totally unaware of it, and may seem not to pay the least attention to the respiratory symptoms. Symptoms suggesting nervous system involvement are common, e.g., dizziness, lightheadedness, blurring of vision, feelings of unreality, impairment of memory, parethesias, and in the most severe form, occasional syncope. Chest pain is common and is usually described as a sharp fleeting twinge about the left nipple or under the left breast. Frequently there are palpations, tachycardia, or premature beats. Musculoskeletal system symptoms include myalgia, carpopedal spasms, twitching and rarely tetany. The patient may complain of a dry mouth and difficulty in swallowing. Aerophagia accounts for the belching, abdominal bloating and gas pains. Fatigue, exhaustion, weakness and lack of ambition are common. These symptoms develop in settings of tension. The anxiety may be overt and obvious even though the patient denies it and claims to be calm. On hyperventilation, the PCO_2 falls rapidly and the pH rises. The hypocapnia is believed to be responsible for the reduction of the cerebral blood flow. This is reflected in the electroencephalogram, which shows the slow wave activity. The reduction in the level of consciousness correlates well with slowing of the EEG. The syndrome may be relieved by having the patient rebreathe into a paper bag. Frequently hyperventilation can be prevented if time is taken to provide the proper explanation and support prior to initiating any dental treatment. Occasionally it may be necessary to prescribe tranquilizers to assist in alleviating the stress and anxiety associated with dental care.

Seizures

The term "epilepsy," refers to many types of recurrent seizures produced by excessive paroxysmal neuronal discharges. Epilepsy is usually divided into two categories: idiopathic and symptomatic. Idiopathic epilepsy is not caused by detectable, specific brain disease or by a metabolic disorder. In the vast majority of patients, the onset of idiopathic epileptic seizures occurs prior to age 30. Symptomatic epilepsy, on the other hand, is due to a structural cerebral lesion or metabolic abnormality, such as hypoglycemia or hypocalcemia. With advancing age and the onset of seizures, the incidence of symptomatic epilepsy rises steadily.

The spectrum of convulsive disorders poses its own baffling problems. Probably no other neurologic condition presents so varied and tangled an assortment of symptoms. Usually, the etiology is unknown, and evidence of structural disease is absent. The group is a large one and methods of classifying the epilepsies are diverse.

Attacks may be frequent or sparse, cyclical or quite capricious, triggered or spontaneous, and of variable intensity on successive occasions. The magnitude of distress may be massive or slight. Patterning of the attack is the rule, but variations are by no means exceptional from individual to individual and attack to attack.

Despite the variations, the vast array of patterns and the seemingly endless clinical types, there is a common denominator—the paroxysmal quality. An abrupt and dramatic change occurs in the person. The word ictus (a stroke blow, sudden attack) defines the phenomenon precisely. So do the terms, seizure and epilepsy, provided that the "seized" one returns to his normal state after the attack.

All convulsive seizures have one or more of the following components:

1. Impairment or loss of consciousness,
2. Amnesia for the episode,
3. Excessive or loss of muscle tone or movement,
4. Distorted sensations,
5. Vegetative and visceral manifestations caused by involvement of autonomic nervous systems or
6. Various psychic phenomena, such as abnormal thought processes or moods.

This section will present profiles of two of the more common types of epilepsy in the convulsive spectrum—grand mal epilepsy (generalized seizures) and petit mal epilepsy.

Grand mal epilepsy

Grand mal is the most conspicuous and severe of all seizures types, affecting more people than any other form of epilepsy. Loss of consciousness, its hallmark, is sudden in onset and brief in duration. Frequently the patient has a history of seizures and may experience an aura (e.g., a disagreeable odor or taste, irritable feeling or sensation of flashing light), which often precedes the seizure.

The grand mal seizure can be loosely divided in two phases—tonic and clonic. During both phases the pulse rate is usually rapid; blood pressure (often difficult to obtain), normal or slightly increased. Respiration may be irregular, with periods of apnea, and with the patient becoming progressively cyanotic.

The presence, prominence and duration of symptoms differ from patient to patient, but the variations are overshadowed by the convulsion itself. Grand mal often co-exists with other types, or it may be the culmination of other kinds of seizures.

The tonic (muscle tension) phase begins when the patient loses consciousness and collapses. At the same time, a massive tonic spasm wracks the body, often accompanied by a loud cry or scream. The back arches and the face grimaces. The limbs are rigidly extended; the ankles and wrists sharply flexed. The head is hyperextended and may rotate from one side to the other. In a fully developed major motor convulsion, a sequence of catatonic movements is very characteristic. Strangulation and death appear imminent. The tonic phase seldom lasts more than 10-15 seconds.

The transition to clonus is gradual. The first rhythmic, jerking movements are barely perceptible. Within seconds, however, the movements mount in magnitude and intensify, but become slower and more distinct until the violent flailings reach a climax in one final, most forceful jerk. The body goes limp. A deep, toneless coma sets in.

In the intervals between muscle contractions, air has begun to enter the lungs, cyanosis clears and apnea gives way to stertorous breathing. The patient gradually regains consciousness.

It is during the "crescendo" phase, particularly in a severe convulsion, that the tongue may be bitten, caught between teeth or fall back occluding the airway. Clonic heavings of the chest propel blood tinged, frothy saliva from the mouth. Voiding of urine may also occur; passage of feces is less frequent.

Prodromes and aura, whether of a sensory, motor, neurovegetative, or psychic nature are precursors of the paroxysm and are now generally viewed as detached portions of the seizure itself. Prodromes are regarded as the warnings that precede the main event by hours or even days and auras by seconds or minutes. About half the patients with recurrent major convulsions experience auras; far fewer report the occurrence of prodromes.

The symptoms heralding the onset of unconsciousness are usually stereotyped for the individual but the variety is large. Motor auras may be confused with focal seizures.

Post-seizure symptoms also are notable for their diversity and depend in large measure on the severity and duration of the attack. Headache may be reported and psychic disturbances are not uncommon. Usually the patient experiences the aftereffects upon awakening from a deep sleep that follows the coma and that may last from a few minutes to hours.

Status epilepticus

Status epilepticus is repeated, generalized seizures without intercurrent recovery. It is thought to be a direct continuation of the tonic, clonic convulsion described above. The difference between the convulsive phase and the generalized seizure in status epilepticus is the duration of the seizure activity. Status epilepticus may persist for hours and is the major cause of mortality directly related to the convulsive disorders.

Clinically, the patient is unconscious, cyanotic, demonstrates diaphoresis and has generalized clonic contractions. As status epilepticus continues, the patients become hyperthermic (body temperature reaches 106°) and the cardiovascular system is greatly overworked (rapid and irregular heart beat, blood pressure elevated significantly).

If the seizure activity continues and is not self limiting, immediate intravenous anticonvulsants are required. The administration of drugs, however, should not supercede the simple supportive measures required to maintain ventilation. A secure airway should be rapidly established. Head position, an oropharyngeal airway and suctioning often are sufficient. Oxygen should be started if the patient appears hypoxic.

Diazepam (valium) has the advantage of prompt action and is the drug of choice when immediate cessation of seizures is indicated. It is administered in doses of 5-10 mg intravenously with a rate not to exceed 5 mg/min. This dosage may be repeated in 15 minutes. The major side-effects of intravenous diazepam are respiratory depression and hypotension. Seizures tend to recur in 30-60 minutes, yet the depression of consciousness and risk of respiratory depression may be cumulative. These effects appear to be potentiated by barbiturates, monoamine oxydase inhibitors and narcotics. When status epilepticus does occur in the dental office, immediate medical assistance should be sought.

Diphenylhydanthoin (dilantin) is a highly effective anticonvulsant in adults and offers a reasonable margin of safety. When dilantin is administered intravenously, therapeutic levels cannot be achieved safely in less than 20 minutes. Therefore the drug is not used initially, when more immediate seizure control is mandatory. In suitable cases, intravenous dilantin offers the significant advantage of not severely depressing consciousness and this permits better neurological evaluation when the seizure has ceased.

Phenobarbital is the most commonly used barbituate in status epilepticus. Respiratory depression and hypertension, though rare, are the main side effects of large intravenous doses. An initial dose of 150-250 mg. is given at the rate of 25 mg/min. Additional doses can be given each 15-20 minutes if the seizure persists, but the cumulative dosage in the first two hours should usually not be greater than 400 mg.

Dental considerations

The dentist must determine the possibility of an acute seizure occurring during dental treatment. This of course is accomplished by eliciting a thorough medical history. A patient with a history of seizure activity should be asked the following questions:

1. What *type* of seizure, grand mal or petit mal
2. Does an *aura* precede the seizure
3. How long does the seizure *last*
4. Is it *self limiting*
5. When did the patient experience the last convulsion
6. What precipitated the last convulsion
7. What medication is the patient taking and when was the last dose taken

In addition to a thorough medical history, steps should be taken to diminish stress and anxiety, which tend to increase the possibility of seizures. Pre-medication with valium, either orally or parenterally, may be helpful, as well as the administration of nitrous oxide and oxygen. It is most important for the dentist and his staff to be prepared to manage any convulsion that may arise.

Treatment

1. If the seizure occurs in the dental chair, the chair should be placed in a supine position. In any case, the patient should be supine and often the floor offers a firm, flat, treatment surface. The pa-

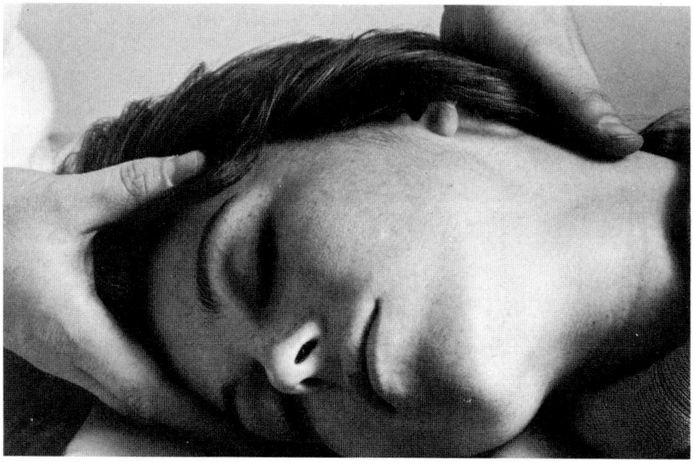

Fig. 5-2 Positioning of head to side to prevent aspiration of oral and nasopharyngeal secretions or vomitus.

tient's head is placed sideways in order to allow saliva and vomitus to exit and thereby prevent the possibility of aspiration (Fig. 5-2).

2. Patients should be protected from injuring themselves. This is accomplished by gently restraining the patient's extremities from uncontrolled movements but still allowing for some freedom of movement.
3. An adequate airway must be maintained. Occasionally during seizure activity there are periods of apnea. (To assist in maintaining a patent airway, the head tilt position may be used as long as all secretions have been suctioned from the patient's mouth so as not to create a situation where the patient may aspirate). At times the use of oxygen may be helpful, via face or nose mask.
4. There is some controversy as to the use of an object such as a tongue depressor covered with gauze to prevent tongue, cheek and lip biting. Many feel that this is not necessary and may cause tissue injury and bleeding due to the improper placement of these devices, as well as compromised airway patency.

Postictal phase

This is the period of time immediately following seizure activity. During this phase the patient is noted to be somewhat depressed and rather fatigued. Blood pressure, pulse and respirations may be somewhat below normal limits during this period. It is during this time that the patient must be observed very carefully to be sure that respiratory depression or airway obstruction does not occur. The emergency situation is not over until all vital signs are normal and patient is alert and oriented.
The patient should not be discharged from the office unaccompanied. It is recommended that the patient relax for the remainder of the day and not carry on any strenuous activity since the potential for a subsequent seizure exists.

Petit mal epilepsy

Petit mal epilepsy is viewed as a triad of minor fits, consisting of "absences," myoclonic jerks and akinetic "spells." They are dissimilar in appearance and seizure pattern but are closely connected by certain common bonds. All occur chiefly in childhood. All are very brief, with abrupt onset and end, have great frequency, and a characteristic spike wave abnormality in the electroencephlogram. Generally, each one of the types presents exclusively in each patient, but combinations do occur. They are more apt to occur when the patient is quiescent or drowsy than during activity. Often these attacks are not recognized as such because the changes are so slight and fleeting. In many cases of petit mal epilepsy it is not unusual for months or even a few years to pass before the parents consult a physician about the child's peculiarities.

The "absence" is by far the most common seizure type in petit mal. A sudden lapse in consciousness brings an abrupt change in appearance. An alert child instantly becomes a child who seems far away. A blank look or a vacant stare lasting several seconds interrupts the ordinary flow of psychic continuity. Simultaneously there may be a few adventitious eye blinks. At times there may be a momentary grimace, occasionally a gulp or two, a rub of the nose or a twitch of the mouth, but mainly the absence in the eyes. Then, just as rapidly, the child returns to normal.

The individual may or may not be aware of the transient blackout. Interruption of consciousness spans so short a time that he may not perceive the lapse. Asking the patient after an attack to repeat rote phrases or a number series spoken to him during the spell can test whether or not consciousness did exist. Having the patient hyperventilate for three or more minutes usually evokes typical "absences" thereby establishing the diagnosis. As a rule, these seizures disappear in adult life. Sometimes major attacks replace them.

Myoclonic jerks are sudden, split-second involuntary jerks of an entire limb, usually involving the muscles of the neck, arms or shoulders. They are massive, but random and isolated movements; sporadic, but most likely to occur in the morning. A pencil, a cup or spoon may be flung out of the child's hand and he is unable to explain the act. Quite often the incident is interpreted as a gesture of petulance. Such seizures are less common than "absences" and are relatively rare in adults.

Akinetic seizures known as "drop" seizures are less common than the other two forms. The child may suddenly drop, sag, collapse or fall to the ground with no perceptible change in consciousness. The fall may be quite forceful and cause injuries. In most instances, the patient gets up immediately and resumes his activity. Usually there is no report of lapse of consciousness.

Treatment

Petit mal seizures are self limiting and rarely is any treatment indicated. The patient should be observed to be sure that the petit mal seizure does not precede a grand mal convulsion. Patients who have petit mal status, where the petit mal seizures are repetitive, require intravenous diazepam.

Hypoglycemia

The maintenance of a constant blood glucose level is an essential part of homeostasis. A blood glucose level below the lower limits of normal reflects a defect in one or more of two kinds of homeostatic processes: 1) those which add glucose to the blood by mobilization of glucose from glycogen stores, formation of carbohydrates from non-glucose stores (gluconeogenesis), or absorption of ingested carbohydrates; and 2) those which remove glucose from the blood through utilization of glucose by liver, adipose tissue, muscle, brain, or other tissues.

Spontaneous hypoglycemia is a symptom complex caused by or associated with a variety of diseases. A precise classification of hypoglycemia, based on etiology and pathologic physiology that is both complete and logical, is difficult to establish, since in some entities the mechanism is still poorly understood, while in others the cause of hypoglycemia may be multifactoral. From the clinical view, patients with hypoglycemia may be grouped according to the usual relation of hypoglycemia to the fasting or postprandial (fed) state, as listed in Table 5-1.

Clinical manifestations

The clinical symptoms and signs of hypoglycemia are the same regardless of the underlying cause. The symptoms which occur in any given patient vary with the degree and rate of decline of blood glucose levels and with the variable and individual susceptibility of the underlying state of the central and autonomic nervous system. Symptoms associated with a rapid decline in blood glucose levels are due in part to activation of the autonomic nervous system and the ensuing release of epinephrine. The symptoms are sweating, shakiness, trembling, tachycardia, palpitations, pyloerection, anxiety, nervousness, weakness, fatigue, hunger, nausea and vomiting. Other symptoms of hypoglycemia result from decreased uptake of glucose and decreased utilization of oxygen by the brain. They usually occur when the decline in blood glucose to low levels is slow and/or when hypoglycemia is severe or prolonged. These symptoms are headache, lightheadedness, disturbances of vision, lethargy, yawning, faintness, restlessness, sense of unreality and difficulty with speech and thinking.

Other manifestations may be agitation, mental confusion, outbursts of temper or queer, bizarre, and psychotic behavior, somnolence, stupor, prolonged sleep, loss of consciousness, fever and hypothermia. Twitching, convulsions, "epilepsy" and bizarre neurologic signs, motor as well as sensory in nature, may occur. Prominent signs observed in patients with alcohol-induced hypoglycemia are hypothermia, conjugate deviation of eyes, extensor rigidity of extremities, positive Babinski signs and trismus. Repeated hypoglycemic episodes may lead to loss of intellectual ability. Extensive and permanent mental or neurologic damage may result from frequent and prolonged episodes of hypoglycemia, particularly in children.

The most commonly encountered form of hypoglycemia is termed Reactive Hypoglycemia. It is frequently associated with diabetes mellitus and in other cases there is no known underlying disease (idiopathic). This category will be discussed in detail.

Functional reactive hypoglycemia

The most frequently encountered hypoglycemic disorder in the adult in whom no demonstrable autonomic lesion can be demonstrated is "functional reactive" hypoglycemia. These patients have normal fasting blood glucose levels. Reactive functional hypoglycemia occurs almost uniformly in tense, striving individuals with some emotional problems. Excessive secretion of insulin in response to the normal rise of blood glucose following meals is seldom found. The mechanism involved in this type of hypoglycemia remains unclear. The diagnosis is suspected by a history of intermittent hypoglycemic symptoms occurring two to three hours after ingestion of a meal of carbohydrates. It is confirmed by an oral glucose tolerance test extended for four to five hours with blood samples being obtained at half hour intervals. Additional samples should be drawn at the onset of symptoms of hypoglycemia. After an initial normal rise in blood glucose, it is not unusual to find blood glucose levels of 30-40 mg per 100 ml between the second and fourth hour of the test. This is associated with reproduction of the patient's postprandial symptoms with a spontaneous return of the blood glucose level toward fasting level shortly thereafter.

The usual symptoms produced by reactive hypoglycemia are transitory and often subside spontaneously in 15-30 minutes.

Table 5-1 Classification of spontaneous hypoglycemia

I Fasting hypoglycemia
  A. Organic hypoglycemia: recognizable anatomic lesion
    1. Pancreatic islet beta-cell disease with **hyperinsulinism** in the adult
      a. Adenoma, single or multiple
      b. Microadenomatosis, with or without macroscopic isle-cell adenomas
      c. Carcinoma, with metastases
      d. Adenoma(s) or carcinoma, associated with adenomas or hyperplasia of other endocrine glands (familial multiple endocrine adenomatosis)
      e. Hyperplasia (rare)
    2. Pancreatic islet beta-cell disease with hyperinsulinism in infancy and childhood
      a. Hyperplasia (leucine-sensitive or -insensitive)
      b. Nesidioblastosis
      c. Adenoma
    3. Nonpancreatic tumors associated with hypoglycemia
    4. Anterior pituitary hypofunciton
    5. Adrenocortical hypofunciton
    6. Acquired diffuse hepatic disease
    7. Severe congestive renal insufficiency in non-insulin-dependent diabetic patients

  B. Hypoglycemia due to specific hepatic enzyme deficiency (infancy and childhood)
    1. Glycogen storage diseases
    2. Glycogen synthase deficiency
    3. Fructose 1,6-diphosphatase deficiency

  C. Functional hypoglycemia: no recognizable or persistent anatomic lesion
    1. Ethanol and poor nutrition
    2. Deficiency of glugcagon
    3. Severe inanition
    4. Ketotic hypoglycemia (infancy and childhood)
    5. Transient hypoglycemia in the newborn of low birth weight
    6. Transient **hyperinsulinism** of the newborn (hyperplasia of pancreatic islet cells reported)
      a. Infant of diabetic mother
      b. Erythroblastosis fetalis
    7. Insulin autoimmunity without previous insulin administration (?)

  D. Exogenous hypoglycemia
    1. Insulin administration
    2. Sulfonylurea administration
    3. Ingestion of ackee fruit (hypoglycin)
    4. Miscellaneous drugs

II Reactive (postabsorptive) hypoglycemia
  A. Functional hypoglycemia: no recognizable anatomic lesion
    1. Reactive functional: idiopathic
    2. Reactive: secondary to mild diabetes
    3. Alimentary hyperinsulinism

  B. Hypoglycemia due to specific hepatic enzyme deficiency
    1. Hereditary fructose intolerance (fructose 1-phosphate aldolase deficiency): infancy and childhood
    2. Galactosemia: infancy and childhood
    3. Familial fructose and galactose intolerance

Weakness, hunger, inward trembling, sweating, palpations, and tachycardia are the most common symptoms in these patients. Severe central nervous system dysfunction, especially loss of consciousness or convulsions, does not occur and the severity of symptoms is not progressive. In patients with functional hypoglycemia, attacks are more frequent when emotional stress and anxiety are greater. A prolonged or 72-hour fast is well tolerated and the concentration of blood glucose rarely drops below 45 mg per 100 ml. A family history of diabetes mellitus is usually absent. Recent publicity in the popular press and in books by some medical authors have led the public and some segments of the medical profession to believe that spontaneous hypoglycemia is a widespread and unrecognized cause of many physical and psychic ills. Promoting such a notion is a mistake. Persistent symptoms such as chronic fatigue, depression, lethargy, loss of vitality or anxiety that affect the population of the United States are not due to hypoglycemia. A definite diagnosis of hypoglycemia is justified only in the patient who has a history of transient symptoms typical of hypoglycemia occurring 2-4 hours after meals and in whom the glucose tolerance test produces both hypoglycemia and synchronous symptoms.

The distressing symptoms experienced by patients with functional hypoglycemia may be prevented by a diet low in carbohydrates, and high in protein, with adequate fat to maintain caloric requirements. An important approach is to improve the psychologic and emotional status of the patient with functional hypoglycemia. The prognosis is good, since usually the disease is self limiting within a few months or years.

Reactive hypoglycemia secondary to diabetes mellitus

The reactive hypoglycemia secondary to diabetes has a different underlying mechanism than reactive functional hypoglycemia and the prognosis is different. Whereas in patients with reactive functional hypoglycemia the pancreatic insulin release is well timed in response to the rising postprandial blood glucose, in patients with mild diabetes insulin release is delayed. It is not until blood glucose rises to frankly diabetic levels that insulin is secreted in excess. Measurements of serum insulin during glucose tolerance tests in such patients have demonstrated that relatively large amounts of insulin are released, albeit late. The blood glucose then decreases from diabetic to normal levels and further to hypoglycemic levels. This type of hypoglycemic response is most likely to occur between the third and fifth hours. It is apparent that these patients have only mild diabetes, since endogoneous insulin is available and their fasting blood glucose is within normal limits. Their carbohydrate intolerance can be detected by postprandial blood glucose determination or an oral glucose tolerance test. Frequently, there is a family history of diabetes mellitus. Treatment consists of a diabetic diet with limitation of carbohydrate intake and frequent feeding. Weight reduction in the obese patient may normalize glucose tolerance, with a disappearance of reactive hypoglycemia. Unlike the relatively benign prognosis of reactive functional hypoglycemia, this disorder is not self limiting, and some patients may eventually progress to a more advanced state of insulin deficiency and the clinical syndrome of diabetes mellitus.

Treatment

The management of a patient experiencing a reactive hypoglycemia episode will be dictated by the patient's state of consciousness.

The Conscious Patient: The treatment of choice for the conscious patient who is cooperative and demonstrates clinical symptoms of hypoglycemia is the adminis-

Abboject disposable single-dose vial and vial injector with needle

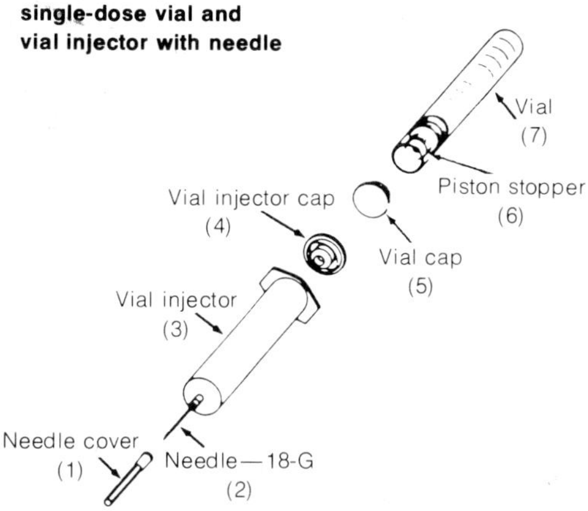

Directions for use

Note: To maintain sterility of needle and piston-stopper, do not assemble vial injector (syringe) or remove needle cover until ready to use.

A) Aseptically remove vial injector cap (4) and vial cap (5).

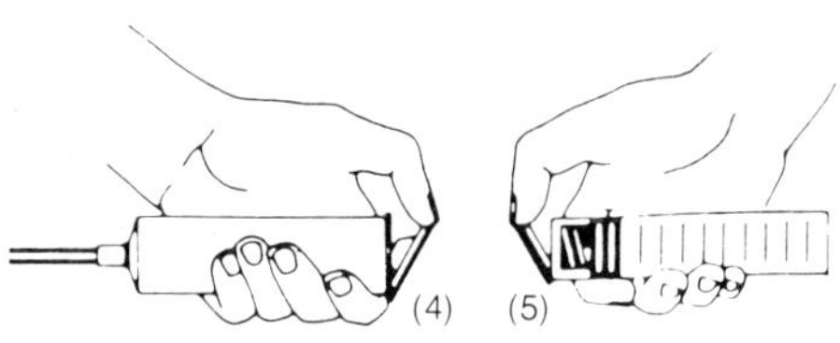

B) Insert glass vial (7) into plastic vial injector (3).

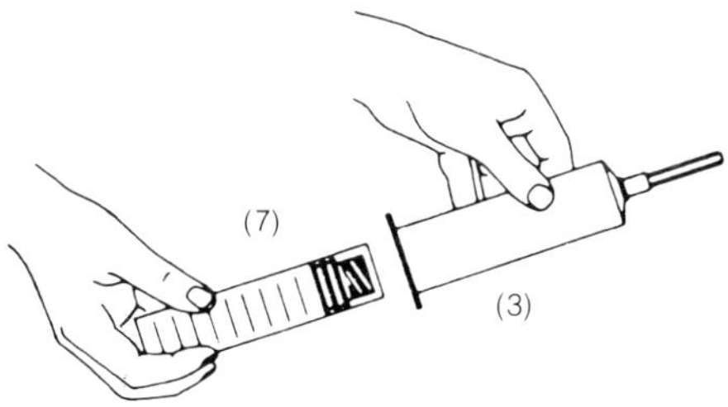

C) Rotate vial (7) three turns clockwise, or until resistance is felt. Needle will then be in contact with medication.

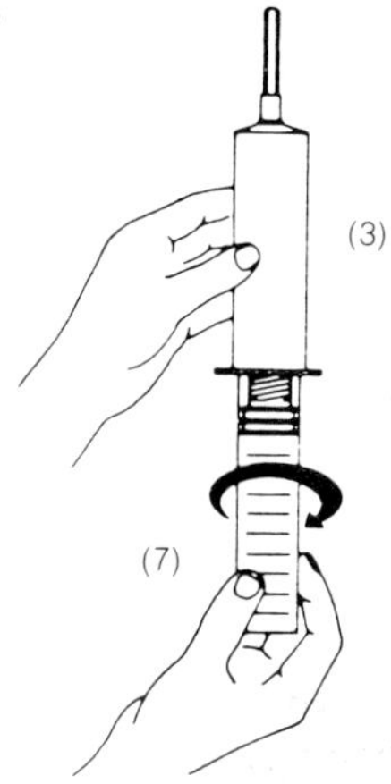

D) Grasp needle cover (1) firmly at the base, twist until loose, then pull off. (To adapt Vial Injector to Luer fitment: Raise needle cover just above the hub. Bend needle back and forth to snap off. Vial injector is now ready for use with any universal female adapter.)

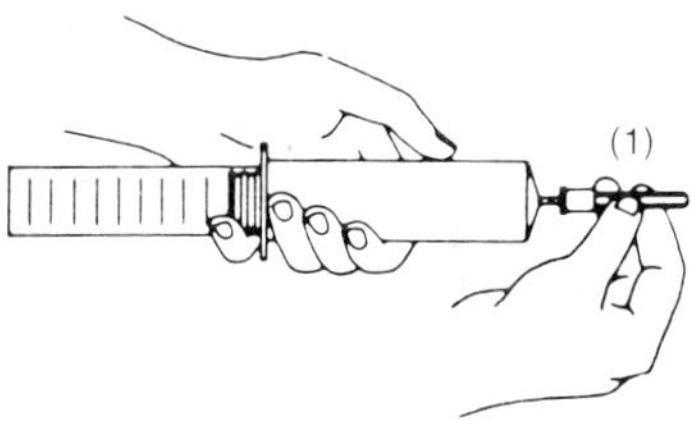

E) Use the assembled vial and vial injector the same as a conventional syringe.
Important: If plunger (glass vial) is rotated during injection, rotation must be clockwise.

(Counterclockwise rotation will prevent needle from maintaining proper contact with medication.)

F) Discard any unused solution and the injector with needle after single patient use. Do not resterilize or reuse.

Fig. 5-3 Directions for use of Abboject disposable single-dose vial (From Schijatschky, M., "Life Threatening Emergencies in the Dental Practice" published in 1975 by Quintessence Publishing Co., Inc.).

tration of a high carbohydrate beverage, such as orange juice, cola, ginger ale or a glucose drink such as glucola. A six to 12 ounce portion of cola soft drink contains 20-40 gm of glucose. The patient will respond almost immediately and should be observed until vital signs are stable and all signs and symptoms of hypoglycemia have disappeared.

Unconscious Patient: In the unconscious individual, 50% dextrose in water (30-50 ml intravenously) should be administered intravenously at once (Fig. 5-3). Within three to five minutes after injection the patient should regain consciousness. Another drug that can be administered is glucagon, 1 mg. intramuscularly. The patient will respond to the glucagon within 10-15 minutes after the injection. Any patient who has experienced periods of unconsciousness should not be permitted to go home, but rather should be taken to a hospital for further evaluation and treatment. In addition to the above, management of the unconscious patient includes airway maintenance, oxygen administration and monitoring of vital signs.

Dental considerations

Following medical and dental evaluation of the diabetic patient, consideration should be given to the patient's management. If any questions arise as to the patient's status, consultation with the patient's physician is encouraged. Dental appointments should be scheduled approximately one and one-half hours after breakfast and administration of the morning insulin. Patients on intermediate and long-lasting insulin dosage must have it adjusted accordingly. This, of course, should be done in consultation with the physician. Common causes of hypoglycemia are omission or delay of meals, excessive exercise prior to meals and overdosage of insulin. Dental therapy may require the patient to alter eating habits for periods of time. The patient may avoid eating either prior to or after a dental appointment.

References

1. Beeson, P.B., McDermott, W., Wyngaarden, J.B.: *Cecil's Textbook of Medicine.* Philadelphia: Saunders, 1979.
2. Chue, P.W.: "Transient Loss of Consciousness: Common Faint or Serious Symptom," *Dental Survey* 51, No. 11, 40-8, November 1975.
3. "Commonly Encountered Neurologic Disorders: the Convulsive Spectrum, Part I: an illustrated overview." No. 4 in a series. Nutley, NJ: Roche Laboratories 1973.
4. McCarthy, F.M. *Emergencies in Dental Practice—Prevention and Treatment.* Philadelphia: Saunders, 1979.
5. Malamed, Stanley, F. *Handbook of Medical Emergencies in the Dental Office.* St. Louis: Mosby, 1978.
6. Schwartz, G.R., et al. *Principles in Practice of Emergency Medicine.* Philadelphia: Saunders, 1978.
7. Thorn, G.W., Adams, R.D., Braunwald, E., Isselbacher, K.J., Petersdorf, R.G. *Harrison's Principles of Internal Medicine.* N.Y.: McGraw-Hill, 19.

Chapter 6

Respiratory Emergencies

Barry H. Hendler, D.D.S., M.D. and Louis F. Rose, D.D.S., M.D.

During normal inspiration, the diaphram descends and the ribs move upward so that the thoracic cavity is enlarged. This creates a negative pressure within the thorax, causing air to enter the upper airway and travel to the lungs which inflate and thereby eliminate this vacuum. Oxygen in the inspired air leaves the pulmonary alveolar spaces and enters the circulation. Carbon dioxide leaves the blood and enters the alveolar air from which it is carried to the atmosphere with exhalation. Interference at any point in this sequence, or with the central nervous system's control of it, may result in respiratory insufficiency requiring respiratory support. Entitites which cause this state of interference range from underlying medical disorders, such as congestive heart failure to simple aspiration of a foreign body.

The respiratory emergencies discussed, which commonly occur acutely in outpatient practice, can be classified as follows: 1) upper airway *obstruction*, 2) acute bronchiolar and upper airway *constriction* and 3) hyperventilation. In treating any patient with respiratory insufficiencies, certain signs become apparent and are keys to the successful diagnosis and management of these problems.

Respiratory rate is normally between 14 and 20 breaths per minute, spaced fairly evenly. An extremely low rate found in some patients with narcotic overdose or brain damage may not allow adequate air exchange. An extremely rapid rate, with a relatively small volume of air moved per breath, may also be inadequate. By itself, respiratory rate is seldom absolutely diagnostic of insufficiency but may afford a clue raising a reasonable doubt of adequacy.

Since normal breathing is mostly diaphramatic the rise and fall of the abdomen is the predominant physical feature. In many pathologic conditions all the chest muscles that control its expansion are called into play. The muscles of the neck which attach to the clavical and upper ribs contract during inspiration raising and stabilizing the thorax. When these *muscular movements* of the neck become plainly visible, this is a sign of respiratory difficulty. When the airway is obstructed the thoracic cavity expands and a partial vacuum is created within the chest, but air cannot pass freely into the lungs to eliminate it. The soft tissues between the ribs and just above the clavical will be drawn inward by this vacuum and this *retraction* may even include the sternum. This sign is most easily seen in young people and is much less prominent in the older individual with a fixed, relatively rigid rib cage.

In anyone with an obstructed airway, this retraction may be seen and its observation provides an immediate insight into the nature of the respiratory problem. After the observation of retraction, inspection of the oropharynx may reveal obstruction due to foreign matter, such as vomitus, blood, dentures, food or other materials. It is surprising how often this simple examination is overlooked, however its importance cannot be overemphasized.

The skin and oral tissues offer additional diagnostic clues. If oxygenation of the blood is so poor that a sufficient amount of hemoglobin is not combined with oxygen to give it a bright red color, the blood becomes dark. The skin and oral mucous membranes transmit this dark color; and the tissues with rich blood supply become noticeably cyanotic.

This is readily seen in the lips, gums and tongue, regardless of the race of the individual. Since cyanosis depends upon the change in color of circulating hemoglobin, the profoundly anemic individual may not show it, since there must be an absolute reduction of five (5) grams.

Another skin sign is related to the accumulation of carbon dioxide in the blood. The release of neurohumoral agents such as epinephrine or norepinephrine cause constriction of small blood vessels under the stimulus of accumulated carbon dioxide. This causes notable pallor of the skin. Perspiration is also stimulated to the extent that moisture can be seen clearly on the skin, and the skin will demonstrate a cold, damp or "clammy" nature. Palpation of the pulses will usually reveal a fast and often irregular beat, caused by circulating epinephrine or norepinephrine. In severe cases brain damage may have ensued and the pulse may be very slow because of central nervous system depression.

When examining the patient, respiratory sound should be noted by the observer. The most ominous sign of all is the silence accompanying complete airway obstruction. This is the gravest of emergencies since death will result very quickly unless the obstruction is relieved. If obstruction is partial and caused by the tongue falling back, occluding the posterior wall of the oral pharynx, a low-pitched snoring sound will be heard. A pure, high-pitched crowing sound may be made by air moving through the cords in partial spasm, rather than widely separated as in normal inspiration. Liquid, such as blood, thick ropy saliva or vomitus in the upper airway will cause a gurgling sound as air percolates through it. In the lungs, bronchiolar spasm causes air to make a wheezing sound during exhalation. Such sounds may also be generated by air moving past a partial obstruction elsewhere in the respiratory tract, through the larynx to the bronchioles. Liquid in fine air passages, such as the terminal alveolar sacs, will cause a variety of sounds, best heard with a stethoscope. These range from crackling noises known as rales to louder, coarser sounds called rhonchi.

Emergency measures are mandatory if signs of severe difficulty are present. Simple manual measures should be taken before complex maneuvers, requiring specialized instrumentation and skills, are performed.

If the patient is attempting to breathe but the airway is obstructed, the site and nature of the obstruction must be determined. The mouth should be opened and the pharynx inspected for foreign material. Any liquid should be removed by suction and solid matter should be extracted manually. During digital exploration of the pharynx, the patient may gag and vomit, so suction should always be immediately available during this maneuver. If vomiting takes place, the patient's head should be turned to the side and the oral cavity evacuated as quickly as possible, to prevent aspiration. If the pharynx is filled with material, this initial clearing will be aided by gravity, if the patient's head is turned to one side and the opposite shoulder is elevated. If the patient is not fully conscious, a rubber bite block or gauze roll should be placed between the patient's teeth before introducing an examining finger or instruments into the patient's mouth.

Other than foreign matter in the airway, the commonest obstruction is caused by the base of the tongue. The tongue has a tendency to fall backward against the posterior pharyngeal wall when the patient is lying on his back. If unconscious, the patient cannot correct this situation, and the base

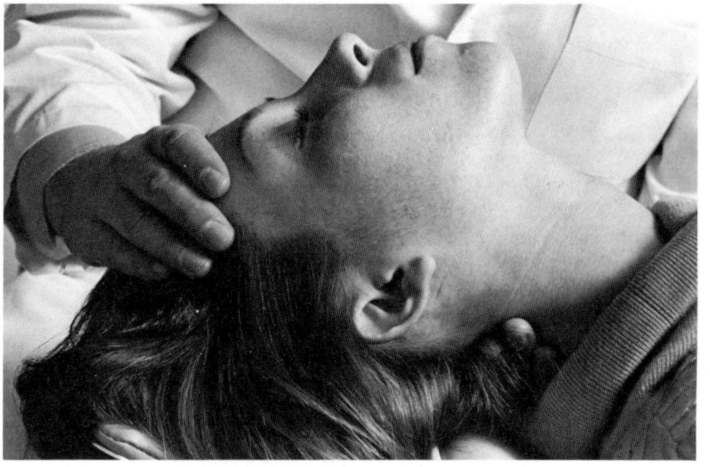

Fig. 6-1 Head tilt—hyperextension of the head is the simplest way of establishing an emergency airway.

of the tongue can completely obstruct the airway at the laryngeal inlet, by closing off all air ingress through the oral and nasal pharynx. By placing one hand behind the patient's neck and one hand on the patient's forehead, the head can be quickly hyperextended (Fig. 6-1).

This hyperextension maneuver will force the mandible forward and help pull the base of the tongue from the posterior pharyngeal wall. If this maneuver is not successful, the mandible can be further displaced forward, by placing pressure behind the angles of the mandible slightly below and in front of each ear, and exerting manual pressure forward (Fig. 6-2). Another simple maneuver involves grasping the symphysis menti with two fingers, controlling the dorsum of the tongue and dislocating the mandible forward (Fig. 6-3).

This should insure an adequate airway, with no obstruction at the base of the tongue. Several other devices have been employed to facilitate resuscitative respiratory care. Oral and nasal airways aid in the anterior displacement of the tongue but do not necessarily eliminate the need for manual mandibular displacement as well (Fig. 6-4). When used in conjunction with a bag and mask these may be found to be quite useful.

Once the airway has been secured, attention must be focused on the patient's respiratory efforts. If the patient is apneic, or breathing is so infrequent that there is doubt about sufficiency, the first thing that must be done is to assume this function for the patient. By controlling respiration, life may be sustained while the cause of respiratory failure is ascertained. If no equipment is available, mouth-to-mouth resuscitation is a satisfactory method (Fig. 6-5). A plastic mouthpiece that is designed to prevent the patient's tongue from falling back into the pharynx facilitates the delivery of mouth-to-mouth resuscitation. A self inflating bag and mask, with a provision for adding oxygen to the inflow of the bag, is a valuable aid to ventilation for patients who experience respiratory failure (Fig. 6-6).

Upper airway obstruction—aspiration of a foreign body

Obviously, foreign body aspiration can occur anywhere. However, the dental operatory, with the patient in a supine position and with the availability of objects and

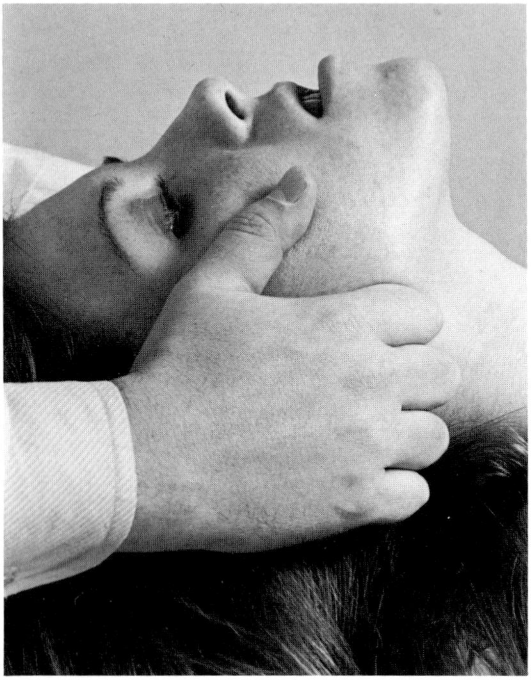

Fig. 6–2 Forward pressure at the posterior border and angle of mandible is exerted with both hands.

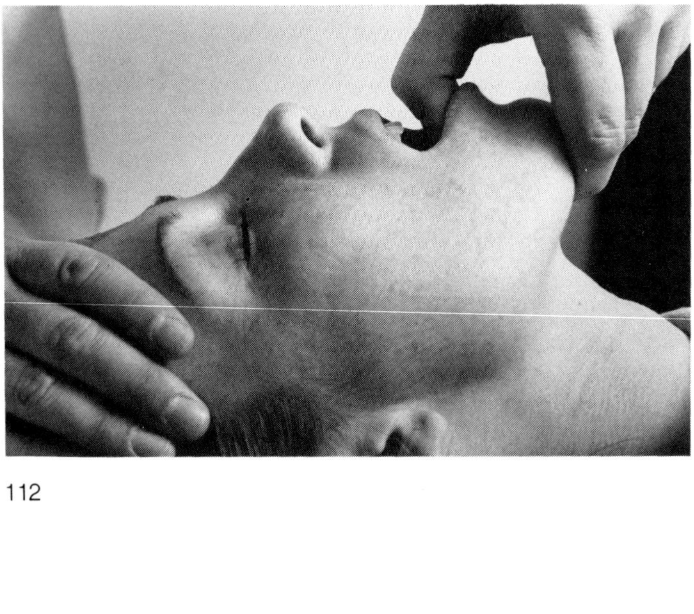

Fig. 6–3 Anterior dislocation of the mandible can be achieved by grasping the symphysis menti.

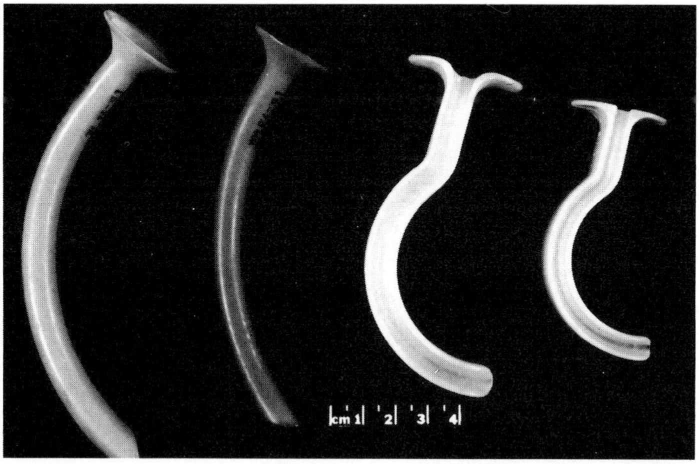

Fig. 6–4a Nasal and oropharyngeal airways, various sizes.

Figs. 6–4b and 6–4c Technique of placing an oral airway.

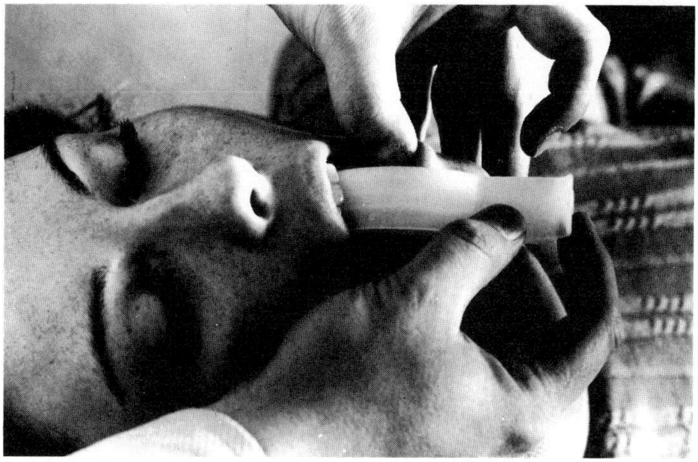

Figure 6–4b

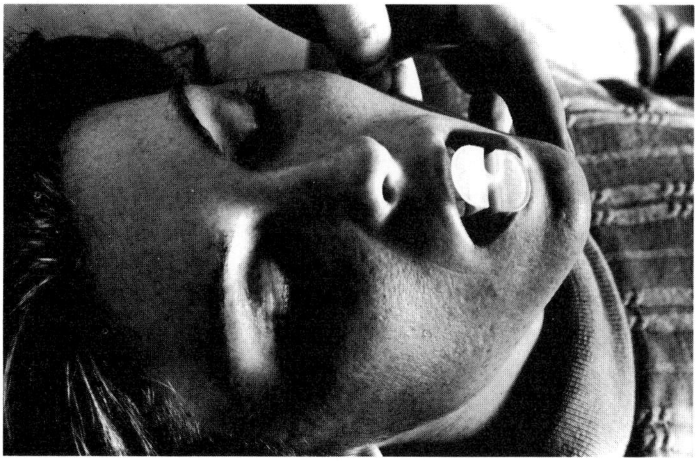

Figure 6–4c

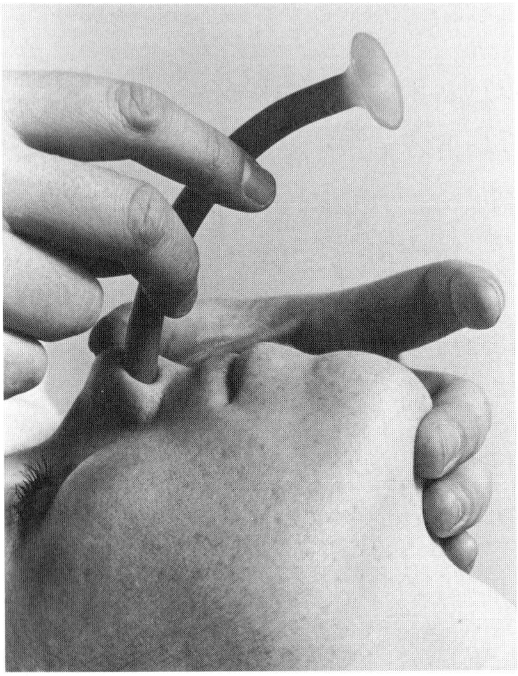

Figure 6–4d

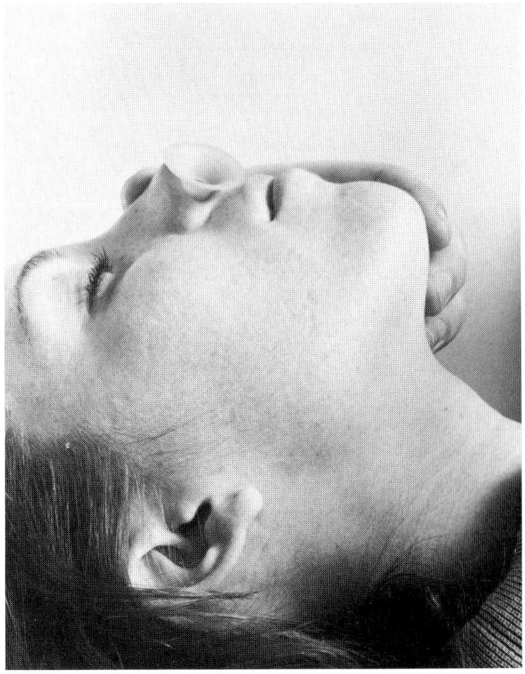

Figure 6–4e

Figs. 6–4d and 6–4e Technique of placing a nasal airway.

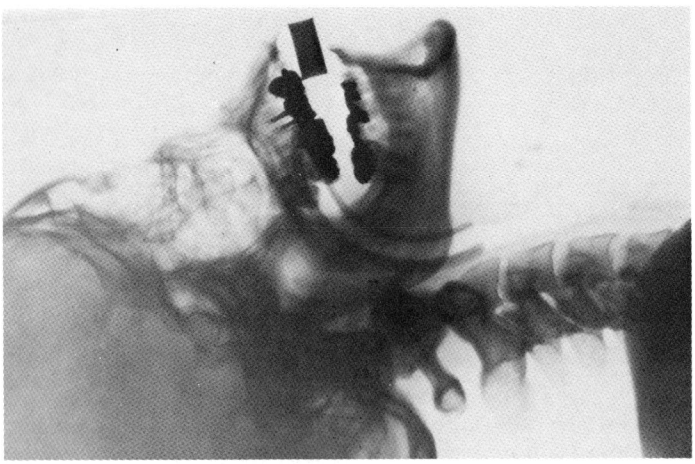

Fig. 6–4f X-ray of improper oral anatomic airway position (From Schijatschky M., "Life Threatening Emergencies in the Dental Practice" published in 1975 by Quintessence Publishing Co., Inc.).

Figs. 6-5a and 6-5b Mouth-to-mouth ventilatory assistance.

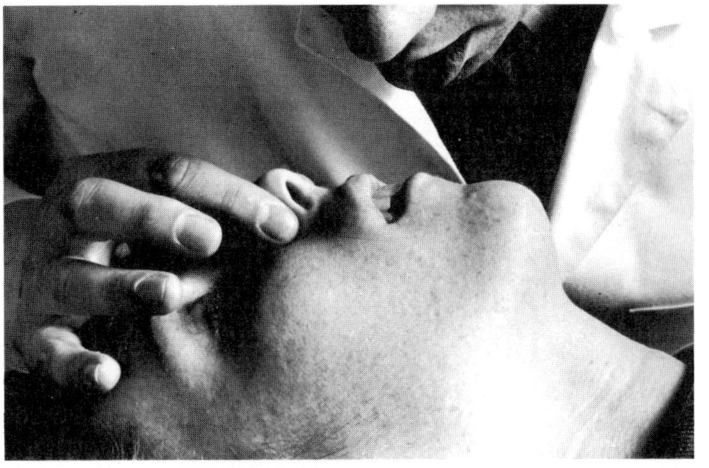

Fig. 6-5a Nose pinched—head hyperextended.

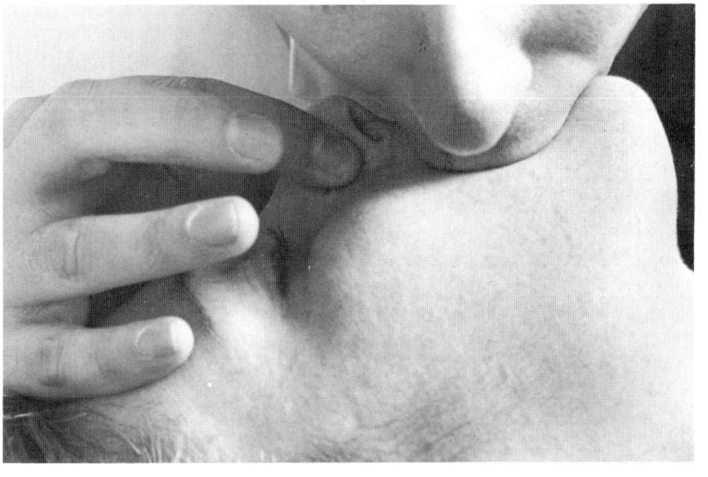

Fig. 6-5b Patient's mouth engulfed by rescuer's, prior to inflation of lungs.

materials in the oral cavity, is a high risk environment for upper airway obstruction and aspiration. Small objects of obstruction are usually coughed out or swallowed by a conscious dental patient. If the object lodges in the tracheobronchial tree or in the larynx, immediate attention is focused on removal of the object. An aspirated foreign body will produce either partial or total obstruction. If partial obstruction has occurred, the patient will usually be able to phonate or make high-pitched, crowing-like sounds and cough effectively. It is important not to interfere with the patient's attempt to clear his throat and upper airway passages. If these initial attempts are unsuccessful, obstruction may be relieved, as described below. The positioning of the patient is extremely important. If the patient is in the supine position, the airway should be opened by hyperextension of the head and placing the mandible forward. The airway should be checked and breathing assessed. If the patient is not breathing, an initial attempt at artificial ventilation is performed by any of the methods described. If the patient cannot be ventilated, treatment is then performed as follows.

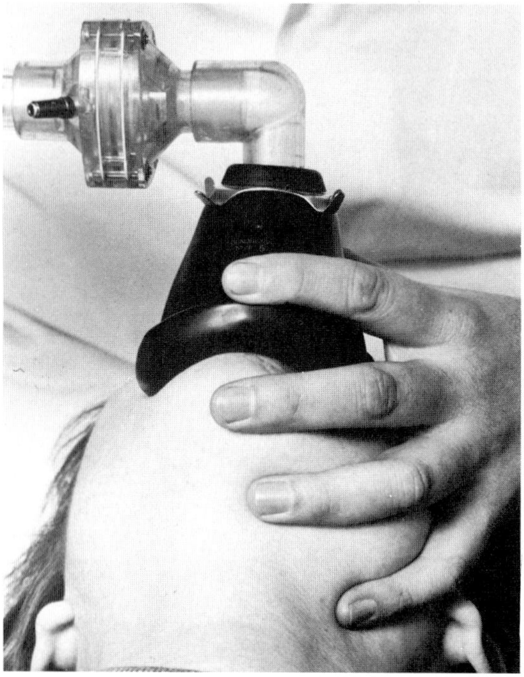

Fig. 6-6 Hand position for bag and face mask ventilatory assistance.

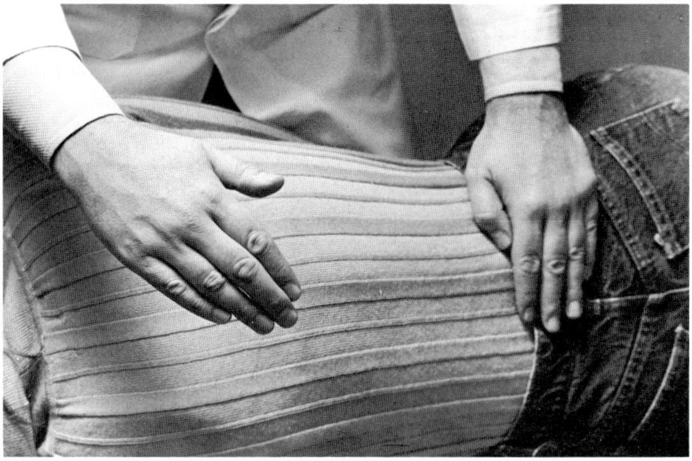

Fig. 6-7 Back slap maneuver.

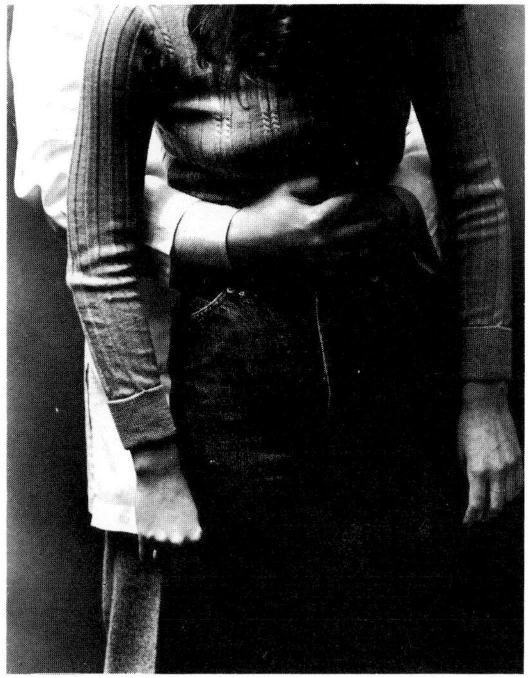

Fig. 6-8 Heimlich maneuver.

Conscious Patient: If the patient is in a supine position and conscious, he should be turned toward the doctor. With the heel of the hand the patient is struck between the shoulder blades several times in rapid succession (Fig. 6-7). As in this and all subsequent maneuvers, an attempt is made to increase intrathoracic pressure and generate sufficient force to expel an object which may be dislodged somewhere along the tracheobronchial tree. After the back blows are delivered the patient is returned to the supine position, the airway rechecked and respiration reassessed. In the conscious patient, if this technique has not been successful, the Heimlich maneuver should be performed (Fig. 6-8). The rescuer is positioned behind the patient, wrapping his arms around the patient's waist. A fist is formed and placed so the thumb side is against the abdomen between the navel and rib cage. With the other hand the fist is grasped and pressure is applied quickly in an inward and upward direction. If necessary, this maneuver is repeated several times. The objective of the Heimlich maneuver is to elevate the diaphragm in order to compress the lungs, an additional technique to increase intrathoracic pressure. A third maneuver is the abdominal thrust. This should be performed if the first two methods have failed and normal respiration has not returned (Fig. 6-9). The rescuer kneels next to the patient and places the heel of one hand in the middle of the abdomen between the navel and the rib cage. This hand is then grasped with the free hand and pressure is applied inward and upward against the abdominal wall. If necessary, these thrusts are repeated several times.

The Unconscious Patient: If the patient is unconscious and breathing has ceased, it is important to first ascertain the cause of the respiratory arrest. If there is total

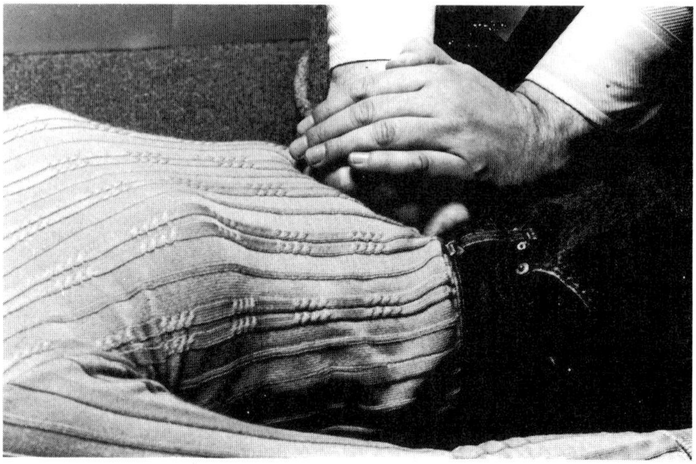

Fig. 6–9 Abdominal thrust.

obstruction by a foreign body the patient will be unable to breathe or make any sound. Interventation must take place immediately. The patient should be placed in the supine position and the airway assessed by head hyperextension. An attempt should be made to restore breathing, using mouth-to-mouth resuscitation or bag mask resuscitation. A back slap maneuver should be performed, as in the conscious patient, by positioning the patient on his side with the chest braced against the legs of the rescuer. The back is struck between the shoulder blades with the heel of the hand, several times in rapid succession. If this is unsuccessful the abdominal thrust maneuver should be performed.

Other Procedures: If the foreign body cannot be removed by any of the aforementioned procedures, then the rescuer has three techniques available: 1) endotracheal intubation, 2) cricothyreotomy, and 3) tracheostomy. Cricothyreotomy is the simplest method to achieve an adequate airway in a patient with diagnosed foreign body aspiration. The cricothyreotomy permits entrance into the upper airway below the obstruction which is usually in the larynx, without the need for a surgical procedure such as tracheostomy, which should be performed by one experienced in the technique.

The laryngeal skeleton is formed predominantly by the thyroid and cricoid cartilages and the hyoid bone. These structures are readily palpated in the midline of the neck anteriorally. The thyroid cartilage is responsible for the visible bulge known as the "Adams Apple." It is composed of two large plates of cartilage that are joined anteriorally and are open in the back. A downward projection articulates with the cricoid cartilage below. The level of the upper border of the thyroid cartilage can be determined by feeling a V shaped notch where the upper borders of the two thyroid plates meet in the midline.

The cricoid cartilage is frequently described as having the shape of a signet ring, with a narrow arch anteriorally and laterally and an expanded portion posteriorally. It is the only complete tracheal ring and in the upper respiratory tract; it is the only rigid structure that completely encircles the airway. The first cartilageous tracheal ring is attached to the cricoid by the cricoid tracheal ligament. The thyroid cartilage is attached above, to the hyoid bone, by the thyrohyoid membrane, and below to

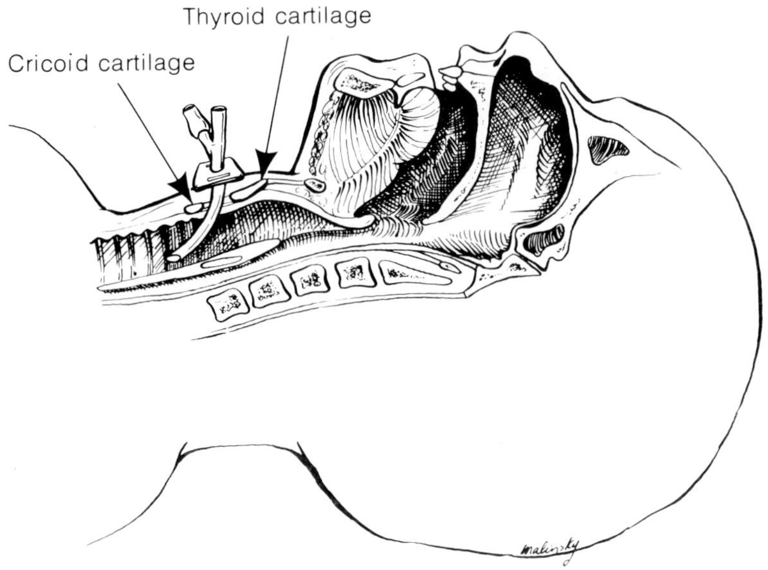

Fig. 6–10 (Schematic drawing) Technique of cricothyreotomy.

the cricoid by the cricothyroid membrane, This membrane occupies a relatively superficial location in the neck and can be easily punctured in an emergency situation for airway management.

The head should be hyperextended to permit easy identification of the thyroid and cricoid cartilages as well as the cricothyroid membrane. The index finger should be placed between the thyroid and cricoid cartilages, in the midline on the membrane, and held steady. A small horizontal incision can be made with a scalpel approximately ½ cm. in length just through the skin and subcutaneous tissue. If a cricothyroid needle is available anesthesia may not be needed, if the patient is unconscious, or can be achieved by local anesthetic infiltration in the area of the incision. The needle is inserted through this incision, through the cricothyroid membrane, until the tracheal lumin is entered. Vigorous coughing by the patient may be noted at this point. The curved nature of the torcar should insure proper passage inferiorly through the trachial lumin. As spontaneous respiration occurs, the victim may soon regain consciousness; however, ventilatory assistance may be instituted immediately through the cricothyroidomy needle's external opening (Fig. 6-10).

Acute bronchiolar and upper airway constriction

Emergencies in Allergy: Both mild and severe allergic reactions have common initial signs and symptoms, i.e., sneezing with rhinorrhea, itching and tearing of the eyes, skin rash, etc. However, they may be differentiated by progression and severity of these clinical manifestations. Mild allergic reactions may be drug-induced or secondary to exposure to allergens. Therapeutic substances such as penicillin and aspirin have often been incriminated in these reactions. However, any new substance to which the patient has been exposed can be potentially dangerous. Clinical manifestations also include nasal obstruction, or hives with intense itching, or swelling of the hands, face and eyelids.

More serious reactions may lead to respiratory difficulty caused by laryngeal edema. Since the patient may have an allergy to a particular drug, caution is required before administering any medications. An important criterion in evaluating the severity of allergic reaction is the period of time between the administration of the drug and the manifestation of the signs and symptoms.

Although a severe allergic reaction is usually rapid in onset, occurring within minutes of ingestion or exposure to the sensitizing agent, it may take hours for the signs and symptoms to become manifest. Generally, the longer it takes for the clinical findings to appear the milder the reaction will be. Though allergic reactions can be immediate or delayed, the immediate type of reaction is of particular significance in outpatient practice.

There are three recognizable forms of severe allergic reactions. These include acute laryngeal edema, acute severe bronchial asthma and acute anaphylactic shock. All three have in common the inherent danger of respiratory tract obstruction by interference with the passage of air, either in the larynx or in the finer branches of the bronchial tree.

Although it is important to distinguish this group of emergencies from the so-called anaphylactoid group, the primary respiratory nature of these, as opposed to the picture of shock and convulsions of the anaphylactoid phenomena, simplifies the rapid decision so necessary in some of these cases. Differential diagnosis should not present a problem except in the case of laryngeal edema when the possibility of a foreign body lodged in the larynx should be considered. Much has been made of the differential diagnosis between acute severe asthma and acute pulmonary edema, but it is our opinion that the resemblance between the two is not sufficient to cause confusion.

Anaphylactic reactions are sudden shock-like and often fatal events most commonly occurring incident to the use of antibiotics, local anesthetics or intravenous die contrast media. The local anesthetics are usually in toxic dose. Anaphylactoid reactions are the result of accidental intravenous injection, drug idiosyncracy, or potentiated toxicity. Recent evidence suggests that some of these may be due to otherwise innocuous genetic traits or enzyme deficiencies. Neither skin tests nor history of allergy is of any value in anticipating anaphylactoid reaction.

Acute Laryngeal Edema: This emergency is a rather localized reaction which is pathologically similar to acute anaphylactic shock, but edema is restricted to the larynx, mouth and lips, and there may be an associated generalized bradycardia. The patient becomes quite frightened and feels that his throat is "closing off." The patient's instinctive alarm is quite justified, although his panic may be out of proportion to the degree of laryngeal obstruction. The clinical picture can appear quite rapidly. However, certain manifestations may take an hour or more to develop.

Cyanosis is a late manifestation and is rare if the acute edema is treated immediately. Characteristic of acute laryngeal edema is the absence of breath sounds, or feeling of air movement within oral and nasal passages. Respiratory attempts are made, but little or no air is moved.

In partial laryngeal obstruction, a high-pitched crowing sound is audible. The patient may rapidly lose consciousness from hypoxia. His condition will respond promptly with treatment of aqueous epinephrine (1:1,000) administered by subcutaneous or IM injection. The adult dose ranges from 0.3 to 0.5 cc. The pediatric dose is 0.01 mg/kg to a maximum of 0.3 mgm. Epinephrine may be repeated whenever there is evidence of recurrence of symptoms regardless of frequency, usually every 5 to 15 minutes.

However, the use of diphenhydramine (Benadryl) 50 mg. IM for its antihistamic effect, or corticosteroid (hydrocordisone succinate) 100-500 mg. IM for its action in curtailing edema, may be of benefit and may obviate the additional use of epinephrine once acute symptoms have subsided. Benadryl and cortisone have long-term effects which will help to prevent relapse of symptoms. Cricothyreotomy may be indicated in the totally obstructed airway which cannot be relieved by epinephrine administration.

There is always the possibility that the trachea may also be as edematous as the larynx, thus cricothyreotomy is more difficult in this type patient. We reserve decision for tracheotomy for those skilled in this procedure.

Acute Bronchial Asthma: Bronchial asthma is defined clinically as paroxysmal shortness of breath, associated with expiratory wheezing. Mechanisms responsible for the various airway obstructions which is the cause of breathlessness are: 1) increased tone of the bronchial smooth muscle, 2) thickening of the bronchial mucosa as a result of edema or hyperemia, and 3) plugging of the smaller airways by viscid secretions.

Major factors which precipitate asthmatic attacks are emotional disturbances, hypersensitivity or allergic reactions, and infection of the respiratory tract. Hypoxemia is a common occurrence even in mild asthmatic attacks. However, severe attacks may cause dangerous hypoxemia which is potentially lethal.

The most striking pulmonary lesion in patients who die from this condition is widespread plugging of the bronchioles and bronchi with inspirated mucous. It is a frequent clinical observation that asthmatic attack terminates with the expectoration of sticky mucoid sputum. Therapy, therefore, is on a broader basis than in years past. A predominant symptom is shortness of breath associated with expiratory wheeze. There is a short, gasping inspiration and a long noisy expiration. There is a history of rapid onset of dyspnea which accelerates in severity. Since the patient has usually had previous asthma his familiar medications have failed to provide relief. These previous similar attacks often date back to childhood or early adult life. There is notably poor chest expansion and the patient may be severely distressed, fatigued and pale. His total efforts are being devoted to the respiratory process. Shock is usually not present; cyanosis is uncommon.

Danger signs indicating that intensive therapy is urgent are: 1) tachycardia, 2) minimum sputum production suggesting the retention of secretions in the bronchial tree further intensifying the airway obstruction, 3) increasing restlessness and confusion suggesting cerebral anoxia, 4) increasing breathlessness with decreased wheezing indicating partial airway obstruction is becoming complete, and 5) exhaustion and the evidence of peripheral circulatory failure.

The most likely condition to be confused with severe bronchial asthma is acute left heart failure, particularly because both frequently cause attacks of breathlessness during the night.

There are some clinical features which aid in distinguishing between these two similiar entities. Congestive heart failure often produces breathlessness for the first time during middle age or after. Wheezing is less noticeable in congestive heart failure. Sputum, if produced, is watery and blood stained, as opposed to the thick mucoid or purulent sputum produced in bronchial asthma. Other signs of underlying heart disease and congestive heart failure, such as ankle edema, are often present.

Management

Patients with acute bronchial asthma attacks are rarely admitted to the hospital. They are commonly encountered in outpatient practice, and even though the attack may be somewhat severe, conventional bronchodilator therapy is usually effective.

1. Oxygen—all patients with severe bronchial asthma require oxygen, and this can usually be given safely in high concentration; however, controlled oxygen therapy may be necessary if there is evidence of co-existing chronic airway obstruction, i.e., chronic obstructive pulmonary disease COPD. In a patient with COPD there is always the possibility of an elevated arterial PCO_2. If any suspicion of this condition exists, when the patient is deteriorating while breathing oxygen in high concentrations, oxygen therapy should at once be discontinued. In any case, humidification of the oxygen is desirable.
2. Bronchodialators—the use of an epinephrine or isoproterenol medihalor is often extremely beneficial, in the outpatient with sudden exacerbation of acute bronchial asthma. If the medihalor does not terminate bronchospasm within several minutes of administration, epinephrine should be given subcutaneously in dosage of 0.5 cc of 1:1,000 solution. (See laryngeal edema). Since epinephrine may produce sinus tachycardia or more serious cardiac arrythmia, it is important to use extreme caution with this drug if the patient has a history of hypertension, hyperthyroidism, or cardiac disease. In these patients, aminophyllin 250-500 mg. is given by slow intravenous injection. This drug is injected over a 15 minute period in order to avoid severe hypotension which, in addition to nausea and vomiting, is a common side reaction to this drug.
3. Corticosteroids—until recently corticosteroids were administered only as a last resort and the condition of many patients was allowed to deteriorate seriously before they were given. It is now apparent that the prognosis of patients with severe bronchial asthma has been much improved by the early drug use. Very little harm is done by the administration of large doses of hydrocortisone intravenously or prednisone orally over a short period of time. The dose can be quickly reduced as the patient's condition improves. Cortisone should not be administered unless the patient has been unresponsive to treatment with a medihalor, epinephrine or aminophyllin, or has already been transferred to a hospital for further evaluation.
4. Sedation—asthmatic patients often tend to be overanxious and acute breathlessness only increases their agitation. However, restlessness in such patients is often an early indication of cerebral anoxia and sedation will further impair ventilation by depression of the respiratory center, and aggravate sputum retention by depression of the cough reflex. Therefore, sedatives should be avoided.
5. Aids to expectoration—progressive obstruction of the peripheral airways by plugs of tenacious mucous is an important and serious feature of severe, prolonged bronchial asthma. Therefore, chest physiotherapy with supervised coughing and postural drainage, and the addition of effective mucolytic agents and steam inhalation are valuable adjuncts in follow-up, long-term therapy of a patient who has experienced an acute attack of bronchial asthma.

Acute Anaphylaxis: This is an acute, potentially fatal reaction, most often due to parenteral drug administration. Penicillin, iodinated contrast media and other drugs are frequently implicated. Atopic individuals are predisposed to anaphylaxis. A negative history of reaction to a drug does not preclude the occurrence of anaphylaxis.

Symptoms begin between five and 60 minutes after parenteral drug administration. Laryngeal edema and hypotension are most often associated with a fatal outcome.

Symptoms may respond rapidly to therapy and may last for a day or more. Cutaneous and respiratory manifestations are the most common, but cardiovascular dysfunction may supervene. Skin lesions include a generalized sensation of warmth or burning, diffuse urticaria and angioedema, especially of the face and tongue. Respiratory distress results from either laryngeal edema with strider or airway obstruction or from bronchospasm which leads to tightness of the chest, tachypnea, cough, wheezes and occasional rales. Hypotension leads to tachycardia, dizziness and syncope. Anoxia due to respiratory tract involvement can potentiate vascular collapse and lead to cardiac arrythmias and cardiac arrest. Occasionally nausea, vomiting, abdominal cramps or diarrhea may be present. Respiratory or cardiovascular patterns may be noted without skin lesions. Early diagnosis and treatment are mandatory to avert death, which can occur within 15 minutes. Constant attention must be given to an adequate airway. Any agent known to cause anaphylaxis should be injected below the deltoid area in the arm. If possible, emergency equipment should be available and the following measures taken:

1. Aqueous epinephrine 1:1,000, 0.3 to 0.5 cc IM. Urticaria, bronchospasm and hypotension usually improve. Epinephrine may be repeated in 5 to 15 minutes, if necessary. If profound hypotension occurs, the aqueous epinephrine dose can be diluted in 10 ml of saline and can be given slowly intravenously, but this method may precipitate cardiac arrythmias.
2. To retard absorption of an injected drug, place a tourniquet proximal to the injection site and infiltrate the area with aqueous epinephrine 1:1,000, 0.3cc. If laryngeal edema progresses, a cricothyreotomy or tracheostomy is necessary. An endotracheal tube may not pass through an edematous larynx. In any event, the maintenance of an airway and respiratory assistance are essential. Persistent bronchospasm after epinephrine therapy should be treated by administering aminophylline 500 mg. IV slowly. Aminophylline may increase hypotension and should only be used in patients not responding to epinephrine.
3. Oxygen and assisted ventilation are helpful. A positive pressure breathing apparatus often helps relieve bronchospasm. Prolonged hypotension may respond to intravenous administration of vasoconstrictors or intravenous fluids.
4. Antihistamines are usually administered to block further histamine binding and target cells. Diphenhydramine (Benadryl) 50 mg. IM should be given early in the course of treatment.
5. Corticosteroids do not act rapidly enough to reverse acute anaphylaxis. Prolonged anaphylaxis and persistent hypotension or bronchospasm should be treated with hydrocortisone succinate 100-500 mg. IV every six hours.
6. Cardiorespiratory arrest should be managed by CPR and assisted ventilation.

Hyperventilation

This may be an inappropriate response to anxiety or an appropriate response to an underlying abnormality. Hyperventilation causes increased elimination of carbon dioxide through the lungs. This shifts the body's acid based balance and causes a decreased arterial PCO_2, causing cerebral vessels to constrict. This diminishes cerebral blood flow and may cause the patient to faint. Lessened flow becomes apparent clinically when the patient complains of numbness and tingling of the hands, fingers and often the feet. Characteristically the circumoral area may also be involved. Hyperventilation most often occurs in those patients who are unable to cope with stresses imposed on them. Outpatient dental procedures are frequent predisposing factors.

As hyperventilation begins, rapid exhalations take place and CO_2 (carbon dioxide) is "blown off," thus reducing CO_2 concentration in the blood. The patient begins feeling lightheaded and may have feelings of giddiness. This may precipitate increased anxiety and apprehension and further hypertension. Tachycardia ensues and the patient may develop tingling sensations or parathesias in the hands and feet as previously noted. It is often described as a "numb sensation." As the patient continues to hyperventilate there may be frank muscle twitching which can occur due to the metabolic derangement caused by release and lowering of CO_2 concentrations, as well as change in ionic calcium balance due to pH change. This results in nerve irritability. Loss of consciousness may ensue.

Treatment

The treatment of hyperventilation initially involves an attempt to calm the patient by eliminating some of the causes which may have triggered the reaction. If any procedure is being performed it should be terminated, the patient placed in a supine position and calmly reassured.

The time honored treatment for hyperventilation secondary to an anxiety reaction is to provide a way for the patient to rebreathe his own carbon dioxide and thus raise his blood PCO_2. This can easily be accomplished by holding a small paper bag over the patient's mouth and nose and by having the patient breathe into the bag slowly 6 to 12 times per minute. Any bag apparatus will suffice as long as the bag does not collapse between breaths, making breathing more difficult.

Oxygen is generally not indicated since the symptoms of hyperventilation are due to a decreased normal blood level of carbon-dioxide and not by an increase in oxygen. If the increase in oxygen occurs simultaneously, however, the major goal in the management of this emergency is to produce an increased blood level of carbon dioxide. Thus the administration of 100% oxygen or any high oxygen content of inspired gas will further decrease the PCO_2 delaying return to normal.

Patients who are known to hyperventilate can be treated with premedication for outpatient procedures. Those in which normal management is not successful can be treated with intravenous agents to reduce anxiety. Valium 10 mg. given by slow injection is a satisfactory drug to decrease anxiety and to reduce hyperventilation.

References

1. "Emergency Management of C-Spine Injuries," Abbott Laboratories, American College of Emergency Physicians Series. 1977.
2. Beeson, P.B. and McDermott, W., Editors. *Textbook of Medicine*. Philadelphia: Saunders, 1979.
3. "Rational Asthma Therapy for the Outpatient," R.K. and Bergner, A. *JAMA*, 235:288, 1976.
4. "Cricothyroidotomy: Elective Use in Respiratory Problems Requiring Tracheotomy,"Bratigan, C.O. and Grow, J.B. , *J. Thorac. Cardiovasc. Surgery* 71:72, 1976.
5. "The Heart as a Target Organ in Systemic Allergic Reaction," Capurro, N. and Levi, R. *Circ. Res.* 36: 520, 1975.
6. Conn, H.F. and Conn, R.B. Editors. *Current Diagnosis 5*, Philadelphia: Saunders, 1977.
7. "The Antigen-Antibody Reaction," Fischell, E.E. *Medical Clin. North Am.* 49:1553, 1965.
8. "Prognosis of Asthma," Galant, S.P. *Lancet* 1:437, 1972.
9. "Anaphylactic Reaction to Oral Penicillin," Geyman, J.P. *Calif. Med.* 114:87, 1971.
10. "Anaphylaxis," Henderson, L.L. *Ann. Allergy* 23:525, 1965.
11. "Common Medical Emergencies: A Dilemma in Dental Evaluation," Hendler, B.H. and Rose, L.F. *J.A.D.A.*, 91:575-582, 1975.
12. "Rise and Fall of Asthma Mortality in England and Wales in Relation to Rise of Pressurized Aerosols," Inman, W.H.W. and Adelstein, A.M. *Lancet* 2:281, 1969.

13. "Immunologic Mechanisms for Release of Chemical Mediators of Anaphylaxis from Human Living Tissue," Kaliner, M. *Can. Med. Asso. J.* 110:432, 1974.
14. "Anaphylaxis," Kelly, J.F. and Patterson, R. *JAMA* 227:1431, 1974.
15. "Immunochemical Mechanisms of Drug Allergy," Levine, B.B. *Ann. Rev. Med.* 17:23, 1966.
16. Malamad, Stanley, F. *Handbook of Medical Emergencies in the Dental Office*, St. Louis: Mosby, 1978.
17. McCarthy, F.M. *Emergencies in Dental Practice,* ed. 2, Philadelphia: Saunders, 1972.
18. *Merck Manual of Diagnosis and Therapy*, Ed. 11 West Point, Pa.: Merck, Sharp and Dohme Research Laboratories, 1966.
19. "Allergic Rhinitis and Sinusitus," Norman, P.S. *Postgrad. Med.* 54:94, 1973.
20. Pallasch, T.J. *Clinical Drug Therapy in Dental Practice,* Philadelphia: Lea & Febriger, 1973.
21. "Drug Allergy," Parker, C.W. *New England J. Med.* 292; 511, 1975.
22. Rose, L.F. *Diagnosis and Management of Medical Emergencies in the Dental Office,* Continuing Education Manual, University of Pa., School of Dental Medicine, vol. 1, no. 3, 1977.
23. Salter, R.H. *Common Medical Emergencies*, Bristol: John Wright and Sons, 1968.
24. Sharp, J.C. and Marx, F.W., Jr. *Management of Medical Emergencies,* ed. 2, New York: McGraw-Hill, 1969.
25. "Pulmonary Effects of Heart Failure," Smulyan, H., Gilber, A. and Rich, R.H. *Surg. Clin. North Amer.* 54:1077, 1974.

Chapter 7

Chest Pain and Hypertensive Emergencies

Scott Ulin, M.D.

Chest pain evaluation and diagnosis

Any discussion of cardiovascular emergencies must begin with a review of chest pain, far and away the most common chief complaint. The interpretation of chest pain is a difficult diagnostic problem because in most instances, the examiner must interpret the patient's subjective perception of pain without being able to analyze it objectively. By definition, pain is a disagreeable sensation resulting from the stimulation of nerve fiber endings. An increase in tissue tensions or hypoxia are common noxious stimuli causing cardiovascular pain.

Chest pain may arise from any of the following systems and structures: the chest wall; the lungs and its vessels; the heart, its lining and great vessels; and the gastrointestinal tract (Table 7-1). Chest pain manifests a spectrum of conditions, some of which are benign and common while others are unusual and catastrophic. The greatest concern of the patient and doctor is whether or not the pain is of cardiac origin, and if it is, the practitioner must then determine whether or not it represents an emergency or urgent situation.

Table 7-1 Some common causes of chest pain

a. Musculoskeletal
   - Costochondritis
   - Intercostal muscle spasm
   - Trauma

b. Lung
   - Pulmonary embolus
   - Pleurisy
   - Pneumothorax
   - Pneumomediastinum

c. Heart and great vessels
   - Coronary artery disease
   - Right ventricular hypertension
   - Valvular disease
   - Pericarditis
   - Aortic dissection and aneurysm

d. Gastro-intestinal
   - Peptic ulcer
   - Esophagitis
   - Gastritis
   - Cholecystitis
   - Pancreatitis

e. Psychogenic
   - Hyperventilation syndrome
   - Anxiety

In evaluating the patient with the complaint of chest pain (Table 7-2), the quickest and simplest maneuver is to palpate the pulse, which allows quick assessment of cardiac rate, rhythm and pulse pressure. If the pulse is irregular, rapid, weak, thready or absent, the insertion of an intravenous life line is indicated. The administration of supplemental oxygen and the initiation of electrocardiographic monitoring are the next priorities. Any patient over twenty-five years of age with chest pain should be con-

Table 7-2 Approach to acute chest pain: Conscious and over 20—25

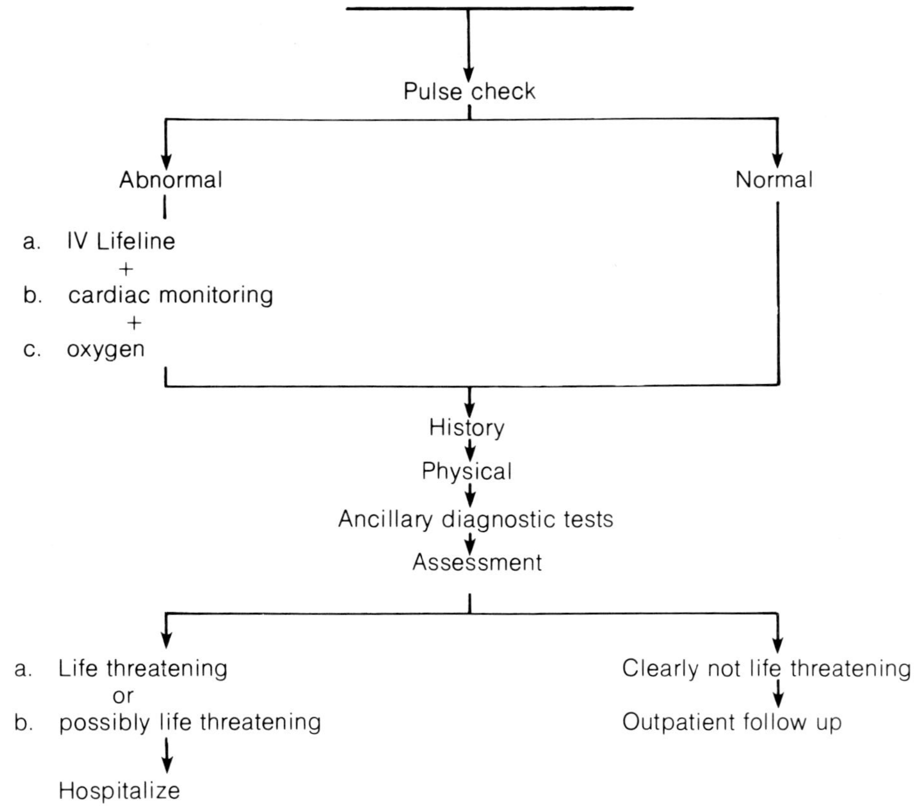

sidered as a candidate for a myocardial problem and given treatment priority.
The evaluation and optimal management of the patient with chest pain depends upon a careful history and physical examination followed by a review of the differential diagnosis.

History

An accurate history is the most important tool in the diagnosis of chest pain. The patient should be allowed time to describe the history in his own words followed by questions to elicit specific data as listed in Table 7-3a.

Table 7-3a Important elements of the history

a. Onset
b. Location
c. Quality
d. Radiation
e. Alleviating Factors
f. Circumstances Surrounding
g. Past Medical History
h. Associated Diseases and Symptoms

Onset: The temporal nature of the pain is important, for instance, is it insidious or sudden? The pain of angina pectoris is usually sudden and brought on by exertion or stress, whereas the pain of myocardial infarction although sudden, often occurs at rest. The pain of aortic dissection or pneumothorax is also sudden; but the pain of musculo-skeletal or gastrointestional origin is usually insidious at the onset and of inexact timing. Characteristically the pain of gallbladder disease is frequently precipitated by food intake.
Pain brought on by inspiration or coughing, called pleuritic pain, suggests a pulmonary or chest wall etiology. Pain of only a few seconds duration is unlikely to be of cardiac origin. Another question to ask is it progressive in severity or maximal from the start? The pain of myocardial infarction, although severe, usually increases over a period of time to maximal intensity, whereas the pain from a dissecting aortic aneurysm is maximal from the start.

Location: Chest pain may be substernal, across the chest, on one side only or radiating into the back. Frequently, the location can alert the clinician to the source of the pain. The pain of myocardial ischemia is usually substernal in origin, while the pain of musculo-skeletal origin is usually localized to a specific area of the thorax such as the pectoral muscles, the costo-chondral junctions, or inframammary area. Acute chest pain radiating to the back is usually due to aortic dissection or pericarditis.

Quality: This characteristic is best explained by the patient since it is subjective; however, descriptive terms such as sharp, dull, penetrating, or burning can help trim the differential. The pain of myocardial insufficiency or infarction is usually not described as a true pain by the patient but as a pressure-like, squeezing sensation, or heaviness substernally. Often, the patient will give the classic sign of coronary insufficiency, the Levine sign, as he subconsciously holds a clinched fist over the sternum while describing the pain (Fig. 7-1). A burning pain suggests the gastrointestinal tract as the source of discomfort and tearing chest pain is typical of aortic dissection.

Radiation: The pain of coronary insufficiency is classically described as radiating down the inner aspect of the left arm, but it may also radiate to the neck, jaw, or epigastrum. Lower quadrant oro-facial pain may be an initial sign, especially in absence of any dental etiology. The pain of aortic dissection usually penetrates through to the interscapular region of the back; while the pain of intercostal muscle

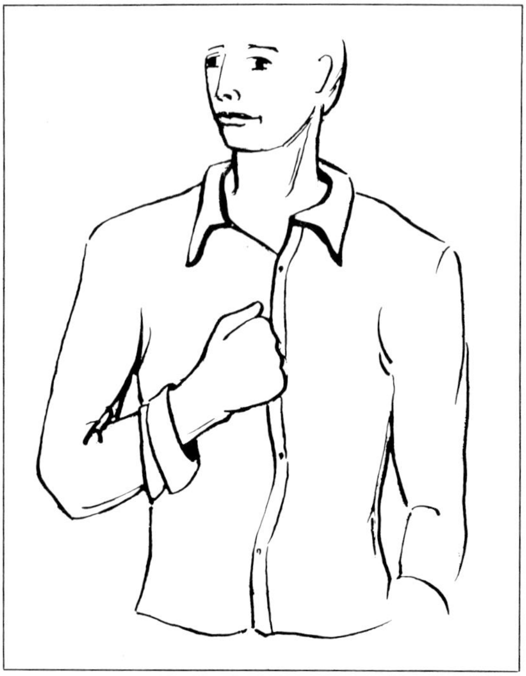

Fig. 7-1 The Levine sign.

spasm radiates around one side of the thorax.

Alleviate or Relieve: The factors which relieve the pain can be vitally important in differentiating the various etiologies. Exertional pain that quickly subsides with rest and relaxation, or the administration of nitroglycerin is characteristic of angina. The pain of esophageal spasm, which closely mimics angina, may also be relieved by nitroglycerin but is not exertional in onset. Burning chest pain relieved by antacids suggests a gastrointestinal etiology.

Circumstances Surrounding: If it is not obvious, the circumstances surrounding the onset of pain should be clarified. As mentioned previously, the pain of angina is brought on during exertion, or by a heavy meal, or stress. The pain noticed the morning after vigorous physical activity is likely to be of musculo-skeletal origin. Nonspecific pain that has been present for several days is unlikely to be of cardiac origin.

Past Medical History: Patients with a history of chest pain may be able to relate past episodes with the current episodes. The person with known angina may state the present episode is similar, but of longer duration, or not relieved by the usual dose of nitroglycerin. The patient with a spontaneous pneumothorax may state his sharp pleuritic chest pain is exactly the same as with previous episodes. As a general rule, individuals with a long history of vague multisystem problems are more likely to be experiencing pain of functional origin.

Associated Diseases and Symptoms: The pain of severe myocardial ischemia is usually associated with nausea or vomiting, profuse sweating, shortness of breath, and pre-syncopal symptoms. It is well known that pre-existing diabetes mellitus, hypertension, and elevated serum lipids are highly correlated with coronary artery disease. Patients with chronic obstructive pulmonary disease (COPD) and chronic bronchitis are more likely to have chest pain from respiratory insufficiency or pneumonia.

Physical examination

The physical examination begins with observation of the patient during the initial interview (Table 7-3b). The general appearance can immediately alert the examiner to the severity and often, the probable etiology. For instance, a young, coughing, cyanotic patient may have pneumonia; while a sweating, pale, acutely distressed patient may have a myocardial infarction. The patient who complains of severe pain, yet laughs and moves without difficulty, is unlikely to have a serious problem.

Table 7-3b Important elements in physical examination

a. General Appearance

b. Vital Signs
    - Temperature
    - Blood pressure
        - lying and sitting
        - both arms
    - Pulse rate and quality
    - Respiratory rate and pattern

c. Neck
    - Jugular venous pressure
    - Carotid pulses

d. Cardiovascular
    - Heart
    - Peripheral pulses

e. Thorax
    - Chest wall
    - Lungs

Vital signs: This includes a temperature, blood pressure, the pulse rate and quality, and the respiratory rate and pattern (As described in chapter 2). The pulse should be evaluated not only for rhythm, but also amplitude. For example, the pulse in hypovolemia is usually weak and thready. An irregular pulse may be indicative of ventricular ectopic beats, from increased myocardial irritability, or atrial fibrillation. A very slow pulse may be an indication of heart block from a myocardial infarction or from drug therapy (See chapter 2). Usually, an unexplained, persistent resting tachycardia, although nonspecific, indicates that a serious disease process may be present. Deep, regular respirations may be indicative of an underlying metabolic cause, while the hyperventilation syndrome will usually produce deep sighs interrupting the normal respiratory rhythm. Periods of apnea alternating regularly with a series of rapid respirations can indicate severe myocardial disease.

Thorax: A complete evaluation of the thorax includes inspection, palpation, auscultation and percussion. By palpation one can identify localized areas of tenderness and the location of the cardiac apical impulse. The lungs can be auscultated for pleural friction rubs, rales, wheezes, and areas of decreased breath sounds which may indicate a pulmonary origin of chest pain.

Cardiovascular: The heart can be ausculated and the quality of the sounds noted. The presence of extra sounds and murmurs, might suggest which myocardial process is the source of pain. For instance a young person with severe pain may have a mitral click indicating mitral valve prolapse as the etiology. The jugular neck veins should be checked for signs of distension, as seen with congestive heart failure, and the carotid pulses evaluated for upstroke or bruits suggestive of valvular heart disease.

On summarizing the physical examination, it should be remembered that a normal physical exam does not rule out acute myocardial processes. On the other hand, a myriad of positive physical findings, without the appropriate frame of reference does not always indicate a serious cardiovascular emergency. It is not unusual for more than one acute process to occur concomitantly or for the same findings to fit two distinctly different problems. Even with the above consideration, a thorough, informed physical examination will significantly narrow the differential diagnosis and often allow the clinician to make a definitive diagnosis.

Ancillary diagnostic aids

Further help in determining the source of chest pain may be obtained from the following adjunctive studies: laboratory, electrocardiogram, chest X-ray and arterial blood gases.

Laboratory: Useful laboratory studies are a complete blood count, serum electrolytes, blood sugar, BUN, and cardiac enzymes. A leukocytosis indicates organic rather than functional disease, and an increase in total neutrophils with an elevation in juvenile or band forms may point towards an infection. An elevated serum potassium can help explain myocardial irritability and arrhythmias. Cardiac enzymes, if available, are very helpful, but may not become elevated for 9 to 36 hours after infarction and will not be elevated in severe ischemia, which can itself be an indication for hospitalization.

EKG: The specificity of the EKG is at best suspect as a completely reliable diagnostic tool. Frequently the electrocardiogram may be entirely normal even during an acute infarction or period of severe ischemia.

CXR: Even though a chest X-ray can be normal in the face of serious cardiovascular disease; certain findings can help define pathologic processes that are taking place. Left ventricular hypertrophy and pulmonary edema indicate severe heart disease. Calcification of the aortic valve can suggest aortic stenosis, and a widened mediastinum may be the first evidence of aortic dissection. Atelectasis, localized infiltrates, pleural effusions, and hyperlucent lung fields are indicative of a pulmonary disease.

ABG: Arterial blood gases can demonstrate hypoxia or acidosis which may not necessarily be of cardiac origin, but can still adversely affect myocardial function and secondarily produce ischemic chest pain.

Cardiovascular emergencies

Angina: This is defined as the pain from an imbalance between the myocardium's demand for oxygen and the supply available. The heart derives its blood supply from the coronary arteries, which are perfused during the diastolic phase of the cardiac cycle. Angina may arise from intrinsic disease of the coronary vessels or from extrinsic factors which decrease the diastolic pressure or filling interval.

Classically, Angina is pain or a disagreeable sensation located retrosternally, brought on by exertion or stress, and relieved quickly by rest. The patient will usually describe the discomfort as a "bad case of indigestion," a "squeezing, vice-like sensation," or as a heaviness or pressure. As mentioned before, they may hold a clinched fist over the sternum and describe a sensation of "impending doom." The pain most commonly radiates down the inner aspect of the left arm, but may also go to both shoulders or arms, into the neck or jaw, through the chest to the back, or into the epigastrum (Fig. 7-2).

This multiplicity of symptoms may be confusing and misleading; however, the most

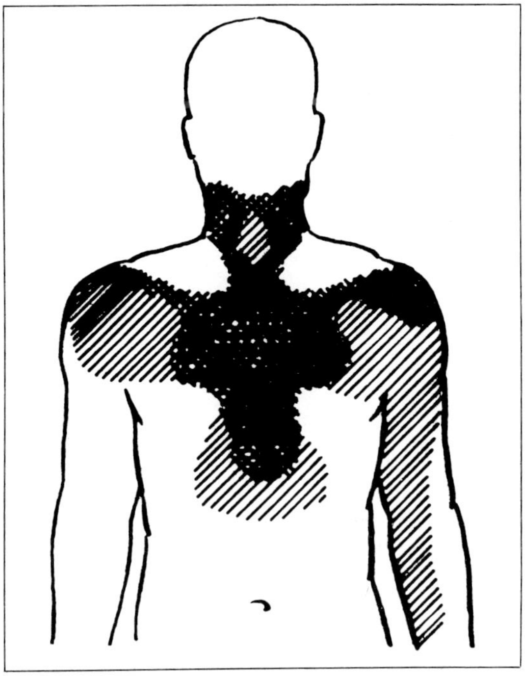

Fig. 7-2 Radiation patterns of chest pain from coronary insufficiency.

important feature for the diagnosis of angina is the constant relationship of pain to exertion. Specific conditions that usually precipitate angina are increased heart rate, elevated systolic blood pressure, diminished diastolic pressure, arrhythmias, and hypoxemia.

Angina pectoris may be divided into three clinical entities; stable angina, unstable or preinfarctional angina, and angina decubitus.

Stable Angina: This is the classic form described above, consisting of exertional pain which lasts for only a few minutes and subsides with rest or nitroglycerin (NTG). For any patient, it is unchanging and totally predictable.

Unstable Angina: This refers to pain patterns that are shown in retrospect to have occurred in patients with myocardial infarction. It is characterized by a change in the patient's previous anginal pattern. Such changes may be an increase in frequency, duration, intensity, or the occurrence at rest or during sleep. Nitroglycerin may be ineffective or larger doses may be required.

Angina Decubitus: This type occurs only at rest or while sleeping. Angina decubitus may arise de novo or develop in a patient with previous exertional angina. In one variant, called Prinzmetal's angina, the pain may paradoxically be relieved by exertion.

The physical examination with any type of angina may be normal, or reveal diaphoresis, tachycardia, pallor, an S4 heart sound, or a systolic murmur of papillary muscle dysfunction. Laboratory studies generally add little to the diagnosis. An ECG taken during an episode of angina may be normal, or demonstrate ST segment elevation or depression.

Management

The emergency management involves maintaining a favorable balance between the myocardial oxygen available and the demand (Table 7-4). Once angina occurs, it reflexly causes an increase in blood pressure, heart rate, and left ventricular pressure, all of which further increase the myocardium's need for oxygen. Treatment should be instituted as quickly as possible. The patient is placed at complete rest and any constricting clothing is loosened; underlying disorders such as heart failure, hypertension, and rhythm disturbances, if found, are corrected; and any medications that aggravate angina, such as bronchodilators, nasal decongestants, and appetite suppressants are discontinued.

If pain does not subside immediately, drug therapy should be instituted. The drug of choice is sublingual nitroglycerin which reduces the oxygen demand on the heart and at the same time augments coronary blood flow. These effects result from its ability to cause vasodilation. The venous return to the heart is decreased, the actual blood pressure is lowered, and the amount of coronary artery spasm is lessened. Nitroglycerin should be placed under the tongue and allowed to dissolve. A positive response is relief of pain within 45 seconds to 2 minutes. If the first dose is ineffective, it may be repeated twice at 5 minute intervals; however, if no relief is then obtained, other therapeutic modalities should be tried. If nitroglycerin is *effective,* it can be administered repeatedly as long as the systolic pressure remains *greater than* 90 mm Hg or drops *less than* 30 mm Hg from the baseline. The most commonly used dosages are 0.4 mg (1/150 gr) and 0.6 mg (1/100 gr). The former is sufficient for most patients; the latter reserved for severe angina. The most common side effects include headache, a stinging under the tongue, and hypotension. The stinging sensation is a sign of freshness. The major drawback of nitroglycerin is its short duration of action.

Once the diagnosis of angina is made, the patient stabilized, and under close medical supervision, newer, longer-acting preparations of nitroglycerin may be used. These include isosorbide dinitrate (Isordil), pentaerythrital tetranitrate (Peritrate), and topical nitroglycerin paste (Nitrol). Another class of drugs gaining in popularity for the treatment of severe angina are the beta adenergic blockers such as propranolol (Inderol). These agents effectively block the increase in myocardial oxygen consumption that results from increased sympathetic activity such as occurs with exercise or stress.

If a patient develops angina de novo or develops a change in the old pattern, it is imperative that the patient be hospitalized for further evaluation and observation. It should be pointed out that if nitroglycerin is not effective, the diagnosis of angina pectoris is not ruled out; severe angina or preinfarction angina may not respond to nitrates alone.

Myocardial infarction

Myocardial infarction is a medical emergency requiring careful, intensive management during the acute phase to reduce morbidity and mortality. It is associated with a high risk of sudden death which may occur within several hours to several days of the initial event. The risk of sudden death is 10-20 times greater in the first 4 hours after infarction and may occur in as many as 60% of cases. The cause of sudden death is usually ventricular fibrillation.

Myocardial infarction implies that a segment of the heart wall has undergone necrosis from anoxia. The most common antecedent process is coronary artery disease, although any process which occludes a coronary artery, such as embolic phenomena or vessel spasm, may result in necrosis. Areas of myocardial necrosis are interspersed with areas of ischemia or injury, and the ultimate extent of infarction de-

Table 7-4 Management of angina

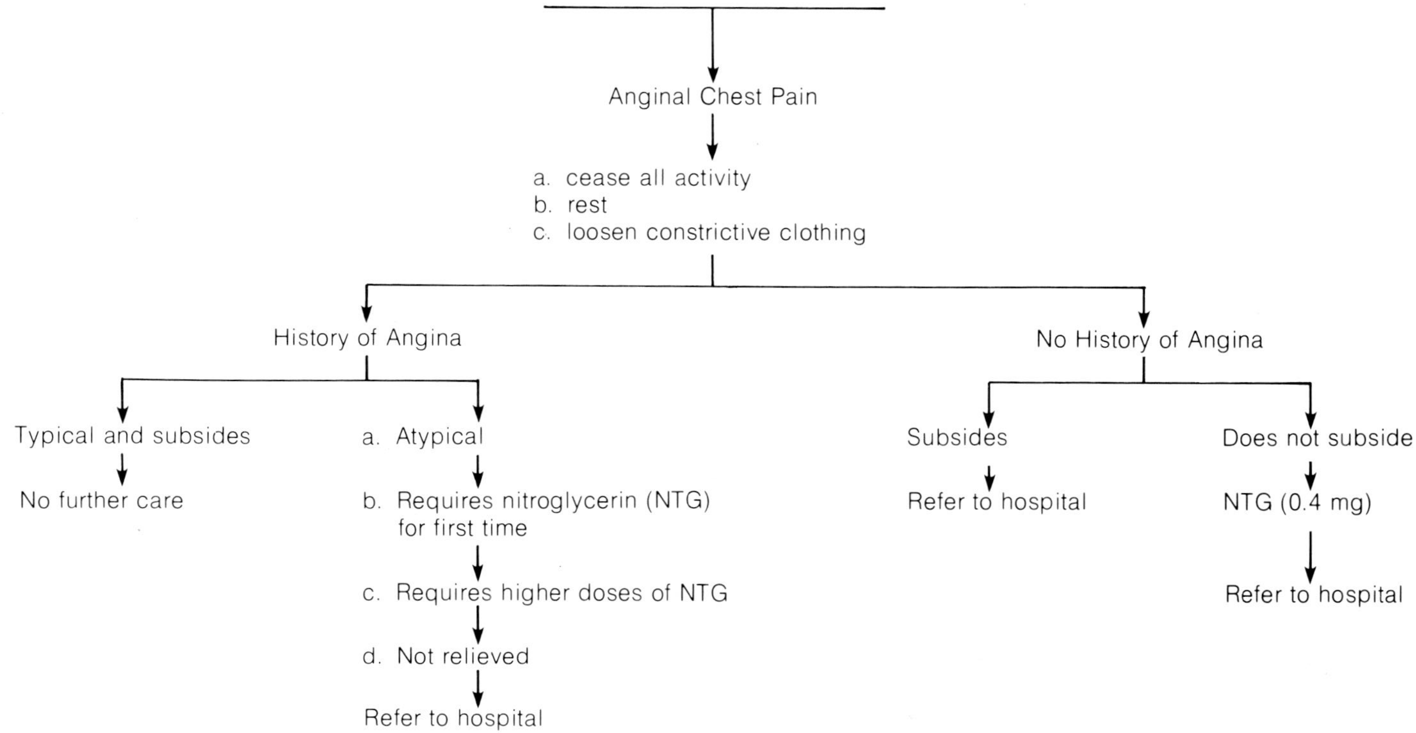

a. Normal
b. Ischemia; I-wave inversion and depression of the J point
c. Injury pattern; elevation of the ST segment
d. Infarction pattern; development of an abnormal Q wave.

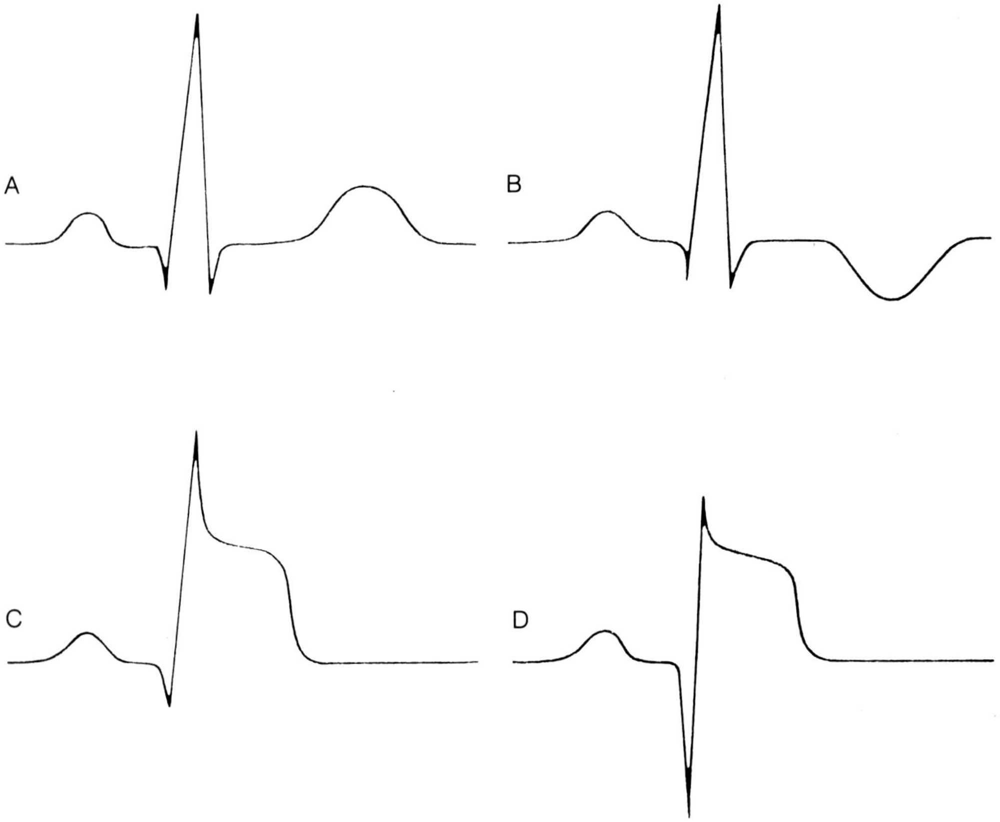

Fig. 7-3 Sequential EKG changes following infarction.

pends upon the balance between myocardial oxygen demand and supply. Thus, infarction is an evolving condition that may improve or deteriorate.

Clinically, the diagnosis is made by the following triad: a history of typical chest discomfort, evolutionary changes on the electrocardiogram in a characteristic pattern, and elevation in the level of enzymes released from devitalized cardiac muscle. Of these three criteria, only the history is reliable in the emergent evaluation and treatment. Electrocardiographic changes may not occur for several hours, and the enzyme changes occur over a period of from 12 hours to several days.

Oppressive retrosternal chest pain that lasts longer than 30 minutes, or chest pain that is not relieved with nitroglycerin suggests acute myocardial infarction. Occasionally, the pain may originate in the epigastrum. The pain may be precipitated by exertion, but just as often it occurs during a period of rest. It may be accompanied by nausea, vomiting, diaphoresis, dyspnea, and syncope. Other entities to consider in the differential are musculo-skeletal chest pain, acute gastrointestinal problems, aortic dissection, and pulmonary embolus. Myocardial infarction should also be considered in individuals presenting with an acute stroke, shock, or syncope of unknown etiology.

The physical examination may be entirely normal. Abnormal findings, when present, include a profuse diaphoresis with cold, clammy skin, hypertension or hypotension, temperature elevation (not usually greater than 101°F) and either an extremely slow or rapid heart rate.

A chest X-ray, if available, may also be entirely normal. Common radiographic abnormalities seen in association with a myocardial infarction include an enlarged heart and pulmonary vascular congestion. EKG abnormalities, when present, consist of ST segment elevation or depression, peaked or symmetrically inverted T-waves, Q-waves, conduction disturbances and various arrhythmias. The hallmark of acute myocardial injury is ST segment elevation with coving, and of infarction, the Q-wave, indicative of an electrically silent area of the heart (Fig. 7-3). The enzymes released from damaged myocardial muscle cells are lactic dehydrogenase (LDH), creatinine phosphokinase (CPK) and serum glutamic oxaloacetic transaminase (SGOT).

In summary, the diagnosis of myocardial infarction should be considered in any patient presenting with prolonged chest pain. Any patient whose pain is suspicious of myocardial ischemia should be treated as if infarction is developing. Myocardial infarction can occur without any previous episode of chest pain or past history of cardiovascular disease, and it can also occur without pain (silent infarct).

The area of damaged myocardium is determined by the coronary artery involved; the prognosis and subsequent management are partially dependent upon this localization. There are three main coronary vessels feeding the heart: the left anterior descending, the left circumflex, and the right coronary artery (Fig. 7-4).

The following is provided for those interested in the electrocardiographic patterns associated with acute myocardial infarction.

The left anterior descending artery supplies the anterior wall of the left ventricle and the interventricular septum. Involvement in this distribution produces the greatest area of infarction and the greatest likelihood of complete heart block. On the ECG, the leads reflecting anterior wall infarction are V1, V2, V3 and V4 (Fig. 7-5).

The left circumflex artery supplies the lateral wall of the left ventricle, and is reflected in limb leads I and AVL. If this vessel feeds the majority of the heart, a posterior wall injury will also involve the left ventricle and manifest changes in leads V1, V2 and V3 (Fig. 7-6).

The right coronary artery feeds the inferior area of the heart and is reflected in limb leads II, III and AVF. This injury usually results in a much smaller area of infarction

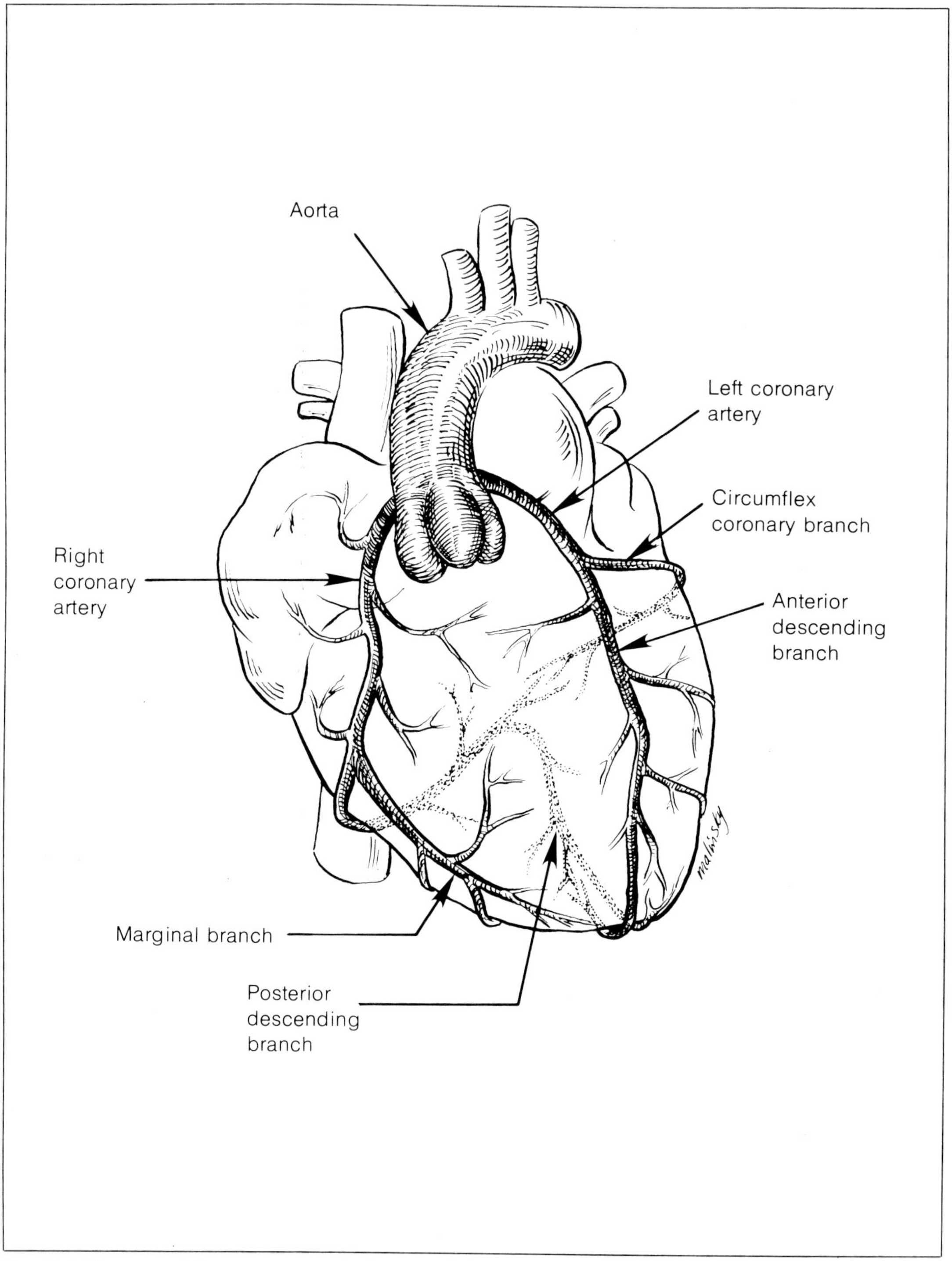

Fig. 7-4 Diagram of the coronary arteries supplying the heart.

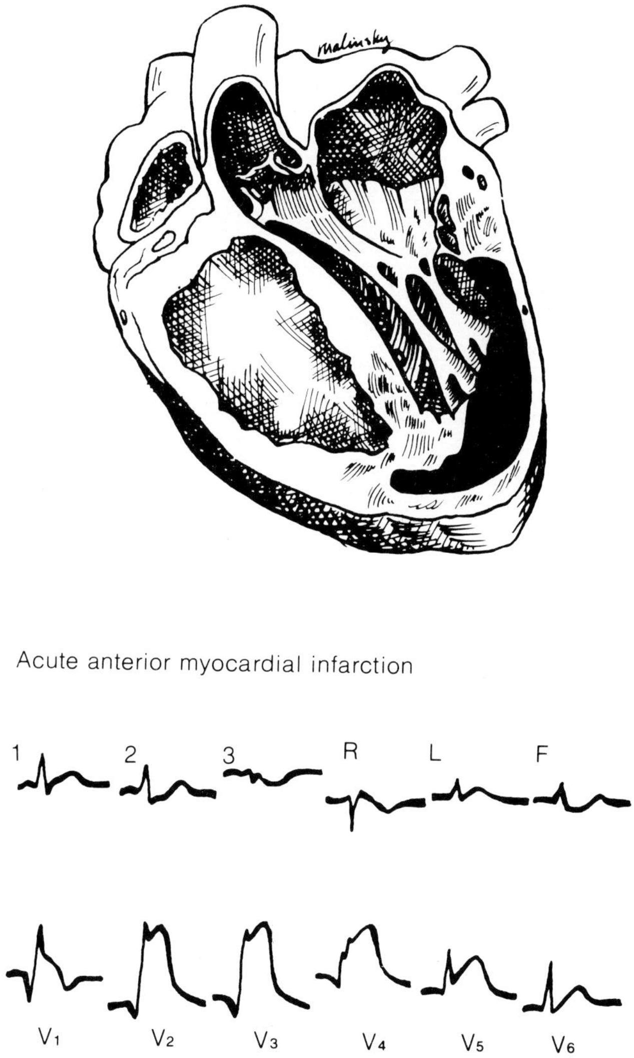

Fig. 7-5 Diagnostic EKG of anterior wall myocardial infarction.

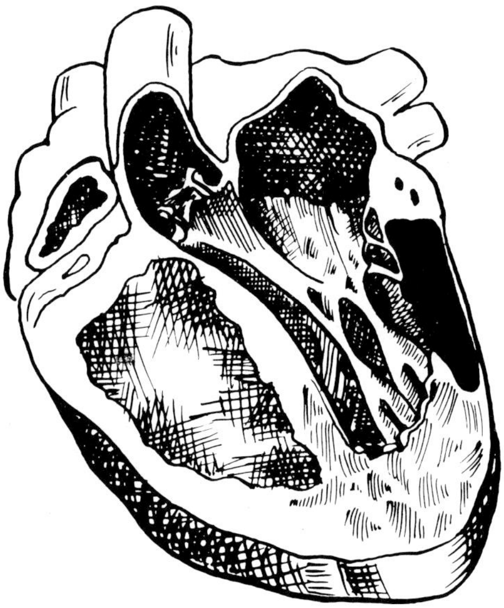

Acute lateral infarction

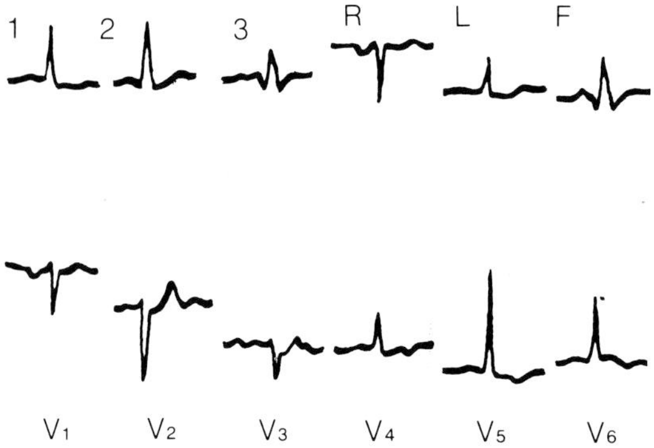

Fig. 7-6 Diagnostic EKG of lateral wall myocardial infarction.

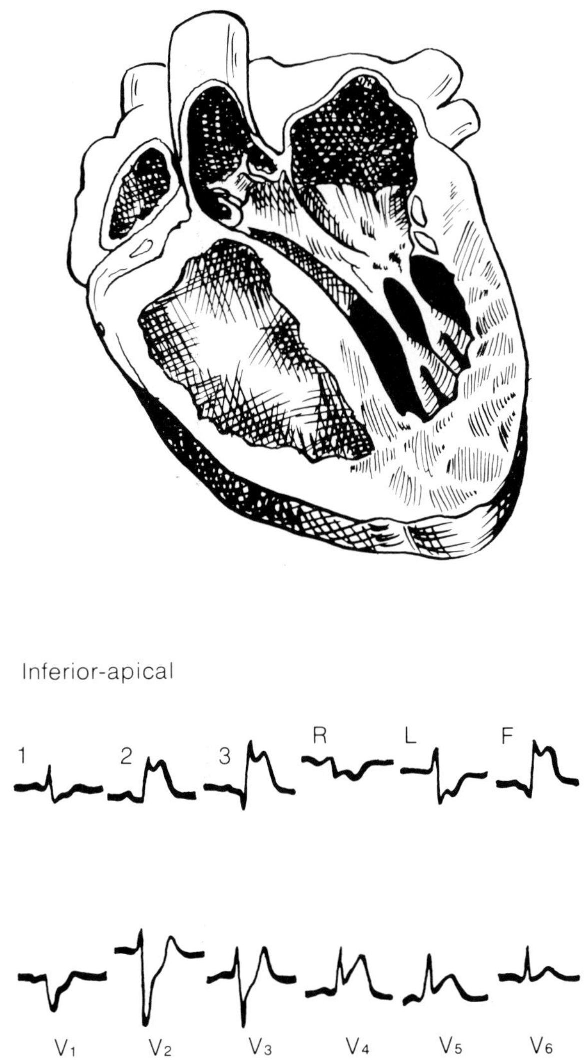

Fig. 7-7 Diagnostic EKG of inferior wall or apical myocardial infarction.

than with occlusion of either branch of the left coronary artery and therefore gives the best overall prognosis. This injury rarely causes complete heart block (Fig. 7-7).

When an infarction occurs, not only are changes seen in the respective leads for that area, but also changes occur in the diametrically opposed area. These are called reciprocal changes and should be recognized. When the anterior wall is involved, these changes occur in II, III and AVF. When the lateral wall is involved, the change will be seen in V1. With inferior infarction, the reciprocal changes are seen in I and AVL.

In assessing the severity of involvement, it is important to remember that only Q-waves are pathognomonic of infarction, and that the infarction may have been old or new. T-wave inversion suggests only ischemia, and ST segment elevation with coving signifies only acute injury that may or may not go on to infarction.

Management

The goals in the management of the acute stages of MI are to relieve pain, prevent and/or treat dysrythmias, attempt to minimize the area of injury, and observe closely for developing complications. The patient should ideally be admitted to a coronary care unit, but management must begin at the time the diagnosis is entertained (Table 7-5). The patient should be put to rest, made comfortable, and reassured. At the very least the pulse should be continuously monitored for changes and, if available, electrocardiographic monitoring should be initiated.

Oxygen is administered immediately and if the patient's systolic blood pressure is greater than 90 mm Hg, sublingual nitroglycerin, 0.4 mg, can quickly be given to alleviate pain while other measures are being carried out. If further pain control is needed, narcotic analgesics such as morphine sulfate or meperidine (Demerol) can be administered, which are not only effective against severe pain, but have a sedative effect as well. All parenteral drugs should be given intravenously or sublingually since intramuscular injections (IM) can cause the release of the same muscle enzymes that are released from damaged myocardial cells; the systemic absorption of IM medications is slower and less predictable. The intravenous administration of analgesics also allows titration of small alliquots until pain control is achieved while minimizing side effects such as respiratory depression. The initial and subsequent doses of morphine should be 2-4 mg and of meperidine 15-25 mg. The goal is not to administer a predetermined amount, but to titrate small amounts, regardless of the total dose, every 3-5 minutes until pain control is achieved. The chance of overdosing a patient with narcotics is thus reduced significantly. If respiratory depression or hypotension occurs, it can be easily reversed with nalaxone (Narcan), which is a specific physiologic antagonist without any adverse effect. The dose is 0.4 to 0.8 mg IV or sublingually.

Up to 85% of acute infarctions are complicated by dysrhythmias. The most common are premature ventricular beats due to increased myocardial irritability. More severe and potentially lethal arrythmias such as ventricular tachycardia and ventricular fibrillation are not uncommon in a significant percentage of patients. The dysrhythmias will be discussed in detail later in this chapter.

As mentioned earlier, sudden death, due to ventricular fibrillation, occurs in a large number of individuals with acute myocardial infarctions. In the hospital, although controversial, intravenous lidocaine hydrochloride given prophylactically has been shown to reduce this incidence. It should be started in patients presenting within four hours of the onset of the acute episode and continued for 12-24 hours. Current dosage recommendations are 1 mg/kg given as a bolus over a few minutes, followed by a continuous drip of approximately 3 mg/minute. Only those patients likely to experi-

Table 7-5 Management of acute myocardial infarction

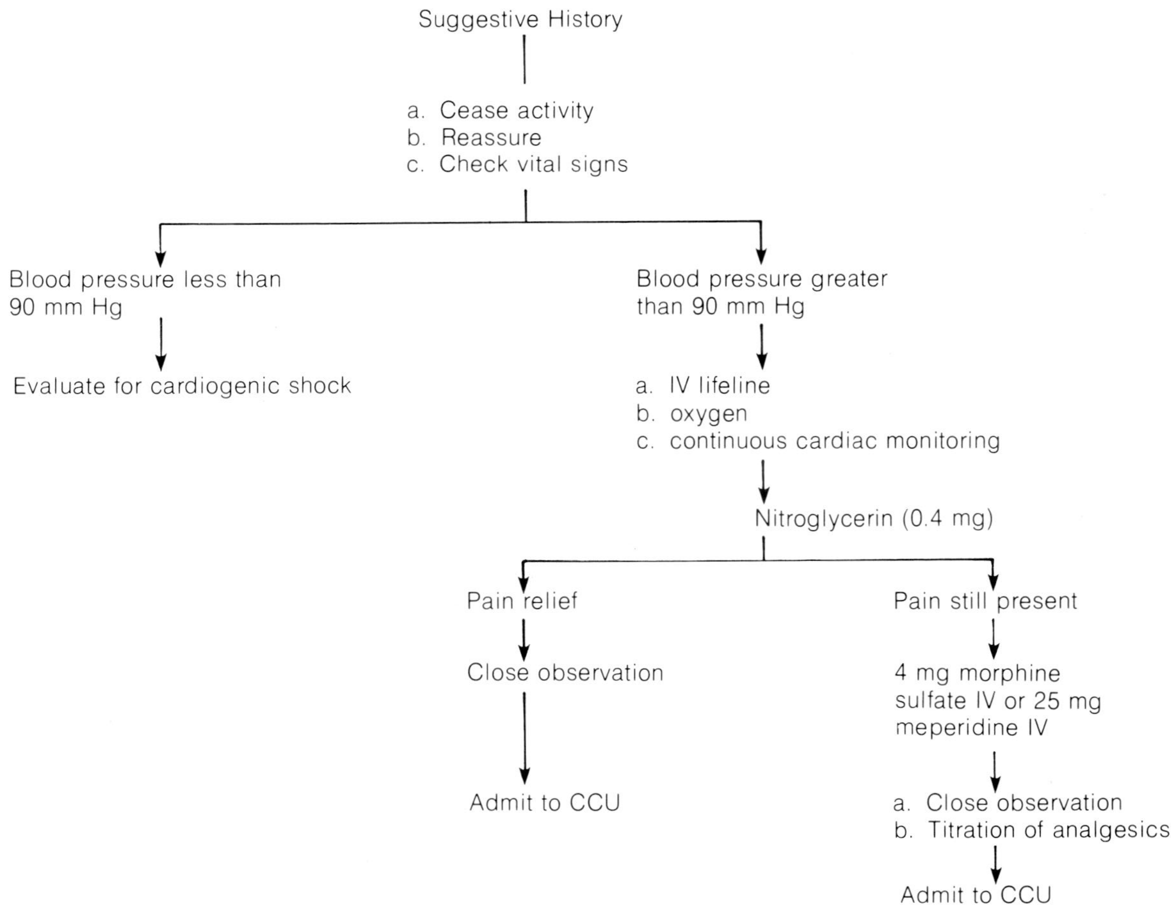

ence severe side effects should be excluded from this regimen. These include patients with liver disease, hypotension or shock, severe heart failure, sinus bradycardia, AV block, known seizure disorder, or allergy to lidocaine.

As we have stated, an acute infarction is an evolving phenomenon. Efforts made to reduce myocardial oxygen demand and increase the amount of oxygen available to the heart can help minimize the ultimate size of the infarct. Heart failure will occur with damage to 25% or more of the left ventricle, and with damage greater than 40%, shock from pump failure will occur.

In summary, the key to the diagnosis of acute myocardial infarction is an accurate history. As soon as the diagnosis is entertained, the patient should be treated as if infarction has occurred. Immediate treatment to minimize extension of the infarct includes: 1) putting the patient to rest, 2) establishing an intravenous lifeline, if possible, 3) continuously monitoring the cardiac rhythm (pulse), 4) administering supplemental oxygen, 5) relieving pain, 6) avoiding drugs which increase myocardial oxygen demand and 7) observing for complications. Abnormal physical, X-ray, or laboratory findings, when present, can support the diagnosis, but these may all be normal during the acute episode.

Acute congestive heart failure

Congestive heart failure (CHF) is not a specific disease entity but a pathologic state secondary to some underlying disease process of the heart. It can have an insidious onset, or it can develop suddenly; it carries an overall mortality of 50%. CHF implies a dysfunction of the ventricles resulting in a cardiac output inadequate to meet the demands of the various organ systems. CHF may be due to failure of the right ventricle, left ventricle, or both. In acute CHF, involvement of both ventricles is the most common clinical presentation. The discussion that follows will be limited to acute congestive heart failure and its most serious presentation, pulmonary edema of cardiac origin.

The pathophysiology of acute CHF revolves around the need for a cardiac output sufficient to keep up with the magnitude of the peripheral oxygen demand. The normal heart is usually able to keep up with an increasing oxygen demand by increasing its output. This occurs by reflex increases in the rate and force of contraction. The diseased left ventricle is not able to respond to the reflex changes and increase the cardiac output, consequently the blood will back up into the heart's chambers and vasculature behind it. When sufficiently elevated, this pressure causes transudation of intravascular fluid across the pulmonary membrane, producing interstitial tissue edema of the lungs. The process interferes with pulmonary compliance and increases pulmonary vascular resistance, causing the symptoms of dyspnea and orthopnea. If the pressure continues to rise, the amount of fluid flowing into the interstitium overloads the lymphatic drainage, and the excess fluid spills into the alveoli, resulting in the auscultatory finding of rales. Fluid-filled alveoli are unable to participate in gas exchange, and thus hypoxemia occurs. If the fluid volume increases even further, it eventually exudes into the lumen of the bronchioles, causing reflex bronchospasm and the physical finding of wheezing. As air flows through the fluid, it produces foaming, giving rise to the characteristic frothy sputum seen with pulmonary edema.

The typical patient with acute CHF is diaphoretic, cyanotic, dyspneic, orthopnic, and anxious. The skin feels cold and clammy. Auscultation of the lungs reveals diffuse rales over both lung fields, with diminished breath sounds at the bases; wheezing may also be present (the so-called cardiac asthma).

The treatment of acute pulmonary edema consists of reducing circulatory demands, improving tissue oxygenation, increasing myocardial contractility, and recognizing and treating the underlying cause. (Table 7-6). Oxygen should be administered to relieve the concomitant hypoxemia and its resultant consequences, decrease the pulmonary vascular spasm, and improve the myocardial function. A mask or nasal cannula may be used at initial flow rates of 4-7 liters/minute. Morphine sulfate has several beneficial effects. It causes pulmonary vasodilation to reduce venous return. It alleviates pain and anxiety, which provides for a more favorable respiratory pattern, and reduces the blood pressure. Small alliquots of 2-4 mg should be given intravenously as long as the blood pressure is greater than 90-100 mm Hg. Potent loop diuretics such as furosemide (Lasix) have multiple beneficial effects also. When given intravenously, furosemide rapidly increases venous capactiance and thoracic duct lymph flow, which causes an immediate decrease in pulmonary capillary pressure. Furosemide then produces a diuresis approximately 20 minutes after administration, thus preventing any further rise in capillary pressure. The recommended dose is 20-40 mg intravenously.

Identifying Precipitating Cause: Although definitive treatment of the underlying causative factors may not be accomplished in the emergency setting, their identification can influence the emergency treatment and permit the initiation of definitive therapy at the earliest possible time.

In summary, the management of acute CHF and pulmonary edema requires an understanding of the pathophysiology of left ventricular dysfunction and the etiologies involved. Immediate therapy required is: the application of supplemental oxygen and proper positioning of the patient. An intravenous lifeline should be inserted and the vital signs continuously monitored. Pharmacologic agents that should be used in the initial phase of management are morphine sulfate, nitroglycerine, and furosemide (Lasix). Laboratory and radiologic evaluation may help diagnose the cause, but contribute nothing to the immediate treatment. Arterial blood gases should be obtained because it is impossible to gauge the severity of acid-base derangements adequately from the patient's clinical condition.

Table 7-6 Treatment of acute congestive heart failure

a. Reduce Circulatory Demands
   1. Preload: body position
      rotating tourniquet
      morphine sulfate
      furosemide (Lasix)
   2. Afterload: morphine sulfate
      ganglionic blockers

b. Improve Tissue Oxygenation
   1. Body position
   2. Oxygen

c. Increase Myocardial Contractility
   1. Inotrophic agents: digitalis
      beta adrenergic stimulants

d. Identify Precipitating Cause
   1. Hypertension
   2. Coronary heart disease
   3. Valvular heart disease
   4. Cardiomyopathies
   5. Constrictive pericarditis
   6. Cardiac tamponade
   7. Volume overload

Cardiogenic shock

Although the heart is involved in all types of shock, cardiogenic shock designates that form of shock precipitated by an acute myocardial infarction. It implies a dysfunction of the left ventricle, which results in a decreased cardiac output and inadequate tissue perfusion. Cardiogenic shock has been defined formally by a set of clinical criteria which are as follows: a systolic

Table 7-7 Criterion to diagnose cardiogenic shock

a. Systolic pressure (<90 mm Hg.)
b. Urinary output (<20 cc/hr.)
c. Decreased cerebral perfusion (altered mental status)
d. Cool, damp, mottled skin

pressure less than 90 mm Hg, or a fall in systolic blood pressure greater than 80 mm Hg in a patient previously known to be hypertensive; a urinary output less than 20 cc/hour; diminished cerebral perfusion as evidenced by mental confusion; and cool, damp, mottled skin (Table 7-7). The mortality rate is in the range of 80-95%. Cardiogenic shock is a complication in approximately 15% of all cases of myocardial infarction; and when it occurs, it indicates that 40% or more of the left ventricle has been involved.

The diagnosis of cardiogenic shock may be recognized prior to a blood pressure drop by closely watching the urinary output and mental status. These two parameters are very sensitive indicators and their alteration occurs in the early, pre-shock phase, at which time therapy can be most effective.

The goal of treatment is to salvage ischemic myocardium and prevent extension of the infarct. The general principles of therapy are the same as for all forms of shock: insuring the adequacy of airway, breathing, and circulation; correction of hypoxemia and acidosis and the elimination of potentially harmful drugs such as myocardial depressants. The specific therapeutic modalities available for the management require a critical care environment, and they are aimed at increasing the cardiac output. Patients with cardiogenic shock are often hypovolemic from a combination of pain-induced reflex vasodilation; sweating; vomiting and previous diuretic therapy. They may benefit from the judicious use of volume expanders; however, it must be kept in mind that these patients have impaired myocardial function, which makes them extremely susceptible to volume overload.

Therefore, invasive monitoring techniques must be available to guide fluid needs. When volume expansion alone does not improve cardiac output adequately, or is not tolerated, a variety of pharmacologic agents may be tried. The drugs currently used are vasodepressors, vasodilators, adrenergic blocking drugs, corticosteroids, and digitalis preparations.

Dissecting aortic aneurysm

The initial event in an acute dissection is a small, intimal tear in the aorta, or erosion through an atheromatous plaque. A stream of blood separates the intima from the media and then continues to dissect apart these two layers of the aorta. The two most frequent sites of origin are: 1) the ascending aorta and 2) the descending aorta distal to the left subclavian artery. The dissection can rupture into the pericardium, the free pleural space, or into a cardiac chamber. The dissecting process can also cause occlusion of a major aortic branch vessel such as the coronary, carotid, renal, or mesenteric arteries with resultant ischemia to their organs, an event just as lethal as hemorrhage itself.

The patient experiencing an acute dissection will often describe a sudden onset of chest pain that is ripping or tearing in quality. The pain may be primarily located in the back, in the front, or both areas, with localization changing as the dissection progresses. The usual physical findings are severe acute distress from pain, and marked hypertension; unless a rupture occurs, producing shock. The chest X-ray will usually show a widened aortic and mediastinal shadow. Often, the calcific deposits located at the edge of the aortic shadow will be found more medial in location as the other wall of the aorta is pushed outward. The goal of treatment is to prevent rupture, or occlusion of the arterial supply to vital organs. This is accomplished by immediately reducing the blood pressure in the hypertensive patient to a systolic pressure of 120-130 mm Hg. The drugs of choice are sodium nitroprusside (Nipride), a vasodilator, or trimethaphan camsylate (Arfonad), a ganglionic blocker. If the patient is hypotensive, volume expanders are used to bring the pressure up to 100 mm Hg. Once the pressure is stabilized, a definitive plan of medical or surgical management can be made. It is obvious that the management of aortic dissection must take place in a critical care unit.

Table 7-8 Pathophysiology of pulmonary embolus

Occlusion of pulmonary artery
↓
Increase right ventricular end—diastolic pressure
↓
Right ventricular failure
↓
Decreased pulmonary venous return
↓
Decreased left ventricular flow
↓
Decreased cardiac output
↓
Decreased coronary and cerebral blood flow

Pulmonary embolus

Another emergency that often is confused with primary myocardial disease is massive pulmonary embolus. Most deaths due to pulmonary embolism occur within minutes to hours after the acute episode and are usually the result of obstruction of the central pulmonary circulation. The most common predisposing factors to the development of pulmonary embolism are prolonged immobilization, venous disease and cardiac disease. The deep veins of the legs are the source of fatal pulmonary embolism in about 90% of patients, but clinical evidence of deep vein thrombosis is present in only about one-half of these cases. Pulmonary embolus causes a spectrum of problems ranging from occlusion of the peripheral pulmonary vasculature without sequale, to obstruction of the main pulmonary artery by a large saddle embolus with shock. This discussion will be limited to emboli that cause hemodynamic compromise.

The sequence of events leading to hemodynamic compromise begins with a large clot occluding a major pulmonary artery. This precipitates a transient rise in pulmonary artery pressure, leading to decreased coronary and cerebral blood flow with hypotension or shock (Table 7-8). Although the amount of pulmonary vascular obstruction appears to be the most critical factor in the clinical significance and hemodynamic effects of pulmonary embolism, a secondary reduction in coronary blood flow and pulmonary vasoconstriction may also play a role.

Common presenting symptoms of massive embolus are chest pain, dyspnea, apprehension and a cough which is often bloody. A small percentage of patients will present with chest pain indistinguishable from the pain of severe myocardial ischemia. The most common physical findings are a respiratory rate greater than 16/min. and a pulse rate greater than 100/min. The absence of these findings, however, does not exclude the presence of severe embolism. The EKG is usually normal or shows nonspecific changes. When present, the classic pattern is due to strain on the right ventricle (Fig. 7-8).

The most accurate method for making the diagnosis is the pulmonary arteriogram; the only limitation to its use being that very small emboli may be missed.

The EKG in patients with pulmonary emboli is usually normal or shows changes that are very nonspecific. The most-characteristic changes, which are very uncommon, consist of a deep S wave in lead I and a deep Q wave in lead III (the so-called S_1Q_3) pattern. These changes are usually associated with T wave depression in III and also often in II. A tendency to right-axis deviation, or right-heart strain, is also suggested here and supports the diagnosis.

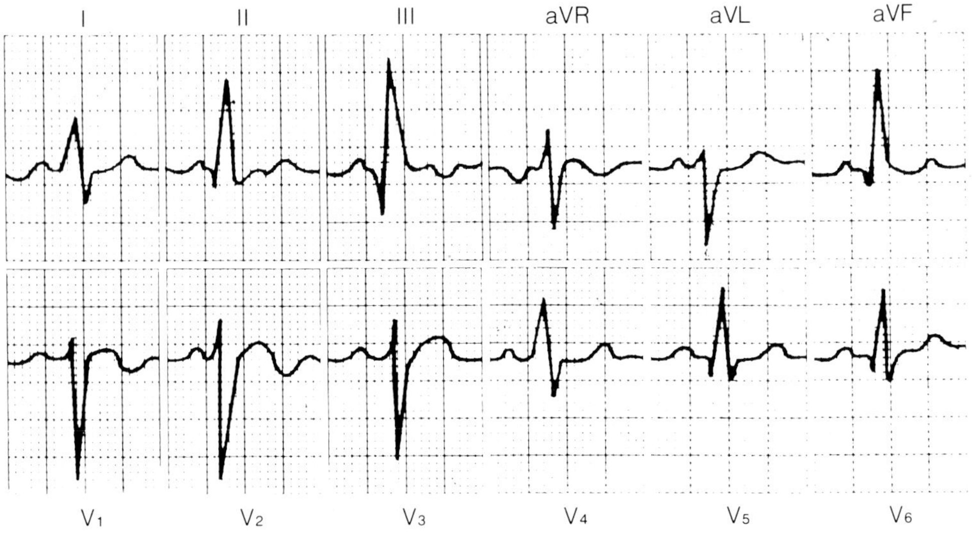

Fig. 7-8 EKG changes of pulmonary embolus.

The treatment of choice is heparin, which has the following beneficial effects: it inhibits coagulation, enhances fibrinolytic activity, and lyses the embolus. It should be given as soon as possible, once the diagnosis is strongly suspected or firmly established. The most efficacious method of administration seems to be by continuous intravenous infusion of 20 units/kg of body weight/hour. Other methods are to give an initial bolus of 15,000 units, followed by intermittent boluses of 5,000-10,000 units every four to six hours. The goal of treatment is to obtain a partial thromboplastin or Lee-White clotting time of 1½ to 2 times the control.

In summary, pulmonary embolus is a disease with nonspecific presenting signs and symptoms that requires a high index of suspicion to make the diagnosis. Massive embolus can be confused with myocardial infarction and must be analyzed differentially. Signs of right ventricular dysfunction, and a supportive history can help in the diagnosis of pulmonary embolus. The most accurate test is the arteriogram. Once the diagnosis is made, heparin therapy should be instituted.

Hypertensive emergencies

More than 15% of the adult population in the United States has elevated blood pressure. Even mild degrees of hypertension have been clearly shown to increase the risk of cardiovascular disease and death from cerebral thrombosis or hemorrhage, heart failure, myocardial infarction, or renal failure. Since only about half of these patients have been diagnosed and not all of them are well controlled, it is not unusual for the practitioner to be confronted with a hypertensive emergency or crisis. These emergencies occur primarily in patients with essential hypertension, as approximately 90% of all hypertensives fall in this category.

A hypertensive emergency is defined as elevation of the diastolic blood pressure to 130 mm Hg or greater. In any given case, it is the *rate of rise* of the diastolic pressure, rather than the absolute pressure rise that is most important. The common hypertensive emergencies, some of which have been discussed elsewhere in this chapter, are the following:

Malignant hypertension
Hypertensive encephalopathy
Pheochromocytoma
Eclampsia
Pulmonary edema
Cerebrovascular syndromes
Subarachnoid hemorrhage

Hypertensive retinopathy

Prior to a discussion of the emergencies, a quick review of retinal changes that occur in hypertension is appropriate because the diagnosis and severity can be accurately estimated from a fundoscopic examination. The retina of the normal eye (Fig. 7-9) has a network of arterioles overlying its surface, which intertwine and cross over the veins returning blood from the retina. Normally when an arteriole crosses over a vein, there is little or no change in the vein; however, when hypertension is present, the vein is pushed centrifically down into the retina, impeding the venous return. This phenomenon is referred to as "A-V nicking" (Fig. 7-10).

The arterioles also undergo sequential changes. The normal vessel is red in color with a thin, central bright yellow line which reflects light. With arteriosclerosis, they become more copper-like in color, with widening of the yellow line, a less distinct light reflex, and increased tortuosity. If the process continues, frank hemorrhage can actually occur (Fig. 7-11).

Other retinal findings associated with hypertension are "exudates," which in actuality are not exudates but degenerative areas of nerve tissue from inadequate blood supply. There are two types of degeneration seen. The soft type appear as fluffy white accumulations on the surface and the hard type appear as small, discrete, yellowish-white plaques lying deep in the retina.

Hypertensive retinal changes are classified on a scale of I to IV (Table 7-9). The emergency syndromes are characterized by at least Grade III or IV changes.

Hypertensive history

In taking a history there are three specific areas of concern: general medical history, neurological syndromes, and cardiovascular syndromes (Table 7-10). It is important to elicit the rapidity of onset of symptoms; for instance, hypertensive encephalopathy develops over a 12-48 hour period, while subarachnoid or intracerebral bleeding occurs over a period of minutes to no more than a few hours. The presence of a headache and its location can help determine the cause; for instance, the headache of hypertensive encephalopathy is severe and generalized, whereas the headache of malignant hypertension is usually occipital and mild.

Cerebral infarction or transient ischemic attacks often occur without any headache.

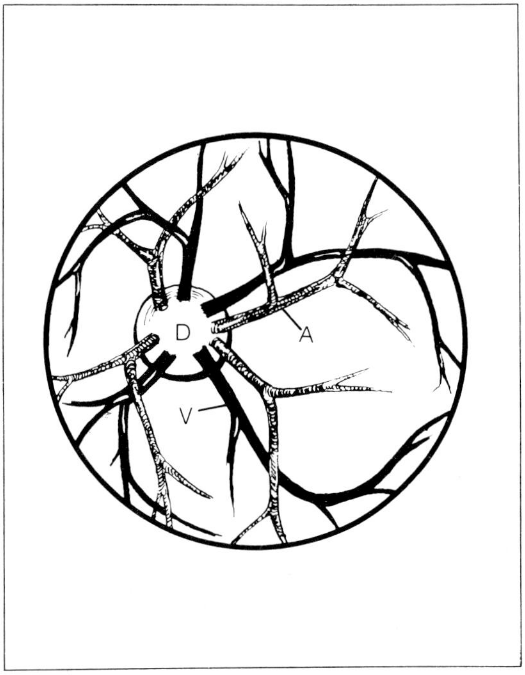

Fig. 7-9 Retina of a normal eye. (A) Arteriole. (V) Vein. (D) Optic Disc.

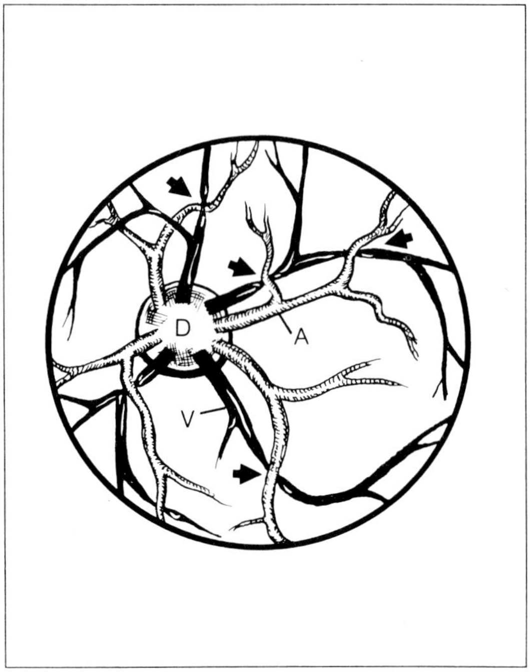

Fig. 7-10 Retina with mild hypertension. (A) Arteriole (V) pushing vein (arrow) down giving appearance of "nicking". The arterioles also have a greater light reflex. The optic disc (D) becomes slightly blurred.

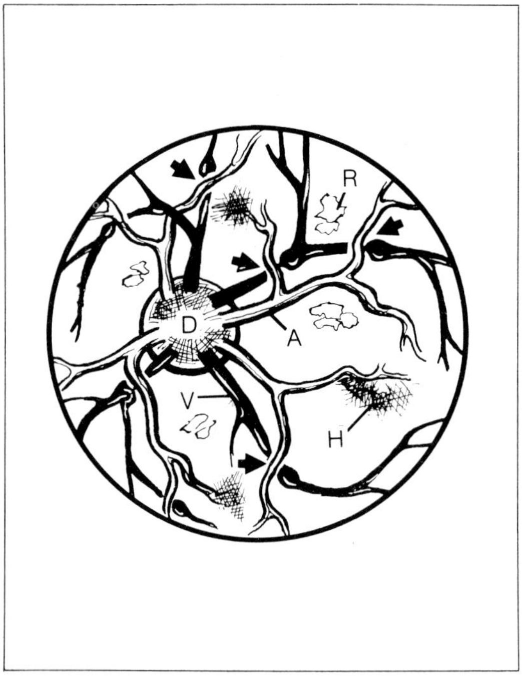

Fig. 7-11 Retina with severe hypertension. The veins (V) appear completely cut in two where the arteriole (A) crosses them. The arterioles (A) are more tortuous with a much larger light reflex. "Cotton wool patches" (R) are present as well as areas of hemorrhage (H). The optic disc (D) is now blurred.

Table 7-9 Classification of hypertensive retinopathy

	General Narrowing A/V Ratio*	Focal Spasm	Hemorrhages	Exudates	Papilledema
Grade I	+	0	0	0	0
Grade II	+	+	0	0	0
Grade III+	+	+	+	0	
Grade IV	++	++	+	+	+

*A/V ration arteriolar/venous diameters—3/4 normal

The progression of symptoms may also be of help. The patient with hypertensive encephalopathy may lose consciousness but this occurs over a longer period of time, and usually the level of coma does not progress to total unresponsiveness. In a subarachnoid hemorrhage there is an extremely rapid deterioration to total unresponsiveness with abnormal respiratory patterns. The patient with a cerebral infarction will rarely lose consciousness unless the infarct involves the brain stem. Associated symptoms contribute to determining the cause, for instance the patient with hypertensive encephalopathy will experience vomiting and transient, migratory focal neurological signs.

The patient with a subarachnoid hemorrhage will also have vomiting plus cranial nerve deficits, aphasia, and a stiff neck. The patient with a cerebral infarction will usually have fixed neurological deficits.

Table 7-10 Hypertensive history

a. General
    - History of hypertension
    - Antihypertensive medications and if currently taking
    - Presence of palpitations, sweating, headache, dizziness
    - History of renal disease
    - Recent sore throat or skin rash if in a child

b. Neurologic
    - Presence of decreased mentation
    - Time frame of evolution of symptoms
    - Previous transient ischemic attacks or localizing neurologic signs

c. Cardiovascular
    - Preexisting CHF
    - Preexisting angina or Myocardial Infarction
    - Preexisting arrythmias

Physical examination

Obviously, baseline blood pressure must be taken on every patient. In doing the physical examination specific attention should be given to the items listed in Table 7-11, but any patient with hypertensive crises must have his blood pressure evaluated in relationship to previous resting levels, understanding that anxiety alone can elevate blood pressure. As a rule, encephalopathy will present with a BP of 250/150 mm Hg or higher, while a subarachnoid hemorrhage or cerebral infarction will not have hypertension of this magnitude. When the history and physical examination suggest a hypertensive emergency, antihypertensive therapy should be started without

Table 7-11 Hypertensive physical examination

a. Blood Pressure
   Check in supine and sitting positions
   Check in both arms and a leg

b. Peripheral Pulses
   Check for presence and symmetry
   Listen for bruits

c. Retina
   Check for hypertensive changes

d. Neck
   Check for stiffness

e. Neurologic
   Define the extent and location of any deficit

waiting for laboratory data. The patient should be transferred to a medical facility immediately.

In summary, it should be emphasized that the diagnosis of hypertensive crisis does not depend as much upon any absolute level of blood pressure elevation as on the rapidity of rise and the clinical status of the patient. The only symptom which can be attributed exclusively to hypertension is a dull occipital headache. Other complaints are due to complications of hypertension or some intercurrent related or unrelated illness.

Management

The ultimate goal of therapy is to reduce the diastolic pressure to 90-100 mm Hg. This level of reduction will reduce the immediate complications of hypertension without compromising the circulation to the brain and heart. There are several types of drugs available to treat hypertensive emergencies, such as diuretics, sodium nitroprusside (Nipride) and diazoxide.

In summarizing the treatment of hypertensive emergencies it is important to reduce the pressure quickly and yet avoid adverse effects. Treatment should be immediate and the drug of choice for all hypertensive crises is sodium nitroprusside (Nipride). Furosemide (Lasix) can be given concomitantly along with supportive care as indicated. The use of other agents should take into consideration their potential for adverse effects and contraindications to their use. Ideally, initial treatment should be performed in an emergency medical facility.

References

1. Burch, G.E.: "Axioms on Myocardial Infarction." *Hospital Medicine*, September, 9-23, 1978.
2. Chung, E.K.: *Cardiac Emergency Card.* Philadelphia: Lea and Febiger, 1978.
3. Engle, T.R.: *Evaluating and Managing the Patient with Angina Pectoris*, Current Topics, vol. 3, no. 2. Philadelphia: The Medical College of Pennsylvania, 1979.
4. Fernandez, P. and Meyerson, R.M.: *Symptomatic Hypertension in the Emergency Room*, Current Topics, Emergency Medicine, vol. 4, no. 10. Philadelphia: The Medical College of Pennsylvania, 1979.
5. Gottlieb, R.S., et al: "Pathophysiology and Medical Management of Angina Pectoris". *AFP*: 16:82-89, 1977.
6. Harvey, A.M., et al: *The Principles and Practice of Medicine*. New York: Appleton-Century-Crofts, 1976.
7. Meister, S.G.: *Diagnosis and Treatment of Congestive Heart Failure*, Current Topics, Family Medicine, vol. 3, no. 8. Philadelphia: The Medical College of Pennsylvania, 1979.
8. Mendlowitz, M.: "Management of Hypertensive Emergencies". *Hospital Medicine*: pp. 63-72, December, 1979.
9. Segal, B.L., et al: "Coronary Risk Factors and Anginal Pain Patterns". *Postgraduate Medicine 61*, 102-125, 1977.
10. Spodick, D.H.: "Acute Cardiac Tamponade: Pathologic Physiology". *Diagnosis and Management, Progress in Cardiovascular Diseases 10*, 64-96, 1967.
11. Stone, J.H.: *Assessment of the Patient With Chest Pain*. Current Topics, Emergency Medicine, vol. 2, no. 5. Philadelphia: The Medical College of Pennsylvania, 1978.

12. Schwartz, G.R., et al: *Principles and Practice of Emergency Medicine*. Philadelphia: Saunders, 1978.
13. Vincent, T.S.: "What You See is What They've Got"! Resident and Staff Physician, pp. 88-90, September, 1979.
14. Wilkins, E.W., et al: *MGH Textbook of Emergency Medicine*. Baltimore: Williams and Wilkins, 1978.
15. Wolf, H.: *Myocardial Infarction.*, Current Topics, Emergency Medicine. vol. 2, no. 6. Philadelphia: The Medical College of Pennsylvania, 1978.

Chapter 8

Acute Cardiac Dysrhythmias and Cardiac Arrest

Richard L. Lammers, M.D.

Introduction

Cardiac dysrhythmias are disorders of the formation and transmission of electrical impulses in the heart, resulting in disturbances of heart rate, rhythm, or impulse conduction. Some of these disorders are benign conditions; others are life threatening, the most serious consequence being cardiac arrest. The sudden onset of a dysrhythmia is not only distressing to a patient but also an anxiety-provoking situation for the practitioner called upon to deal with the problem. There are many possible dysrhythmias from which to differentiate, each requiring specific therapy or no therapy at all. In many cases, time is an additional complicating factor; many dysrhythmias must be corrected as expeditiously as possible. Hence, a prepared, systematic plan of action must be initiated to rapidly and accurately identify and properly treat a dysrhythmia of acute onset.

The seriousness of any dysrhythmia depends upon its effect on cardiac output. Cardiac output is the product of heart rate and stroke volume. In normal hearts, rates ranging from 40 to 160 contractions per minute have little or no effect on cardiac output because of compensatory changes in stroke volume. However, cardiovascular disease states limit this ability to compensate and thus render the person more vulnerable to changes in rate. Dysrhythmias that depress stroke volume beyond the heart's ability to compensate by increases in rate will also decrease cardiac output. The manifestations of a sudden drop in cardiac output include reduced coronary artery perfusion with ischemic cardiac pain, pulmonary congestion, syncope, various neurologic impairments, and shock. Patients with such manifestations of hemodynamic instability during dysrhythmias require immediate therapy.

Most dysrhythmias are consequences of organic heart disease—atherosclerotic, hypertensive, rheumatic, valvular, inflammatory, or congenital. However, any dysrhythmia may be a manifestation of a noncardiac pathologic process, a process often requiring diagnosis and treatment before the dysrhythmia can be terminated. Management of dysrhythmias includes a search for precipitating factors (Table 8-1) and underlying cardiac disease.

Initial evaluation

In a patient suffering from an acute dysrhythmia, treatment of life-threatening conditions—hypoxia, hypotension, pulmonary edema, cardiac or cerebral ischemia, or cardiac arrest—takes precedence over a thorough evaluation. The patient's airway, breathing and circulation is evaluated first. If these are inadequate or absent, cardiopulmonary resuscitation (CPR) is initiated, as described later in this chapter.

Supplemental oxygen is given by nasal prongs or mask to those patients appear-

Table 8-1 Precipitants of dysrhythmias

a. Organic heart disease

b. Hypoxia

c. Hypercapnia

d. Electrolyte disturbances (K+ & Ca++)

e. Acidosis/alkalosis

f. Sudden hypotension

g. Endocrine disorders
   Thyrotoxicosis
   Myxedema
   Pheochromocytoma
   Adrenal disorders

h. Systemic infections

i. Stimulants (caffeine, theophylline, alcohol, tobacco)

j. Physical/emotional stress

k. Pulmonary disease (chronic obstructive pulmonary disease, pulmonary embolism infection)

ing even slightly dyspneic. An intravenous line should be secured, continuous electrocardiographic monitoring started, and resuscitation equipment arranged prior to diagnostic maneuvers. At this point, preterminal or terminal (lethal) dysrhythmias are immediately recognized and treated, should they be present. Blood pressure, apical and peripheral pulse rates, and respiratory rate should be determined. Severe hypotension necessitates immediate therapy, whereas mild hypotension (systolic blood pressure 80-100 mm Hg in the absence of chest pain or disordered mentation) or normal blood pressure allows a more careful appraisal of the problem.

History and physical examination

Precise diagnosis of dysrhythmias is based on the interpretation of electrocardiographic (EKG) tracings. A rhythm tracing can be obtained immediately by placement of "quick look" defibrillator paddles or monitoring electrodes on the chest wall. However, the interpretation is made easier by a selective history and brief physical examination. An adequate initial history and physical examination can be performed within a few minutes (Table 8-2).

EKG interpretation

Systematic evaluation of an electrocardiographic tracing should then be undertaken. First, determine the rate. Either the disorder is a tachyarrhythmia (rate greater than 100) or a bradyarrhythmia (rate less than 60). Second, determine the QRS duration. Either the QRS complex is narrow, (less than 0.12 seconds) or wide (more than 0.12 seconds). Using these two criteria, almost all of the dysrhythmias can be divided into four manageable categories (Table 8-3).

Tachyarrhythmias

The first step in evaluating tachyarrhythmias is to distinguish rhythms of supraventricular from those of ventricular origin. All of the "fast and narrow" rhythms are supraventricular, whereas the "fast and wide" rhythms may be either ventricular or supraventricular. Supraventricular rhythms originate above the bundle branches, from the sinoatrial node to the bundle of His. If bundle branch block or aberration is present, a supraventricular impulse will result in a wide QRS. Ventricular rhythms originate below the bundle branches. They carry a more serious prognosis and have the potential for rapid deterioration into terminal rhythms.

Though not always available to the dental practitioner, past EKG's are invaluable for comparison with the present tracing. Previous ectopic beats may be compared to unusual patterns on the new EKG. The find-

Table 8-2 Initial history and physical examination

History

a. Shortness of breath?

b. Chest pain

c. Previous similar episodes?

d. Known heart or vessel disease?
 WPW syndrome
 Enlarged heart
 Heart murmur
 Rheumatic heart disease
 Heart attacks

e. Known lung disease?

f. Known endocrine disease? (thyroid problems)

g. Medications?
 Digitalis
 Procainamide
 Quinidine
 Disopyramide
 Propranolol
 Diuretics
 Sympathomimetic preparations (cold relief medications, asthma medications, diet pills, amphetamines)
 Thyroid medications

h. Hypertension?

Physical Examination

i. Mentation
j. Skin color (for the adequacy of perfusion)

k. Jugular venous pulse (for Cannon A waves)

l. Auscultation of lungs (for evidence of pulmonary congestion)

m. Cardiac exam:
 a) Displacement of apical impulse
 b) Basic rhythm
 c) Varied intensity of the first heart sound
 d) Murmurs (for evidence of structural disease)
 e) Gallops
 f) Clicks, opening snaps
 g) Friction rubs

n. Pulse deficit (apical pulse rate greater than peripheral pulse rate)

o. Evidence of chronic congestive heart failure

Table 8-3 EKG evaluation of dysrhythmias

1. Recognize terminal dysrhythmias
   1) ventricular fibrillation
   b) asystole
   c) electromechanical dissociation

2. Differentiate other dysrhythmias

QRS | Rate

Tachyarrhythmias (QRS Duration): Narrow QRS	Tachyarrhythmias (QRS Duration): Wide QRS	Bradyarrhythmias (QRS Duration): Narrow QRS	Bradyarrhythmias (QRS Duration): Wide QRS
1. Sinus tachycardia	1. Sinus tachycardia with bundle branch block	1. Sinus bradycardia	1. Atrioventricular nodal block (3°)
2. Paroxysmal supraventricular tachycardia	2. Supraventricular tachycardia with aberrancy	2. Sinus arrest	2. Fáscicular blocks (bundle branch blocks)
3. Atrial tachycardia with block	3. Type A WPW syndrome	3. Sinoatrial block	3. His Purkinje system block (slow idioventricular rhythm)
4. Non-paroxysmal junctional tachycardia	4. Ventricular tachycardia	4. Atrioventricular block	
5. WPW (preexcitation) syndrome	5. Accelerated idioventricular rhythm		
6. Atrial flutter			
7. Atrial fibrillation			
8. Multifocal atrial tachycardia			

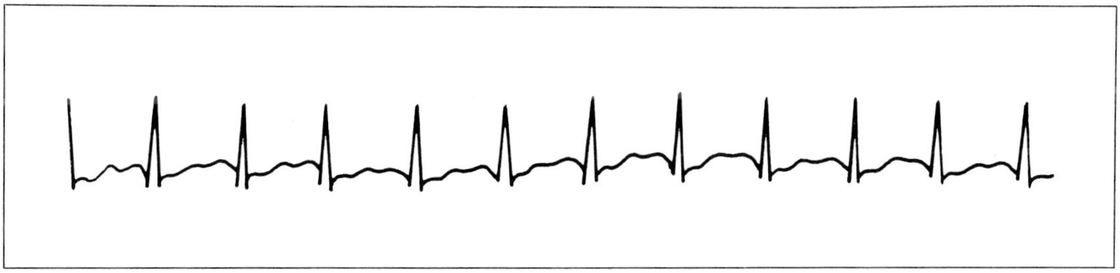

Fig. 8–1 Sinus tachycardia.

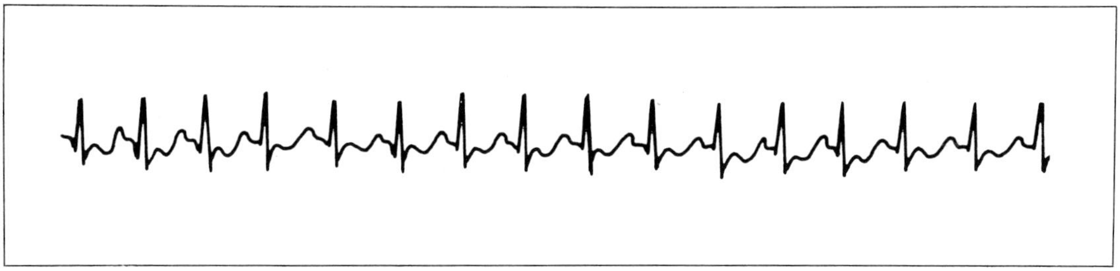

Fig. 8–2 Paroxysmal supraventricular tachycardia.

ing of pre-existing bundle branch block or Wolff-Parkinson-White syndrome on a previous EKG may explain the appearance of or the reason for a bizarre dysrhythmia.

Fast rate and narrow complexes

Sinus tachycardia (Fig. 8-1) is a regular rhythm in which normal P waves precede each QRS complex at a fixed and normal PR interval and each P wave is followed by a QRS. The rate is greater than 100 but is seldom higher than 160/min. in adults or 200/min. in children. Sinus tachycardia is usually a physiologic response to situations such as physical exertion, anxiety, emotional stress, or fright. It may be caused by pain, hypoxia, hypovolemia, congestive heart failure or can occur in hypermetabolic states such as fever, infection, thyrotoxicosis, delerium tremens, or pheochromocytoma. Drugs such as atropine, isoproterenol, or epinephrine may also cause this tachycardia. In almost all cases, treatment should be directed toward correcting the underlying disorder.

Paroxysmal supraventricular tachycardia

Paroxysmal supraventricular tachycardia (Fig. 8-2) is a regular tachyarrhythmia of sudden onset usually caused by a reentry mechanism located in the sinoatrial node, atrium or atrioventricular node. The patient may experience palpitations, lightheadedness, dizziness, chest pain, or even cardiovascular collapse. In normal, young adults, however, there is usually little hemodynamic impairment. The rate is commonly 150-200 beats per minute. If this dysrhythmia is suspected, further history might be helpful. The patient should be asked if similar attacks have occurred in the past. Although paroxysmal supraventricular tachycardia can be associated with organic heart disease or preexcitation syndromes, it is often precipitated by excitement, emo-

Table 8-4 Management of paroxysmal supraventricular tachycardia

1. Establish intravenous line; cardiac monitoring
2. Identify rhythm, if possible
3. Exclude digitals—toxic rhythms
4. Place patient in recumbent position
5. Sedation (diazepam or phenobarbital)
6. Determine hemodynamic status
   - → stable ↓ (continue to 7)
   - → unstable ↓ immediate cardioversion
7. Vagal stimulation
   - A. Gagging ↓
   - B. Valsalva maneuver x 10 seconds ↓
   - C. Immersion of face in cold water ↓
   - ausculate carotid arteries for bruits
     - → present bilaterally → (go to 8)
     - → absent ↓
   - D. Right—side carotid sinus massage x 10 seconds ↓
   - Left—side carotid sinus massage x 10 seconds ↓
   - E. Repeat carotid massages with simultaneous valsalva maneuvers ↓
8. Determine blood pressure

mildly hypotensive or normotensive

↓

9. Metaraminol: 200 mg in 250 cc D5W delivered IV at 10 ug/min

↓

increase delivery rate until a response is achieved or systolic BP = 160 mm Hg

↓

Carotid massage → [to edrophonium step]

hypertensive

↓

edrophonium 10 mg IV test dose of 2 mg (0.2 cc) IV injected over 30 seconds; if no cholinergic reaction.

↓

inject remaining 8 mg (0.8 cc) IV

↓

Carotid massage

↓

repeat the dose in 10—13 minutes

↓

history of bronchial asthma?
pulmonary congestion?
bronchospasm?

No

↓

Propranolol 1 mg/min IV to a maximum of 0.15 mg/kg monitor blood pressure → [No response to above]

Yes

↓

a) young patient?
b) past EKG's document the absence of WPW syndrome?

No → No response to above

Yes

↓

Digoxin 0.5—0.75 mg IV, then 0.25—0.5 mg IV in 60-90 minutes

↓

Carotid massage → [No response to above]

No response to above

↓

Transport to hospital

↓

Cardioversion

Table 8-5 Characteristics of untreated tachyarrhythmias

Tachyarrhythmias	Atrial Rate:	Atrial Regularity: (P—P Intervals)	Ventricular Rate:
Sinus Tachycardia	100—160	regular	100—160
Paroxysmal supra-ventricular Tachycardia	140—250	precisely regular	140—250
Atrial Tachycardia with Block	120—250	regular	70—120
Non-paroxysmal Functional Tachycardia	f waves as in atrial fibrillation or retrograde P wave at 70—250	irregular	70—250
Atrial Flutter	250—350	regular	120—180 (may be 250—350)
Atrial Fibrillation	f waves 350—600	irregular	100—160
Multifocal Atrial Tachycardia	120—200	irregular	120—200

tional upset, fatigue, alcohol, tobacco, or caffeine. A suggested protocol for the management of this disorder is provided (Table 8-4). One should begin with the least dangerous and advance to the most complicated therapeutic modality until a response is achieved.

This rhythm must be differentiated from sinus tachycardia, atrial tachycardia with block, and atrial flutter with 2:1 block (Table 8-5). With rapid ventricular rates, the P waves may be buried in the QRS complexes or in the T waves. Carotid massage may slow these various dysrhythmias by increasing vagal tone, allowing identification of P waves. P waves that are "lost" in either the QRS complexes or the T waves may be identified when there are notches or small peaks altering QRS or T wave configurations. The paper speed of the EKG machine may be increased to expose hidden P waves. Also, moving the right and left arm electrodes of the EKG machine into various positions on the chest may magnify P wave activity.

Carotid sinus massage is performed with

Table 8-5 (Continuation)

Ventricular Regularity: (R—R Intervals)	AV Conduction: (P wave/QRS complex)	P wave Configuration:	Ventricular Response to Carotid Sinus Massage:
regular	1:1	sinus	slight transient slowing
precisely regular	1:1	if seen, differs from sinus	no response or gradual slowing prior to sudden termination
usually regular	2:1 or variable	unusual and spiked in shape; upright in 2, 3 AVF	sudden, transient decrease in rate (as block increases)
regular	(junctional) or 1:1 (retrograde)	atrial fibrillation or retrograde P waves	no effect, or abrupt return to sinus rhythm
usually regular	usually 2:1 or 3:1 (may be 1:1 or variable)	sawtooth pattern inverted in leads 2, 3 AVF	transient slowing in jerky fashion (as block increases)
irregular	variable	not distinct or regular	slight transient slowing
irregular	variable	3 or more different morphologies; varying PR intervals	slowing

the patient's head slightly hyperextended and turned 20-30° to the opposite side. The portion of the artery opposite the larynx is massaged with the fingertips in a direction parallel to the course of the vessel. Vagal maneuvers as well as cardioversion should be avoided in patients suspected of having digitalis toxicity since ventricular fibrillation may result. Atrial tachycardia with block and non-paroxysmal junctional tachycardia are commonly digitalis-toxic dysrhythmias.

If these vagal maneuvers are unsuccessful, pharmacologic vagal stimulation may be tried. Either the rapidly-acting cholinergic drug Edrophonium chloride (Tensilon, Roche Laboratories) or a vasopressor, metaraminol (Aramine, Merck Sharp and Dohme) or phenylephrine, may be used. Edrophonium may cause severe cholinergic reactions in the hypersensitive individual. The patient should be tested for hypersensitivity before the total dose is given. A syringe containing 1 mg of atropine should be available in the event of a severe cholinergic reaction (cardiac or respiratory arrest). Vasopressors should not be used in hypertensive patients because they may precipitate a stroke. If the patient develops chest pain or severe headache with the use of a vasopressor, the drug should be stopped immediately. Propranolol (Inderal, Ayerst) is another drug useful in terminating supraventricular tachycardia. It should not be used in patients with a history of congestive heart failure, compromised left ventricular function, or bronchial asthma. If unwanted side effects develop from the use of propranolol, atropine can be given to counteract the bradycardia and dopamine to counter the hypotension.

Rapid intravenous digitalization is an effective means of treating this dysrhythmia. However, its use before cardioversion should probably be reserved for hemodynamically-stable, young persons with normal renal function. Digitalis may worsen a paroxysmal supraventricular tachycardia in a patient with a WPW syndrome and should not be used in such cases. The cardiac glycoside with the most rapid onset of action (3-10 min.) is Ouabain. Ouabain is preferred if digitalization is urgently needed. This is accomplished using 0.2-0.5 mg. intravenously, then 0.1 mg. every 30 to 60 minutes until 0.5-1.0 mg. has been given or the dysrhythmia has been terminated.

In hemodynamically unstable patients, immediate cardioversion in the office is the treatment of choice. In stable patients, if no other therapeutic modality has been successful, cardioversion is also indicated. Since elderly patients with cardiovascular systems already compromised by disease are less likely to tolerate carotid massage, vasopressor drugs, propranolol, or prolonged therapeutic trials, cardioversion is often an early form of treatment for them. In patients toxic with digitalis, cardioversion can precipitate more serious dysrhythmias. Otherwise, cardioversion has few serious complications (which occur in less than 1 per 100,000 procedures), but preparation should be made for serious bradyarrhythmias and tachyarrhythmias. After the patient is sedated, an external DC cardioverter is set in the synchronous mode and 25 joules is delivered.

Following successful conversion to normal sinus rhythm by any method, most patients should be hospitalized to undergo studies that determine the precipitating cause of the dysrhythmia. A healthy, young person with recurrent episodes of paroxysmal supraventricular tachycardia should be cautioned to avoid various precipitating stimulants already mentioned. Antiarrhythmic drugs or digitalis are given to some patients to prevent further attacks.

Atrial tachycardia with block

This dysrhythmia (Fig 8-3), unlike paroxysmal supraventricular tachycardia, is usually caused by abnormal atrial automaticity. Its characteristics are listed in Table 8-5. The presence of P waves not followed by a QRS complex will distinguish this rhythm from sinus tachycardia and paroxysmal supraventricular tachycardia. Confusion arises when blocked P waves remain hidden in the previous T waves and the abnormality is not recognized. Atrial tachycardia with block must also be distinguished from atrial flutter; digitalis toxicity is a cause in over one half of cases of paroxysmal tachycardia with block, whereas it is rarely a cause of atrial flutter. The treatment in most cases of atrial tachycardia with block is directed toward the underlying cause—digitalis toxicity. This includes stopping the administration of digitalis and delivering potassium chloride 10-15 mEq/hour intravenously under careful monitoring of the electrocardiogram and electrolyte levels. Intravenous Phenytoin (Dilantin, Parke-Davis) 250 mg given at a rate of 50 mg/min under EKG monitoring to a maximum dose of 1 gram may be used to abolish the dysrhythmia. Xylocaine (Lidocaine, Abbott) can be used to treat ventricular irritability. Cardioversion is contraindicated.

In contrast, atrial tachycardia with block proven not to be related to digitalis toxicity is treated with digitalis.

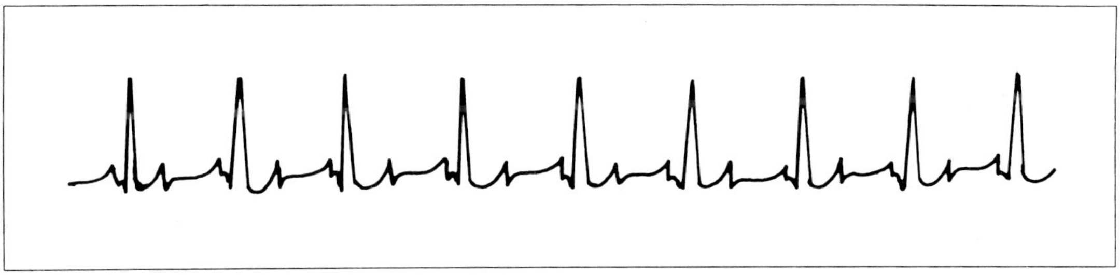

Fig. 8–3 Atrial tachycardia with block.

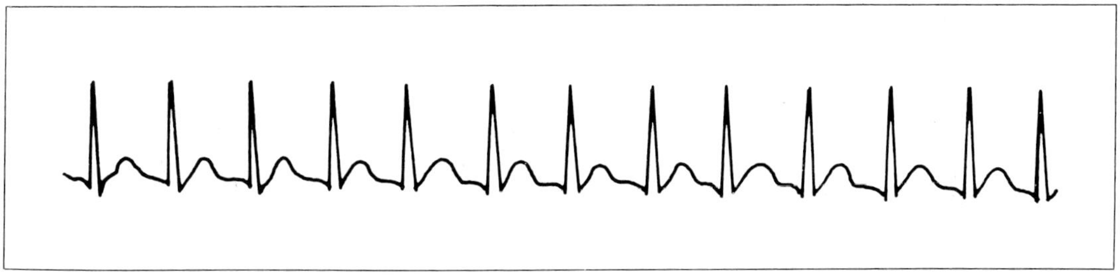

Fig. 8–4 Junctional tachycardia.

Non-paroxysmal junctional tachycardia

This dysrhythmia (Fig. 8-4) is characterized by regular, narrow QRS complexes usually superimposed on atrial fibrillation waves. It is commonly associated with digitalis toxicity, and is occasionally associated with an acute inferior wall myocardial infarction or other heart disease. Treatment is similar to that for paroxysmal supraventricular tachycardia, with the following exceptions:

1. If this dysrhythmia is digitalis-induced, the drug is discontinued.
2. If it is associated with myocardial infarction, the dysrhythmia does not require treatment if the patient is asymptomatic.

Wolff-Parkinson-White syndrome

The preexcitation syndromes (Fig. 8-5) are entities in which there is premature activation of a portion of the ventricles by conduction of an impulse from the atrium through an accessory pathway to the ventricles. The most common of these is the Wolff-Parkinson-White Syndrome (WPW). The WPW syndrome is characterized on the EKG by normal P waves, a shortened PR interval of less than 0.12 seconds, and QRS duration increased by a slurring of the initial upstroke of the complex (called a delta wave). Patients with this disorder are prone to develop atrial and ventricular tachyarrhythmias; atrial tachyarrhythmias include paroxysmal supraventricular tachycardia, atrial flutter, and atrial fibrillation. If a regular supraventricular tachyarrhythmia with narrow QRS complexes develops, the delta wave is not present, and this dysrhythmia is indistinguishable from paroxysmal supraventricular tachycardia. Atrial flutter or fibrillation is uncommon in the WPW syndrome. However, if they occur, the resulting dysrhythmia may end catastrophically. Wide, aberrant QRS com-

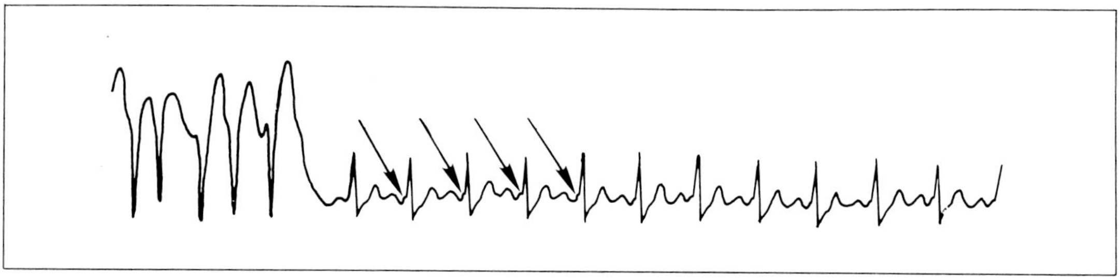

Fig. 8–5 Wolff-Parkinson-White Syndrome: tachycardia with aberrant, conduction converting to sinus tachycardia.

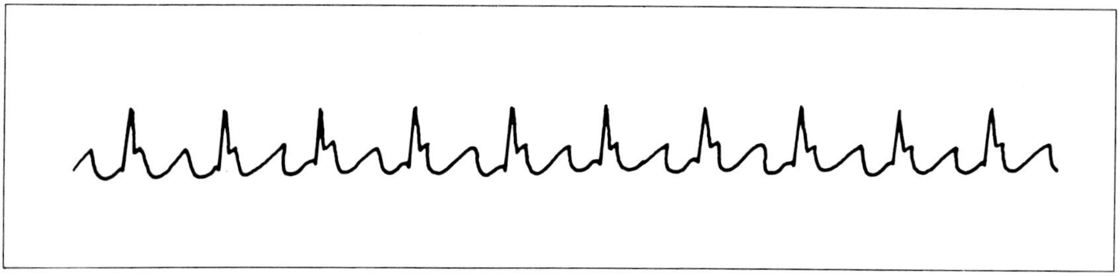

Fig. 8–6 Atrial flutter with a 2:1 AV block.

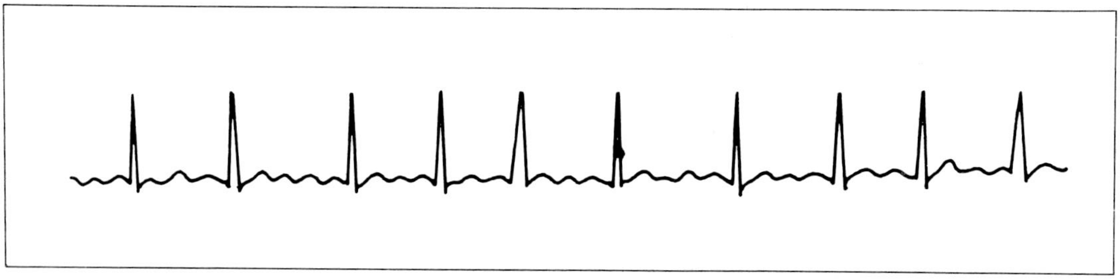

Fig. 8–7 Atrial fibrillation.

plexes may result from conduction antegrade through the anomalous pathway, producing a rapid ventricular response of 250-300/min and a rhythm similar to, but more irregular and bizarre than, ventricular tachycardia.

Vagal maneuvers are sometimes effective in terminating this rhythm. The treatment of choice of a narrow regular tachyarrhythmia in the WPW syndrome is propranolol. Lidocaine is the drug of choice for tachyarrhythmias with anomalous conduction and wide, bizarre QRS complexes. The most effective measure in either tachyarrhythmia associated with the WPW is DC cardioversion—certainly indicated in urgent situations when patients are hemodynamically unstable. Though at times it may be effective in terminating the dysrhythmia, digitalis may enhance anomalous AV conduction and so is contraindicated in the WPW syndrome.

Unless the diagnosis of the WPW syndrome was previously established, the narrow supraventricular tachycardia will probably be undifferentiated and managed as described in the section on paroxysmal supraventricular tachycardia, and the aberrant ventricular conduction will be managed as an undifferentiated fast and wide rhythm.

Atrial flutter

Atrial flutter (Fig. 8-6) is a dysrhythmia characterized by "sawtooth" atrial flutter waves at a rate of 150-300/min and a ventricular rate that is usually regular at 120-180/min. Though the associated AV block can be variable, it is most often a 2:1 block. In two unusual situations, atrial flutter may occur with a 1:1 atrial-to-ventricular conduction and thus a dangerously rapid ventricular response:

1. In association with the WPW syndrome, or
2. In patients treated with quinidine but without concomitant use of digitalis or propranolol.

At a ventricular rate of 140-150/min each blocked P wave may be hidden in a QRS-T complex, making the rhythm identical to other atrial tachycardias. The typical flutter waves may become more apparent with carotid massage, which will increase the degree of AV block.

There are two options for the treatment of atrial flutter. If the patient appears unstable in any way, synchronized direct current cardioversion is the treatment of choice. This may be performed in the dental office. Cardioversion may convert the patient to either sinus rhythm or to the more manageable atrial fibrillation.

If atrial flutter has been present for some time and the patient is hemodynamically stable, the patient may be hospitalized, and rapid "digitalization" over a 24 hour period is tried. Propranolol or quinidine may be added if digitalis does not slow the ventricular response. Cardioversion may be necessary if pharmacologic measures are unsuccessful.

Atrial fibrillation

Atrial fibrillation (Fig. 8-7) is a dysrhythmia in which there are no organized contractions of the atria. The ventricles receive a rapid but irregular series of atrial impulses, since many of these impulses are blocked out at the AV node. In untreated atrial fibrillation, the ventricular rate ranges from 100-160/min. Ventricular rates less than 100/min suggest the presence of conduction system disease; rates of 200/min or greater may be seen with the WPW syndrome or thyrotoxicosis. An "irregularly irregular" rhythm is a hallmark of atrial fibrillation. On the EKG, there are no discernible P waves. This dysrhythmia is associated with a variety of cardiac, pulmonary, and infectious diseases and drug intoxication states.

The clinical significance of atrial fibrillation is that its presence may:

1. Reduce cardiac output by 25%,
2. Predispose to the development of thrombi in the heart with resultant pulmonary and systemic embolization, or
3. Cause the unpleasant sensation of palpitations.

Only atrial fibrillation of acute onset with a rapid ventricular response that is hemodynamically compromising to the patient requires treatment outside the hospital setting. If there is an extremely rapid tachycardia or associated severe chest pain, pulmonary edema, or cardiovascular collapse, synchronized cardioversion is necessary. Otherwise, digitalis is the treatment of choice, given intravenously to patients who are relatively unstable though not in extreme cardiac decompensation. If digoxin is used, a dose of 0.50 mg intravenously is given initially, supplemented by later doses until a complete loading dose of 1.0-1.5 mg in a 24 hour period is given. Intravenous bolus doses must be given slowly. Patients in no distress may be given digitalis in oral doses. The goal of digitalization is to achieve a resting ventricular rate in the range of 70-90/min. Digitalis should not be used if the ventricular rate is less than 100/

min in a patient with the new onset of atrial fibrillation, or if the WPW syndrome is the underlying etiology. In a relatively unstable patient with atrial fibrillation and a fast ventricular response that is not easily controlled by digitalis, intravenous propranolol can be used, if no contraindications to its use exist (congestive heart failure, bronchospasm, hypotension).

Pure atrial fibrillation is rarely a digitalis-toxic rhythm. Digitalis toxicity in the presence of atrial fibrillation will appear with:

1. A slow ventricular rate (usually less than 50/min),
2. A regular ventricular rate, governed by a junctional tachycardia, or
3. Frequent premature ventricular contractions, especially ventricular bigeminy.

Multifocal atrial tachycardia

Multifocal atrial tachycardia, also known as chaotic atrial rhythm, is a rapid and irregular atrial dysrhythmia with distinct P waves of varying configurations (three or more different configurations in the same EKG lead.) Other conduction system disorders are usually present. Underlying disorders include severe cardiac or pulmonary disease, hypoxia, infection, or digitalis toxicity. If warranted, digitalis or cardioversion can be used; however, this dysrhythmia responds poorly to specific antidysrhythmic therapy. Treatment should be directed toward the underlying disorder.

Fast rate and wide complexes

Five tachyarrhythmias produce an EKG tracing with wide QRS complexes. Sinus tachycardia with bundle branch block and supraventricular tachycardia with aberrancy have the same clinical significance as their counterparts with narrow QRS complexes. Both are regular. Prior EKG tracings demonstrating a bundle branch block pattern will make recognition of the former dysrhythmia easy. Aberrant conduction is often a rate-related phenomenon. At rapid rates, the supraventricular impulse finds one of the bundle branches incompletely recovered from the previous depolarization. As a result, the impulse is conducted slowly. Measures that slow the rate might abolish the aberrancy and make the underlying rhythm apparent.

The WPW syndrome with aberrant conduction was described previously.

Ventricular tachycardia

Ventricular tachycardia (Fig. 8-8) is defined as the occurrence of three or more consecutive premature ventricular contractions (PVC's) at a rate of 150-250/min. Multifocal PVC's and more than 6 PVC's/min are premonitory signs of ventricular tachycardia. A premature ventricular contraction, as well as ventricular tachycardia itself, is characterized by a QRS complex of greater than 0.12 seconds duration, lack of a preceeding, associated P wave, and an ST segment and T wave directed opposite to the major QRS deflection of a sinus beat.

Ventricular tachycardia is only slightly irregular. It is the most serious tachyarrhythmia, since it is one step away from ventricular fibrillation. Patients with ventricular tachycardia may have a normal blood pressure. However, they are more likely to develop angina pectoris, congestive heart failure or pulmonary edema, hypotension, syncope, seizures, or cardiovascular collapse. Various causes or precipitating factors include the multiple etiologies of organic heart disease, especially acute myocardial infarction, digitalis, quinidine or procainamide intoxication, electrolyte or acid-base abnormalities, hypoxia, cardiac trauma, or severe infections. Frequent premature ventricular contractions, very slow bradyarrhythmias, or rapid supraventricular tachycardias may predispose a patient to ventricular tachycardia.

Another type of ventricular "tachycardia,"

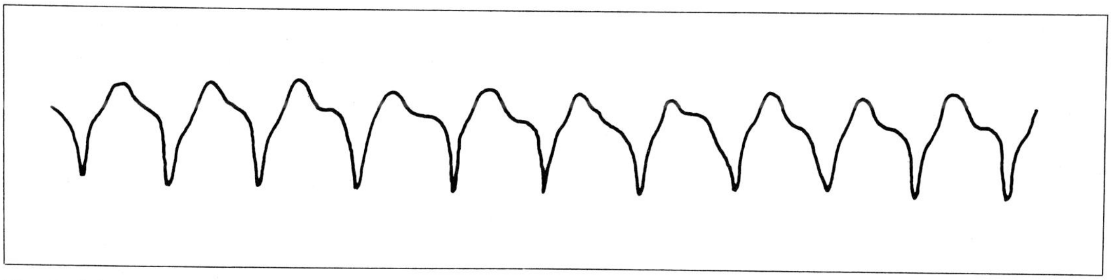

Fig. 8–8 Ventricular tachycardia.

Table 8-6a Characteristics of ventricular ectopy

a. Carotic sinus massage: ventricular rate unchanged; retrograde conduction of P waves blocked
b. Irregular cannon waves in jugular veins
c. Atrioventricular dissociation (regular atrial activity with no relation to the QRS complexes or R to retrograde P interval 〉 0.10 seconds)
d. Capture or fusion beat
e. Left axis deviation (−90° to +180°)
f. Wide mono or biphasic QRS complexes in lead V1 (LBBB pattern)
g. PVC's with similar configuration on previous EKG's

Table 8-6b Characteristics of aberrant supraventricular conduction

a. Carotid sinus massage: AV conduction slowed; P waves more apparent
b. P waves present that precede each QRS by a fixed interval
c. Grossly irregular rhythm (atrial flutter or fibrillation with aberrancy or WPW syndrome with aberrant conduction)
d. R to retrograde P wave interval 〈 0.10 seconds
e. Wide triphasic QRS complexes in lead V1 (RBBB patterns)
f. Previous EKG's demonstrating bundle branch block or WPW syndrome

similar to the above in morphology, but with a rate of about 70-130 beats/min, is "accelerated idioventricular rhythm." This dysrhythmia also occurs in the presence of ischemic heart disease. In general, there is an effective blood pressure present. The dysrhythmia is usually transient, and it seldom deteriorates into ventricular fibrillation. It can occur simultaneously with a sinus bradycardia. It should be recognized and differentiated from the other four tachycarrhythmias described. Lidocaine should not be used in the presence of accelerated idioventricular rhythm, as it may cause asystole. If perfusion is inadequate, atropine may be given to accelerate the idioventricular rhythm, or if present, the sinus rhythm.

In many cases, the origin of a tachyarrhythmia with wide QRS complexes of sudden onset cannot be easily determined on EKG. Some of the criteria for differentiating ventricular ectopy from aberrant supraventricular conduction are listed in Tables 8-6a and 8-6b. Capture or fusion beats are especially helpful in marking a rhythm as ventricular in origin. These are narrower beats among wide QRS complexes that result when the P wave fortuitiously depolarizes the ventricles ("capture") or depolarizes them simultaneously with the ectopic impulse ("fusion").

Little time should be wasted in trying to make this differentiation, however, especially if the patient is unstable. The protocol listed in Table 8-7 should be followed. Such a rhythm is assumed to be ventricular tachycardia until proven otherwise.

No harm is done in giving lidocaine to any of the tachyarrhythmias with wide QRS complexes (except the more easily distinguishable and slower accelerated idioventricular rhythm). In ventricular tachycardia and WPW syndrome, lidocaine will convert the dysrhythmia to a normal sinus rhythm in most cases. In supraventricular or sinus tachycardia with aberrancy or block, no response will be observed. If drugs are ineffective in reversing ventricular tachycardia, immediate cardioversion is indicated.

Cardioversion

If the patient is relatively stable but requires cardioversion, the patient should be transferred to the hospital where a number of preparations can be made that decrease the incidence of complications. These are all forfeited if the situation is urgent. In the office or emergency unit setting, cardioversion should be performed in hemodynamically unstable patients with the following dysrhythmias:

1. Paroxysmal supraventricular tachycardia,
2. WPW syndrome with supraventricular tachycardia,
3. Atrial flutter,
4. Atrial fibrillation with rapid ventricular response,
5. Undifferentiated tachyarrhythmia with wide QRS complexes, or
6. Ventricular tachycardia.

Preparations for cardioversion should be made in the following sequence:

1. Exclude digitalis-toxic rhythms,
2. Explain the procedure to the patient,
3. Place the patient in a supine position,
4. Secure an intravenous line,
5. Provide oxygen by nasal cannula or face mask,
6. Obtain a 12-lead electrocardiogram if the patient's condition permits,
7. Prepare an intravenous solution of isoproternol; have syringes of atropine and lidocaine available; arrange resuscitation equipment,
8. If the patient is awake, give diazepam (Valium, Roche) (3-5 mg intravenously, increasing the dose as necessary until the patient is lightly asleep), or
9. If the patient has been taking digitalis, give lidocaine 75-100 mg iv bolus. This may be given routinely before attempting cardioversion,
10. Charge the cardioversion equipment; set the cardioverter on the synchronized mode, and if there is time, test the synchronizer. The discharge should occur on the R wave but away from the vulnerable period of the T wave, and
11. Coat the paddles with electrode paste; place the posterior paddle just inferior to the left scapula and the anterior paddle at the level of the 3rd intercostal space just to the right of the sternum.

    Initial energy settings are:

atrial flutter or fibrillation	25 joules
paroxysmal supraventricular tachycardia	25 joules
WPW syndrome with supraventricular tachycardia	25 joules
ventricular tachycardia	50 joules
undifferentiated tachyarrythmias with wide QRS complexes	50 joules

12. If this amount of delivered energy produces no effect, increases in the setting in a sequence of 50, 100, 200, and 400 joules can be tried. If digitalis toxicity is a possibility, start with test

Table 8-7 Therapy of undifferentiated tachyarrhythmias with wide QRS complexes

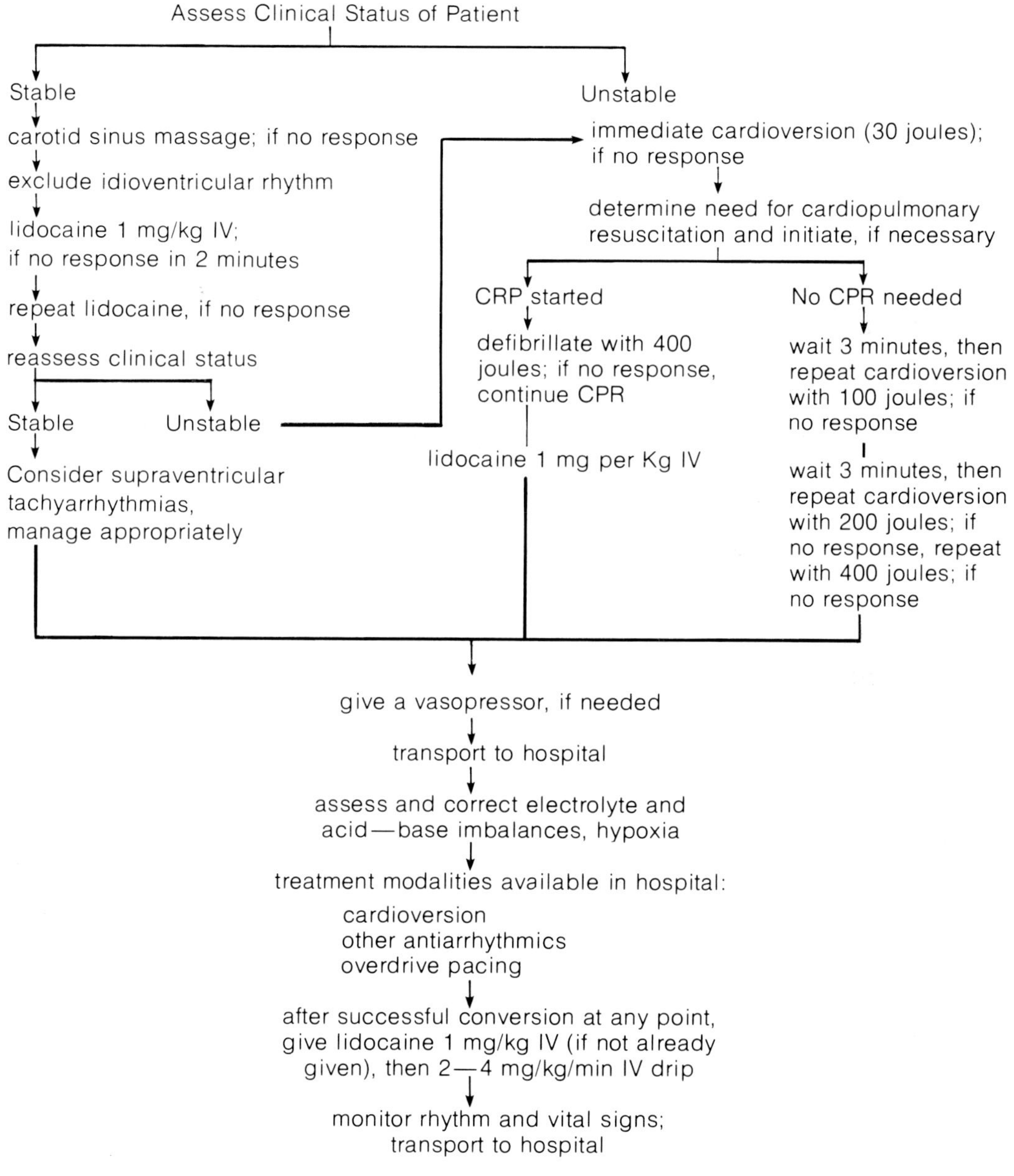

doses of 5-10 joules, observing for ventricular irritability, and

13. Once cardioversion is achieved, the patient's vital signs are closely observed for at least 30 minutes.

Any subsequent dysrhythmias, such as ventricular irritability, bradycardia, ineffective junctional rhythms, or hypotension should be treated as necessary. If ventricular fibrillation occurs after cardioversion, a second shock (at 400 joules) invariably terminates this dysrhythmia.

Bradyarrhythmias

The rhythm disturbance may be a bradyarrhythmia, with a QRS rate of less than 60/min. Most of these dysrhythmias are disturbances of impulse conduction. Bradyarrhythmias can also be divided into two categories, based on the duration of the QRS complexes (Table 8-3). These rhythms are differentiated by determining the location of the block in the conduction system.

Sinus bradycardia

Sinus bradycardia is characterized by a slow, regular sinus rhythm with a rate of less than 60/min. It occurs with atrioventricular conduction abnormalities, increased intracerebral pressure, myxedema, hypothermia, carotid sinus hypersensitivity, as a consequence of the effects of digitalis, quinidine, propranolol, reserpine, and with acute inferior and posterior myocardial infarctions. Although sinus bradycardia may have no clinical significance, it is important if it decreases cardiac output or precipitates chest pain. In the presence of chest pain, this dysrhythmia should be treated: 1) if the heart rate is less than 60/min and the systolic blood pressure is less than 90 mm of mercury, or 2) at any blood pressure if the heart rate is less than 40/min.

Sinus block and sinus arrest

Sinus arrest (sinoatrial arrest) is a failure of impulse formation in the sinus node. Sinoatrial block is a failure of tranmission of an SA impulse through the atria. The result of either abnormality is a delay in the next P-QRS-T complex. These entities are caused by excess digitalis, myocardial disease, vagal stimulation, or hyperkalemia. Treatment is indicated only if the patient is symptomatic.

Atrioventricular nodal block

Heart block is a manifestation of delayed conduction or failure of conduction through the atrium, AV node, His bundle, or bundle branches. The more distal the block, the more serious the prognosis.

In atrioventricular (AV) nodal block, the site of the block may be in the AV node itself or in myocardial tissues surrounding the node. AV block is divided into three categories. First degree block (Fig. 8-9) is characterized by a PR interval of more than 0.20 seconds. All of the P waves are conducted to the ventricles. It is usually the result of impairment of conduction through the AV node itself. Common causes include digitalis excess, acute myocardial infarction, or myocarditis.

In second degree block, some of the P waves fail to conduct to the ventricles in two ways, termed Mobitz type I and Mobitz type II blocks. In type I block (Wenckebach phenomenon) (Figure 8-10), the PR interval progressively elongates until the conduction of an impulse through the AV node is blocked entirely. At this point on the EKG, a P wave appears but no QRS complex follows. The progressive lengthening of the PR interval then repeats itself. Usually two out of three or three out of four atrial impulses are conducted to the ventricles and the QRS complexes manifested on EKG are normal. As the PR intervals elongate, the RR intervals shorten. This results in a bunching of QRS complexes,

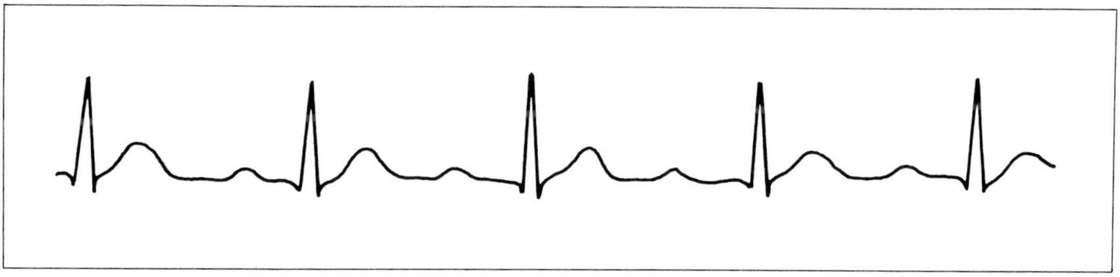

Fig. 8–9 First degree heart block.

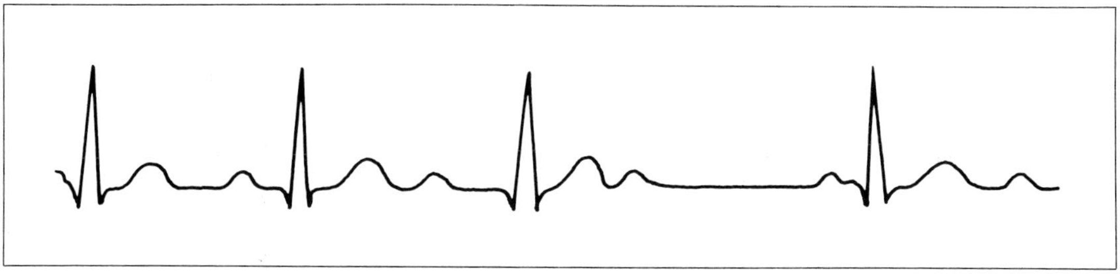

Fig. 8–10 Mobitz type I second degree heart block (Wenckebach's phenomenon).

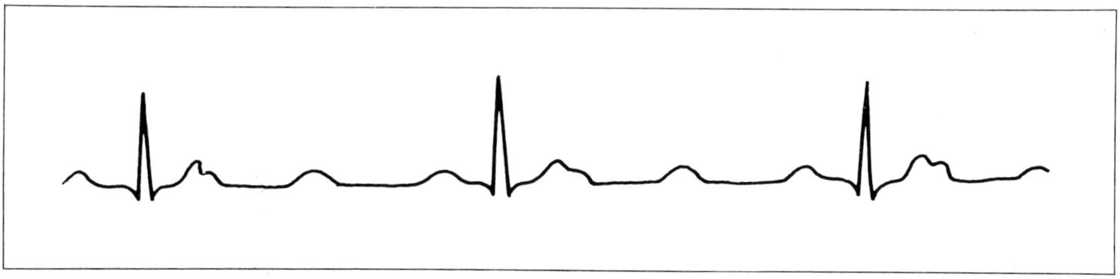

Fig. 8–11 AV conduction with Mobitz type II second degree heart block.

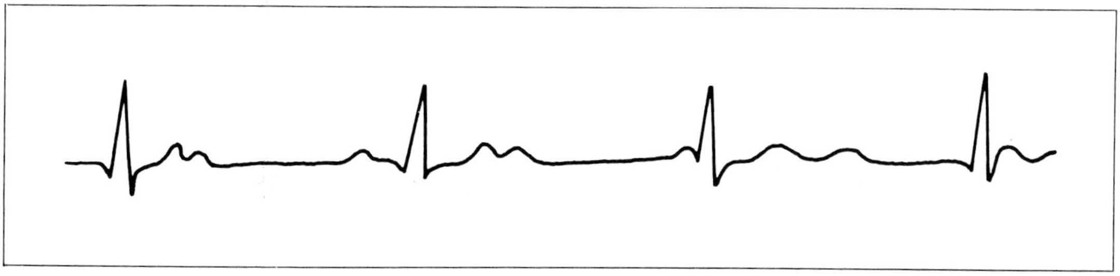

Fig. 8–12 Complete AV dissociation with third degree heart block.

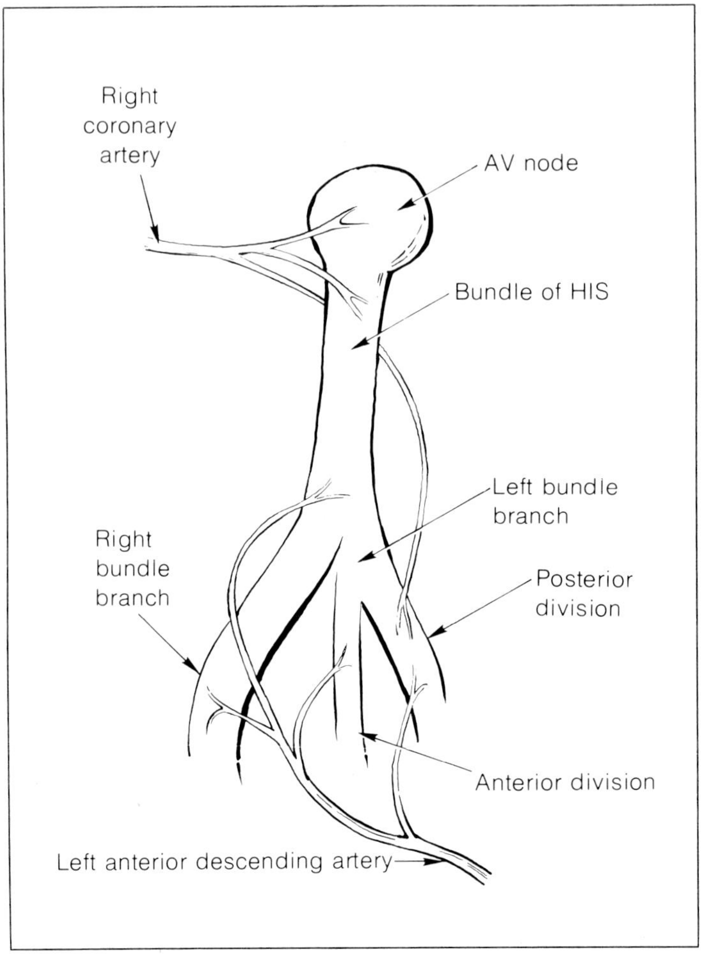

Fig. 8–13 The cardiac conduction system.

making the type I block apparent on cursory examination of a rhythm tracing. This block is often a complication of inferior myocardial infarction, myocarditis, of digitalis, morphine, quinidine, or procainamide toxicity, or it can result from increased vagal tone. This dysrhythmia is not treated unless the patient becomes symptomatic, and it is often transient.

Type II block (Fig. 8-11) is the more serious form of second degree AV block, characterized by fixed and usually normal PR and RR intervals with "dropped beats," i.e., P wave without accompanying QRS on the EKG. Because type II block is the result of a block in the fascicles or the His bundle, the QRS complex may be wider than normal. This block may be caused by anterior myocardial infarction or myocarditis. An abrupt appearance of type II block with an anterior myocardial infarction is cause for concern, because it may suddenly progress to a third degree heart block. Although type II block may be transient, most people with persistent type II block will eventually develop third degree heart block.

Third degree AV block (complete heart block) (Fig. 8-12) is the most advanced form of AV block. In this block, no atrial impulses activate the ventricles. The atrial and ventricular rates may be independent of each other. This condition, AV dissociation, occurs because the impulses from the ventricles are also blocked from traveling in a retrograde direction to the atria. The ventricle acts as its own pacemaker, the rate usually being 45 beats/min. or less, and the QRS complexes are widened. In congenital third degree heart block or in third degree heart block accompanying an acute inferior myocardial infarction, a junctional pacemaker provides a faster rate of 40-60/min, and the QRS complexes are of normal configuration. Other rhythms, from escape rhythms to terminal dysrhythmias, may develop in the presence of third degree heart block. Myocardial infarction is the most common cause of acute AV block.

Each type of block is associated with an infarct of a particular location. The right coronary artery, supplying the inferior and posterior aspects of the ventricles, also supplies the AV node, whereas the left anterior descending artery, a branch of the left coronary artery, supplies the anteroseptal sections of the ventricles, the right bundle branch and left bundle branch (Fig. 8-13). Since the various blocks result from impairment of particular sites in the conducting system, sudden loss of blood supply by occlusion of a coronary artery has predictable consequences for the conducting system (Table 8-8).

Table 8-8 Atrioventricular blocks commonly associated with myocardial infarctions

Inferior and Posterior Anteroseptal Infarctions	Infarctions
1° heart block	2° heart block, Mobitz type 2
2° heart block, Mobitz type 1 and 2 with ventricular pacemaker	3° heart block
3° heart block with junctional pacemaker	

Bundle branch block (fascicular block)

Conduction disturbances may involve any one of the three fascicles conducting impulses from the bundle of His to the Purkinje fibers. If a fascicle is blocked, one ventricle (or part of a ventricle) is activated before the other. Fascicular blocks are the result of myocardial infarction, fibrosis, or inflammation. Right bundle branch block (Fig. 8-14) may be associated with pulmonary hypertension or pulmonary emboli, and left bundle branch block (Fig. 8-15) with many varieties of organic heart disease. In themselves, the bundle branch blocks rarely cause symptoms. The characteristics of the various fascicular blocks (Figs. 8–16 and 8–17) are listed in Table 8-9.

Slow idioventricular rhythm

Slow idioventricular rhythm (Fig. 8-18) not associated with third degree heart block is a preterminal dysrhythmia that eventually progresses to asystole. The QRS is wide, usually more than 0.16 seconds, and the ventricular rate is 10-40 beats/min. Causes of this rhythm include acute myocardial infarction, cardiac tamponade, depleted intravascular volume from hemorrhage, and electrolyte disturbances.

Bradycardia—tachycardia syndrome

This syndrome, known as the "sick sinus syndrome," is characterized by a disorganized sinoatrial rhythm with sinus block or arrest, atrial ectopic beats, and multiple dysrhythmias resulting in both slow and

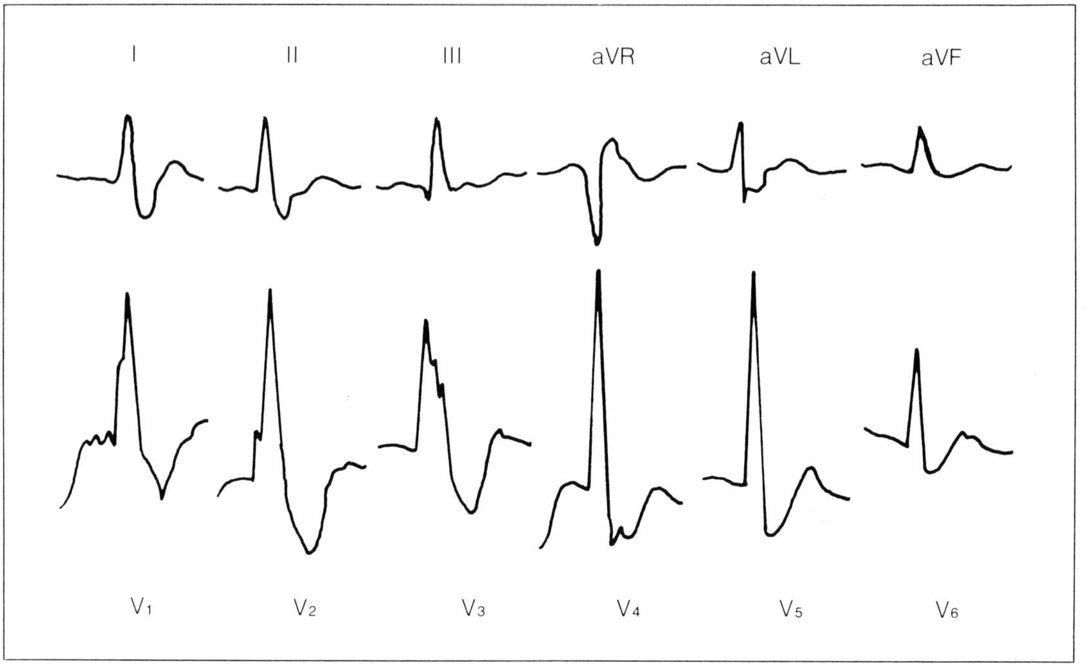

Fig. 8–14 Right bundle branch block (RBBB).

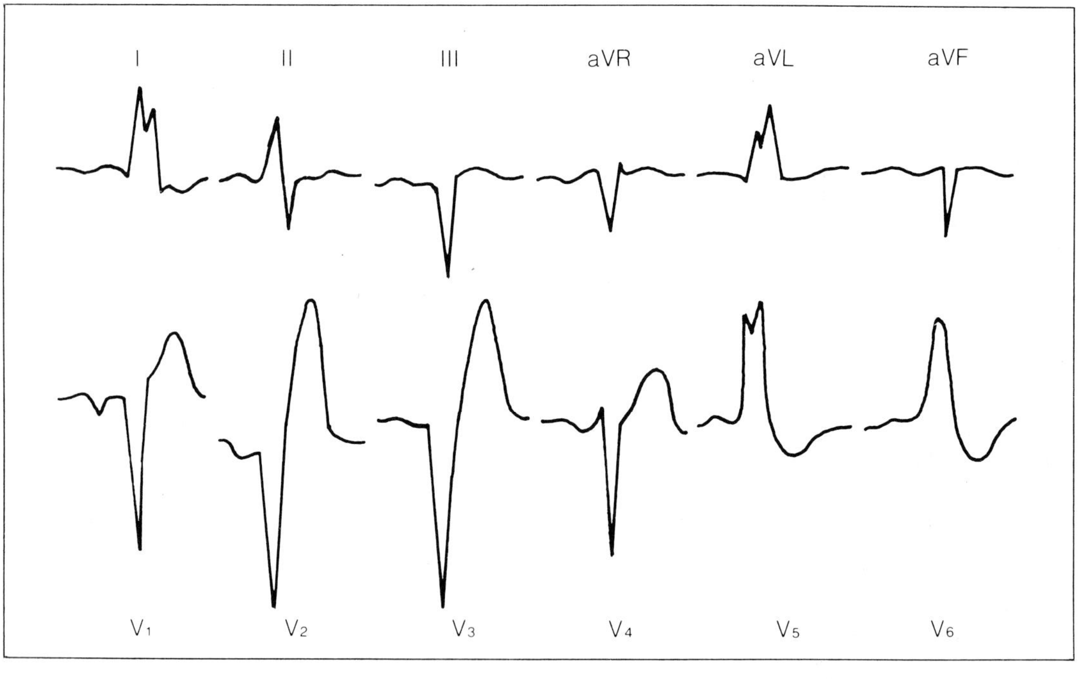

Fig. 8–15 Left bundle branch block (LBBB).

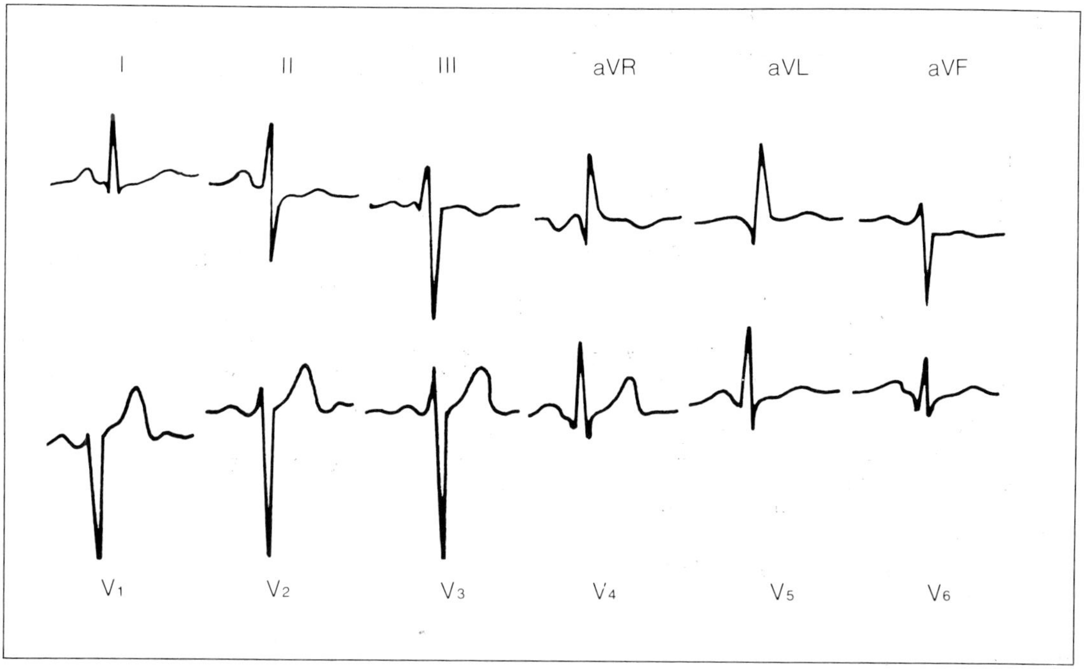

Fig. 8–16 Left anterior hemiblock (LAH).

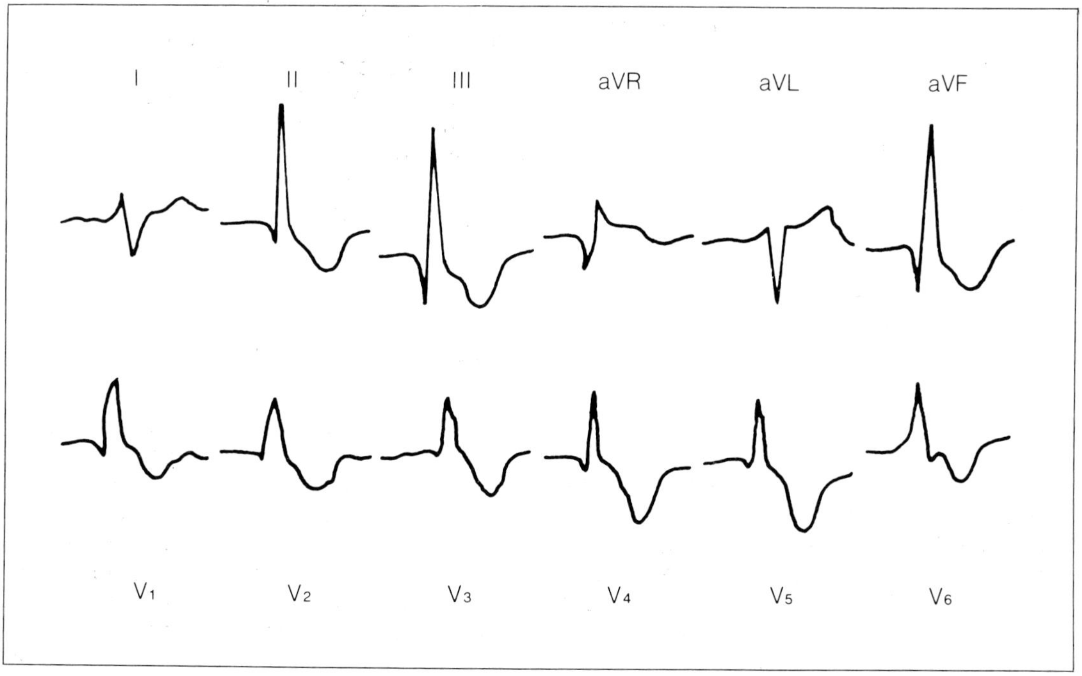

Fig. 8–17 Left posterior hemiblock (LPH).

Table 8-9 Characteristics of fascicular blocks

Unifascicular Blocks:

a. Left Anterior Hemiblock
   1. axis ⟩ −45°
   2. R wave in lead I ⟩ R wave in leads II and III
   3. lead AVL—tall R wave, small q wave

b. Left Posterior Hemiblock
   1. axis ⟩ +120°
   2. lead I—small r wave, deep S wave
   3. lead III—small q wave, tall R wave

c. Right Bundle Branch Block
   1. QRS complex width ≥ 0.12
   2. RSR or qR in V_1
   3. leads III and V_1—main deflection is positive
   4. leads I and V_6—main deflection is negative

Bivascicular Blocks

a. Left Bundle Branch Block (anterior and posterior fascicles)
   1. QRS complex ≥ 0.12 sec.
   2. Q wave absent in lateral precordial leads
   3. leads III and V_1—main deflection is negative
   4. leads I and V_6—main deflection is positive

b. Right Bundle Branch Block with Left Anterior Hemiblock

c. Right Bundle Branch Block with Left Posterior Hemiblock

fast heart rates. Sinus bradycardia is the predominant rhythm. This disease has been found in all age groups but is most common in elderly patients. These patients may present with unexplained dizzy spells or syncope and on EKG may have no more than sinus bradycardia. There are multiple etiologies. In the presence of the syndrome, (i.e., with disease of the sinoatrial node,) digitalis given to treat a tachyarrhythmia may cause sinus arrest.

Pacemaker malfunction

The malfunction of permanent, implanted pacemakers results in a variety of rhythms that will not be discussed in depth. When a pacemaker fails completely, the diseased conduction system must again take over the function of pacing the heart. The usual underlying dysrhythmia is a profound bradyarrhythmia often secondary to heart block.

Terminal dysrhythmias

Cardiac arrest can be defined as a state in which myocardial contractions are ineffective in producing cardiac output or have ceased entirely, and without direct intervention, will result in death. Three dysrhythmias are always associated with cardiac arrest: ventricular fibrillation, asystole, and electromechanical dissociation. Dysrhythmias that are often but not always a cause of cardiac arrest are ventricular tachycardia and idioventricular rhythm.

Ventricular fibrillation

Ventricular fibrillation (Fig. 8-19) is an asynchronous and disorganized electrical activity of the ventricles appearing on an EKG as an irregular, undulating rhythm without P waves or QRS complexes. The usual cause of this rhythm is acute myocardial infarction; other causes include coronary artery disease, digitalis intoxication, cardiac trauma, electrolyte abnormalities, quinidine or procainamide toxicity, hypothermia, or thyrotoxicosis.

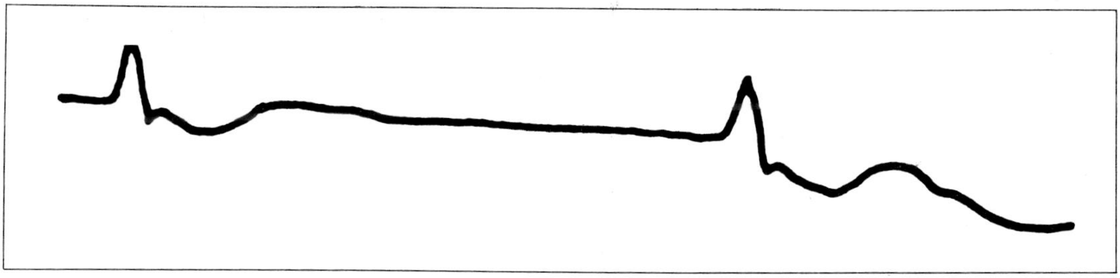

Fig. 8–18 Slow idioventricular rhythm.

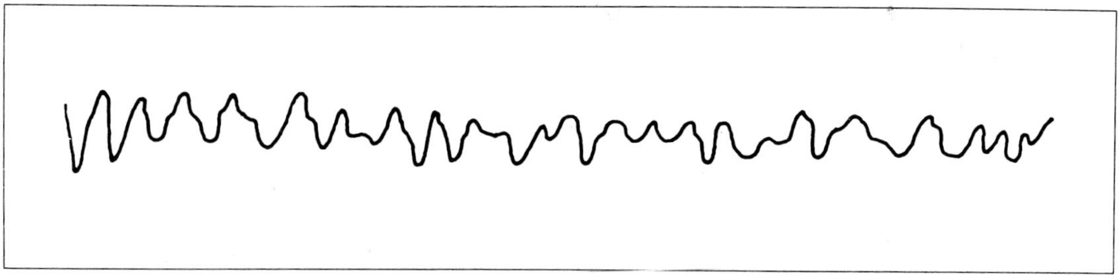

Fig. 8–19 Ventricular fibrillation.

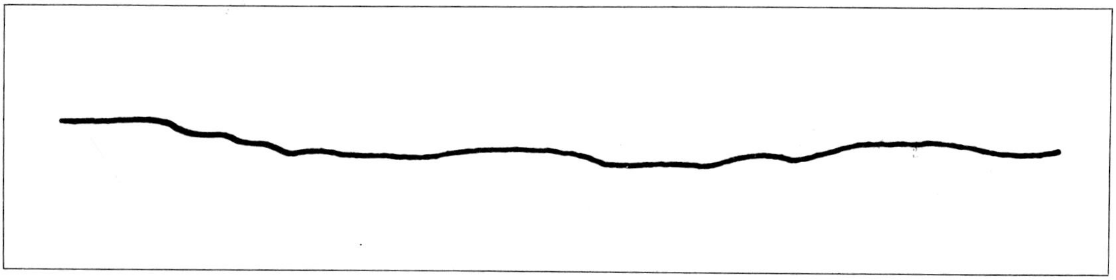

Fig. 8–20 Asystole.

Asystole

Asystole (FIg. 8-20) is the absence of cardiac electrical activity.

Electromechanical dissociation

Electromechanical dissociation is the absence of myocardial contractions in the presence of any electrical rhythm; idioventricular rhythm is usually the associated electrical activity. Important treatable causes of electromechanical dissociation include cardiac tamponade, hypotension and pnemothorax.

Treatment of bradyarrhythmias

The initial treatment of all the bradyarrhythmias is the same, and it is based on the clinical condition of the patient. A heart rate that is too slow to adequately perfuse vital organs is increased with atropine. The recommended dose is 0.6 mg intravenously, repeated at 5 min intervals until the desired rate (around 60 beats/min) is achieved. The maximum dose allowed is 2.0 mg.

If atropine does not improve cardiac output, the sympathominetic amine, isoproterenol (Isuprel, Breon) can be used. An intravenous solution is prepared by adding 1.0 mg of isoproterenol to 250 cc of 5% dextrose in water, producing a concentration of 4 μg/cc. The recommended infusion rate is 2-20 μg/min (0.5-5 cc/min), titrated to achieve the desired heart rate and blood pressure. Because of its potent cardiac stimulating properties, isoproterenol can worsen cardiac ischemia and extend necrosis in acute myocardial infarction or trigger serious dysrhythmias.

In many cases of bradycardia, a temporary and eventually permanent cardiac pacemaker is the definitive treatment. Temporary transvenous pacemakers may be employed in the emergency unit or after hospitalization in the following situations:

1. When the conduction block is progressive,
2. When the bradyarrhythmia leads to impaired cardiac output,
3. When the bradyarrhythmia allows ectopic ventricular dysrhythmias to surface, or
4. When the bradyarrhythmia is symptomatic and unresponsive to drugs.

In the event of an acute anterior myocardial infarction, heart blocks have unpredictable and often sudden progression, resulting in third degree AV block with inadequate cardiac output or terminal dysrhythmias. The presence of various heart blocks with acute anterior myocardial infarction necessitates placement of a prophylactic temporary pacemaker.

Cardiac arrest—treatment

The clinician's response to a patient in cardiopulmonary arrest should be rapid, automatic and sequential. This implies that an organized approach has been well thought out and rehearsed prior to such an unexpected event. The American Heart Association has provided the most widely accepted recommendations for managing the patient in cardiopulmonary arrest. The following protocol is based on those recommendations as applied to the adult patient suffering a witnessed cardiac arrest in the office setting.

Victim collapses:

1. Establish unresponsiveness by shaking and calling to the victim; if no response, continue.
2. Call for additional help; place the victim in a supine position.
3. Kneel adjacent to the victim's shoulders.
4. Lift the neck with one hand and push down on the forehead with the other, tilting the head back and opening the airway (Fig. 8-21).
5. Place your ear next to the victim's mouth and listen for air movement while watching for chest movement; if no response, (Fig. 8-22) continue.
6. Use the mouth-to-mouth technique (pinching nose shut with one hand, covering entire mouth with the lips) give four, quick, full breaths in rapid succession which will visibly expand the chest (Fig. 8-23). If the chest does not expand, recheck the airway and head position; if there is no response after repeating this step, the airway is obstructed and a different set of maneuvers is then necessary. Reaching into the mouth and hypopharynx with the fingers, remove any foreign materials (dentures, packing, food, vomitus, etc).
7. Palpate the carotid pulse for 5-10 seconds; if the pulse is not present, continue.
8. If a defibrillator is not readily available within 1-2 min of the arrest, proceed to #9. Using "quick look" defibrillator paddles, (Fig. 8-24) identify the rhythm. If ventricular fibrillation is present (as in most cases), defibrillate

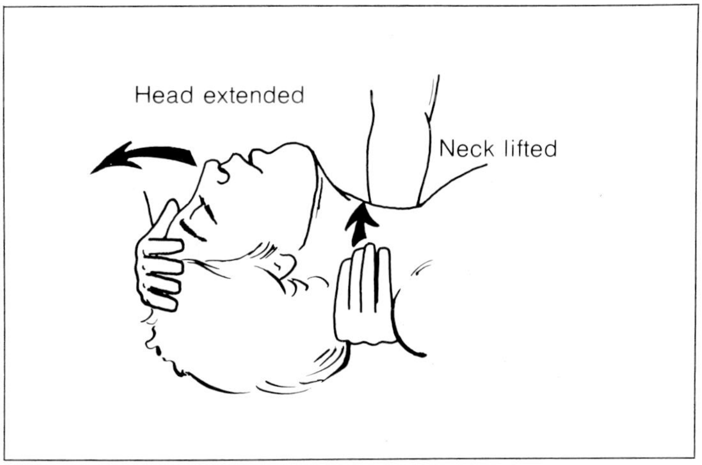

Fig. 8-21 Establishment of airway.

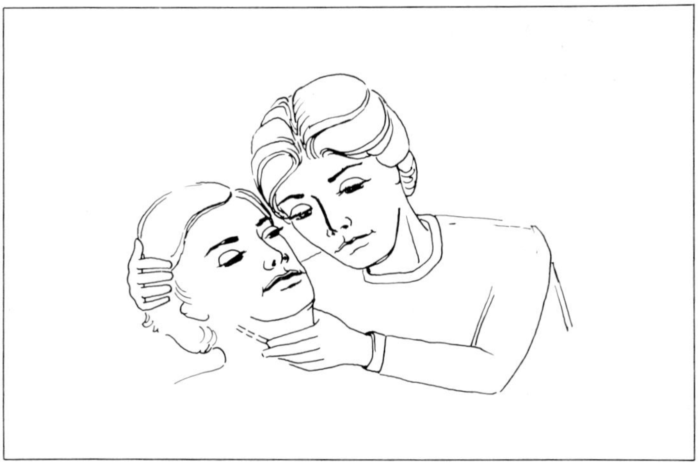

Fig. 8-22 Checking for air and chest movement while feeling for carotid pulse.

with 400 joules. If the "quick look" type paddles are not available, perform "blind" defibrillation. Palpate for the carotid pulse. If there is no response, continue.

9. Begin cardiac compressions and ventilations:
   a) Place the patient's back on a hard surface,
   b) Place the heel of the hand directly over the lower one half of the sternum at a point two finger breaths superior to the xiphoid process,
   c) Place the other hand directly over the first without touching the chest wall with the fingers of either hand (Fig. 8-25),
   d) Bring the shoulders directly over the sternum, keeping the arms straight,
   e) Compress downward on the sternum about 1½-2″ in the adult in a rhythmic and sustained pattern so that compression and relaxation are of about equal duration,
   f) If there is one rescuer, compress the chest 15 times, at a rate of 80 times/minute; then give two ventilations for each 15 chest compressions (Fig. 8-26). If there are two

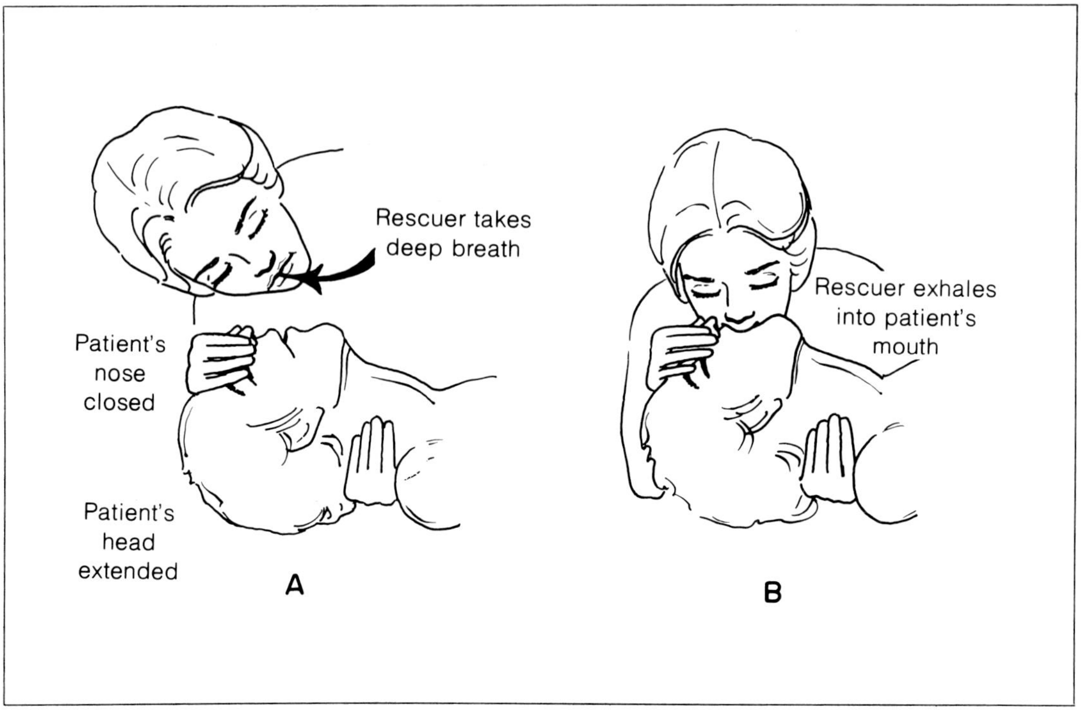

Fig. 8–23 Mouth-to-mouth ventilation.

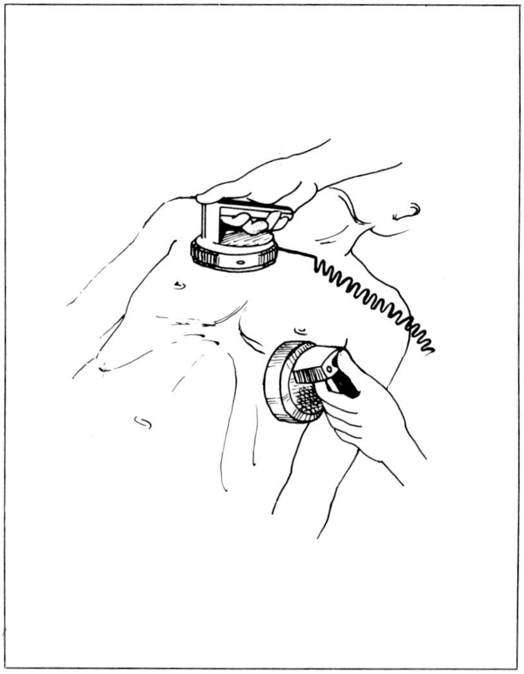

Fig. 8–24 Standard paddle placement.

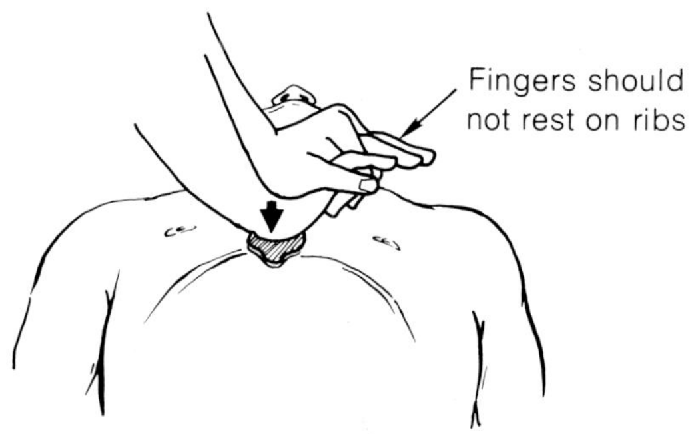

Fig. 8–25 Correct hand position for closed chest cardiac compression.

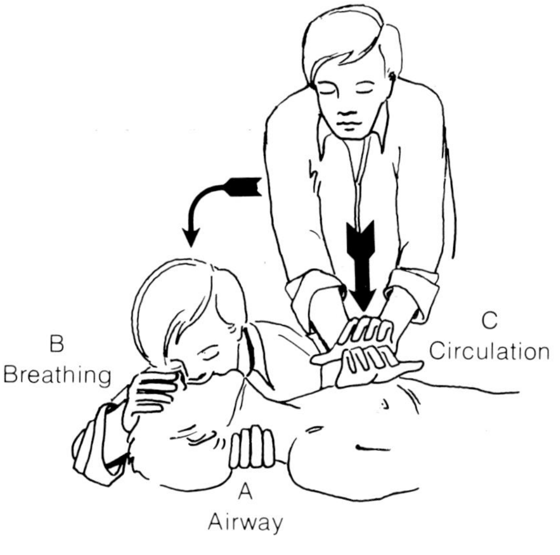

Fig. 8–26 One rescuer cardiopulmonary resuscitation (CPR).

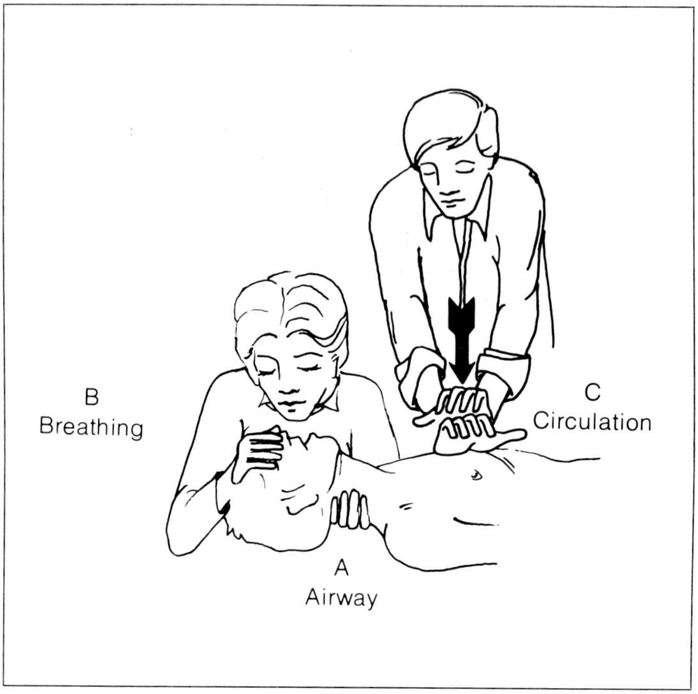

Fig. 8–27 Two rescuer cardiopulmonary resuscitation (CPR).

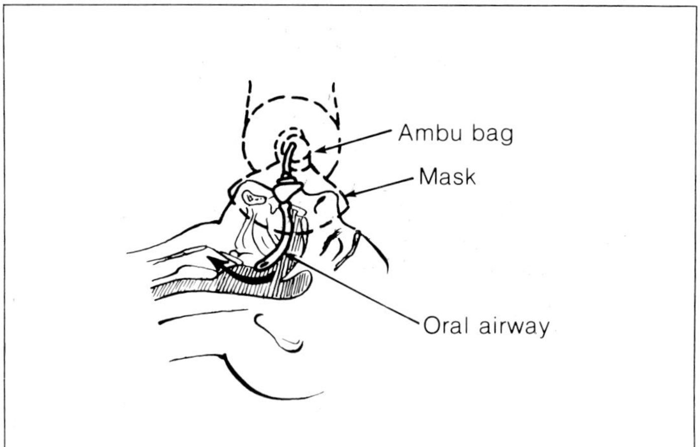

Fig. 8–28 Ventilation with bag-mask unit and oral airway.

rescuers, compress the chest 5 times, at a rate of 60 times/minute, and give one ventilation for each five chest compressions (Fig. 8-27),

g) Check for return of breathing and carotid pulse every 1-2 minutes; have a third rescuer palpate the femoral artery to detect perfusion with the cardiac compressions,

h) A MAST trousers, if available, may be utilized during the resuscitation; this serves to increase aortic diastolic pressure and thus increase coronary perfusion,

10. Establish an intravenous line,
11. Attach an electrocardiographic monitor to determine the rhythm,
12. As soon as it is available, insert an oropharyngeal airway and switch to Ambu bag/mask ventilation, using supplemental oxygen (Fig. 8-28). (A practitioner skilled in intubation may insert a cuffed endotracheal tube after a short period of bag/mask ventilation; the Ambu bag is then attached to the endotracheal tube), and
13. Recognize the rhythm and treat appropriately (Table 8-7).

If resuscitation is successful at any time:

1. Stop CPR,
2. Check pulses,
3. Observe for spontaneous, adequate ventilations; assist if absent,
4. Determine rhythm,
5. Monitor pulse and EKG continuously,
6. Treat hypotension:
   Dopamine (Intropin, Arnar-Stone) 200 mg in 250 cc 5% dextrose and water (800 μg/cc) delivered at 5-10 μg/kg/min, adjusted to blood pressure response, and
7. Transport to hospital. If unsuccessful, basic cardiopulmonary resuscitation should not be discontinued at any time for longer than 10-15 seconds.

Note that these recommendations are based on current knowledge of cardiac resuscitation. New information is constantly being acquired and revisions are to be expected.

Modification for pediatric resuscitation

Cardiopulmonary resuscitation:

Infants—the tips of the index and middle fingers compress the mid-sternum about 1/2-3/4″ at a rate of 80-100/minute,

Children—The heel of the hand compresses the midsternum 3/4 to 1½″ at a rate of 80-100/minute.

Drug dosages:

Sodium bicarbonate
2mEq/kg initially, then 1mEq/kg

Epinephrine 1:10,000
0.01 mg/kg (0.1 cc/kg)

Defibrillating dose
2 joules/kg, using pediatric paddles

Atropine . . . . 0.01 mg/kg

Calcium chloride 10%
10 mg/kg initially, observe, then repeat the dose

Isoproterenol—1 mg, in 500 cc
0.1 μg/kg/minute

Dopamine . . . 5 μg/kg/minutes initially

Fluids . . . D5¼NS or D5½NS or LR soln.

In most cases, cardiac arrest in children is a consequence of respiratory arrest and usually results in asytole.

Summary

Dysrhythmias are one of the most difficult cardiovascular emergencies for dental practitioners to manage. There is a large number of dysrhythmias from which a particular rhythm must be differentiated, yet in some cases differentiation is impossible even for cardiologists. Approaching dysrhythmias systematically makes the evaluation process quick and simple. The approach is based on three basic steps in reviewing the EKG:

1. Recognizing terminal dysrhythmias,
2. Determining heart rate (QRS rate),
3. Determining QRS duration.

This divides most dysrhythmias into four smaller categories. Thereafter the P waves and their relation to QRS complexes are studied to make a final determination of the rhythm.

Dealing with undifferentiated tachyarrhythmias is a matter of following a protocol step-by-step until a therapeutic response is achieved. All symptomatic bradyarrhythmias are treated in similar fashion; drugs are given to speed up the heart rate. Any dysrhythmia, fast or slow, is given special consideration if it occurs in the presence of an acute myocardical infarction. Dysrhythmias resulting from digitalis toxicity have modified treatment plans. In tachyarrhythmias, if the ventricular response to the rapid barrage of atrial impulses is too fast for effective cardiac output, the patient may experience signs of hemodynamic instability—cardiac or cerebral ischemia, syncope, pulmonary congestion, or shock. A bradyarrhythmia with a ventricular rate too slow for effective cardiac output has the same effect. Dysrhythmias that compromise a patient's hemodynamic status require immediate therapy in the office.

Cardiac arrest is the ultimate emergency. Immediate action by the practitioner is required to save the victim's life; there is no time to obtain medical consultation. It is the responsibility of every health professional to be trained in basic cardiopulmonary resuscitation, and it is incumbent upon the dental practitioner to be knowledgeable in some of the techniques of pharmacologic resuscitation and defibrillation. In cardiac arrest, the situation is potentially very stressful and chaotic. The resuscitator should follow a prepared algorithm such as the one discussed until success is achieved or until the patient can be transported to a medical facility.

The most common reasons for failure in a resuscitation are:

1. Poor oxygenation of tissues because of errors in providing proper ventilation or perfusion,
2. Acid-base imbalance because of errors in under- or overcorrecting the metabolic acidosis,
3. Cardiac "pump failure" because of infarction of myocardium to an extent that is incompatible with life.

These problems must be assessed in the hospital setting. The office practitioner can do little more than be certain that ventilations and cardiac compressions are effective and drug therapy is correct. However, the number of lives that can be saved by dental practitioners initiating cardiopulmonary resuscitation in their offices is substantial.

References

1. Chung, E.K.: "Wolff-Parkinson-White Syndrome Current Views." *American Journal of Medicine* 62:252-266.
2. Costrini, N.V., Thomson W.M. "Cardiac Arrythmias." *Manual of Medical Therapeutics.* 22nd ed., pp. 99-124.
3. Ekong, E. *Cardiac Arrhythmias. Medical Emergencies: Diagnostic and Management Procedures from Boston City Hospital.* Boston: Little, Brown, 1977.
4. Hodgkin, J.E., Foster, G.L., Nicolay, L.I. "Cardiopulmonary Resuscitation Development of an Organized Protocol." *Critical Care Medicine* 5:93-100.
5. Jordon, J.L., Yamaguchi, I., Mandel, W. J. "The Sick Sinus Syndrome." *Journal of the American Medical Association* 237:682-684.
6. Moe, G.R., Farah, A.E. *Digitalis and Allied Cardiac Glycosides. The Pharmacologic Basis of Therapeutics.* N.Y.: Macmillan, 1970.
7. Moser, R.H., ed. "Standards for Cardiopulmonary Resuscitation (CPR) and Emergency Cardiac Care (ECC)." *Journal of the American Medical Association* 227 (supplement): 833-868.
8. Peters, R. W., Scheinman, M.M. "Emergency Treatment of Supraventricular Tachycardia (Cardiac Emergencies)." *The Medical Clinics of North America* 63(1):73-92.

9. Redding, J.S. "Cardiopulmonary Resuscitation: An Algorithm and Some Common Pitfalls." *American Heart Journal* 98:788-797.
10. Sobel, B.E. Braunwald, E. *Cardiac Dysrhythmias. Harrison's Principles of Internal Medicine.* N.Y.: McGraw-Hill, 1980.
11. Tintinalli, J.E. "Cardiac Arrhythmias and Their Management. A Study Guide in Emergency Medicine." *American College of Emergency Physicians.* pp. 59-184.
12. Warner, H. "Therapy of Common Arrhythmias." *Medical Clinics of North America.* 58:995-1016.

Chapter 9

Cerebrovascular Disease

Richard L. Lammers, M.D.

Introduction

Cerebral vascular disease includes a variety of pathologic processes involving blood vessels supplying the brain. The "stroke syndrome" is one of the cardinal manifestations of this disease. When one considers the incidence of this common health problem, the mortality rate of 40% within thirty days of the development of a stroke, and the total disability of half of the survivors, the implications of cerebral vascular disease are awesome.

A stroke, also known as a "cerebral vascular accident," is the sudden development of a focal and essentially irreversible neurologic deficit, varying in severity from a disorder that may not interfere with the activities of a person to total incapacitation, coma, or death. The "neurologic deficit" represents an area of infarction or hemorrhage in the brain tissue. The three most common etiologies of strokes are atherosclerotic thrombosis, embolism, and hemorrhage (Table 9-1). Although strokes seem to be unpredictable, those resulting from atherosclerotic thrombosis are the end result of a progressive and potentially recognizable process. A stroke is one of those disorders in which prevention is far more important than treatment. The presence of an asymptomatic bruit or the occurrence of "transient ischemic attacks" are proven warning signals of a stroke (Table 9-2). If these signs are recognized and proper evaluation and treatment are promptly initiated, the practitioner can actually prevent the costly, disabling and often lethal stroke syndrome. Once the stroke has occurred, only supportive treatment can be offered to the patient. However, the severity of the damage caused by infarction or hemorrhage or the threat of recurrence of embolism can be minimized with proper management.

Table 9-1 Common types of strokes

a. Atherosclerotic Thrombosis

b. Embolism
- Cardiac origin
- Intra-arterial origin
- Pulmonary origin
- "Paradoxical" embolism from peripheral venous system

c. Hemorrhage
- Hypertensive intracerebral hemorrhage
- Ruptured saccular aneurysm
- Ruptured angioma
- Trauma
- Hemorrhagic disorders
- Hemorrhage into brain tumors
- Hemorrhagic infarction
- Miscellaneous causes

d. Lacunar Infarctions

Table 9-2 Manifestations of cerebral vascular disease
(In order of severity)

a. Asymptomatic bruit—a vascular murmur heard with a stethoscope.

b. Transcient ischemic attack (TIA)—a focal neurologic deficit of sudden onset that completely resolves within 24 hours.

c. Reversible ischemic neurologic deficit (RIND)—a focal neurologic deficit of sudden onset persisting beyond 24 hours but not indefinitely.

d. Progressing stroke—a focal neurologic deficit of relatively sudden onset which is actively worsening.

e. Completed stroke—a stable, focal and essentially irreversible neurologic deficit of relatively sudden onset.

Table 9-3 Symptoms of TIAs in the carotic artery distribution
(approximate order of frequency)

a. Localized contralateral* sensory loss and/or motor weakness

b. Headache

c. Ipsilateral* monocular blindness (amaurosis fugax) or other sudden visual disturbances

d. Difficulty in understanding language

e. Confusion

f. Difficulty with calculation

g. Veering to one side

*"Ipsilateral" indicates same side as the lesion in the brain; "Contralateral" indicates opposite side.

Transient ischemic attacks

Transient ischemic attacks (TIA) are also manifestations of cerebral vascular disease. By definition, a TIA is a neurologic deficit of sudden onset that completely resolves within an arbitrary time period of 24 hours. Actually, many TIAs last seconds to minutes, and most resolve within two minutes to one hour. Anything from a single TIA to multiple TIAs can precede a stroke. However, TIAs may cease without resulting in a stroke. The course of this illness in a given patient is impossible to predict.

Initially one cannot distinguish a TIA from a completed stroke. Symptoms and signs are identical to those of the various stroke syndromes until a clearing of the episode marks it as a TIA. TIAs in themselves cause no damage. The neurologic deficit of a TIA represents an area of brain ischemia. Depending on the population studied, 20 to 60% of patients experiencing TIAs will subsequently suffer a completed stroke. The risk of a stroke in a patient having TIAs is four to ten times that in a control population and is greatest in the first few months.

It is thought that most TIAs are the result of microemboli composed of platelet-fibrin aggregates or atheromatous debris. These microemboli form on an atherosclerotic plaque in an artery supplying the brain, float free of the plaque, and temporarily lodge in a cerebral vessel.

Goals in the evaluation of a patient with TIAs are:

1. Establish the diagnosis by history and physical examination.
2. Establish the anatomic location of the causative lesion.
3. If the lesion is at the carotid bifurcation, establish whether the lesion is a hemodynamically-obstructing lesion or a non-obstructing but embolizing plaque.

The second and third goals are accomplished during hospitalization.

Manifestations: The ischemic symptoms and signs occurring during an attack reflect the artery that is diseased. It is important to determine by history and/or by physical examination whether the event originates from a lesion in the carotid or the vertebro-basilar artery system and whether the lesion is on the right or left side. Ischemia in the carotid artery distribution involves the cerebral hemispheres and visual system, producing disorders of motor and sensory function, vision, mentation, and communication (Table 9-3). In the vertebro-basilar system, the ischemia involves the brain stem, cranial nerves III-IX, inferior temporal and occipital lobes, the cerebellum and cerebral hemispheres (Table 9-4).*

History: The patient should be questioned about the presence of any of these symptoms (Tables 9-3 and 9-4), the abruptness of their onset, and their duration. The examiner should ask the patient if these same symptoms or any other symptoms have occurred in the past, how frequently they occur, and how long they persist. Determine if the patient has been medically evaluated for TIAs and if he or she is taking anti-platelet or anticoagulant medication. A history for other medical illnesses is useful in determining the risk TIAs represent to a particular patient and in differentiating TIAs from other intracerebral disorders (Table 9-6). Inquire about disorders that may produce emboli responsible for the TIAs, including past myocardial infarctions and valvular heart disease (rheumatic heart disease, artificial valves, endocarditis). The history should also uncover disorders that mimic cerebral vascular disease (Table 9-7). TIA-like symptoms may be associated with sudden changes in neck or in body position. Syncope as a consequence of decreased cardiac output should not be confused with TIAs; focal neurological symptoms would not occur in this situation. Cardiac dysrhythmias are far more likely to cause syncope or dizziness than produce cerebral embolism and consequent focal neurologic symptoms.

*While the symptoms listed in these tables are important to diagnosis, it is well to note that the presence of isolated symptoms must often be considered insufficient evidence for the diagnosis of TIA (Table 9-5).

Table 9-4 Symptoms of TIAs in the vertebro-basilar artery distribution:
(in approximate order of frequency)

a. Dizziness or vertigo
b. Diplopia
c. Drop attacks (sudden weakness in the lower limbs not associated with loss of consciousness)
d. Dysarthia
e. Weakness of part of one side, one half of one side, both sides, or alternating between both sides of the body
f. Crossed sensory loss (one side of face and opposite extremities)
g. Bilateral dimmed or blurred vision, or scintillating scotomatas
h. Tunnel vision
i. Partial or complete blindness
j. Pupillary change
k. Ptosis
l. Pavesis of gaze
m. Difficulty communicating
n. Dysphagia
o. Headache
p. Disorders of equilibrium (ataxia, clumsiness, unsteadiness)
q. Transient global amnesia
r. Tinnitus

Table 9-5 Symptoms that alone cannot be diagnosed as TIA:

a. Dizziness, lightheadedness, giddiness
b. Vertigo
c. Syncope
d. Dysarthria
e. Diplopia
f. Confusion

Table 9-6 Risk factors of strokes:

a. Hypertension
b. Hyperlipidemia
c. Atherosclerotic cerebral vascular disease
d. Atherosclerotic heart disease (coronary artery disease)
e. Polycythemia
f. Diabetes Mellitus
g. Cardiac dysrhythmias (especially atrial fibrillation)
h. Cigarette smoking
i. Emotional stress
j. Hyperuricemia
k. Obesity
l. Oral contraceptives

Physical Examination: The physical examination performed by the practitioner first caring for the patient is crucial because the neurological findings in TIAs are evanescent.

A cardiac examination is of obvious importance since most patients with cerebral disease die of acute cardiac disorders. Life-threatening dysrhythmias must be identified and treated immediately. Blood pressure and other vital signs should be obtained as soon as possible.

The examination should include palpation of the carotid arteries. Reduction of pulse strength on palpation is a hallmark of atherosclerotic occlusive disease. Palpation of the superficial temporal arteries is also useful. A prominent or increased pulsation transmitted through the superficial temporal artery (as a collateral channel) indicates occlusion of the internal carotid artery of the same side. The practitioner should auscultate over the carotid bifurcation for a well-localized bruit that extends throughout systole. Palpation of a thrill is useful in localizing a bruit. Presence of a carotid bruit indicates at least a moderate and probably a severe stenosis of that vessel. The site of a lesion causing the TIAs correlates with the bruit in 60% of cases.

A neurological examination, which includes level of consciousness, cranial nerves (including visual fields), sensory, motor, reflex, and cerebellar function, should be done to detect resolving or residual focal neurological signs.

A fundiscopic examination may reveal retinal changes of atherosclerosis, diabetes mellitus, and hypertension. Retinal vessel emboli, old retinal infarction, hemorrhages, or discrepancy of hypertensive changes between the two eyes are findings indicative of cerebral vascular disease.

Management: All patients with TIAs of new onset should be hospitalized for further investigations. When facilities are available in the office, a blood sugar level can be drawn to exclude the possibility of hypoglycemia. An electrocardiogram can be obtained to detect acute cardiac disorders.

It is best to delay giving anticoagulants prior to admission; intracranial hemorrhage must first be excluded. If the patient is receiving anti-platelet or anticoagulant therapy for TIAs and has an increase in frequency of TIAs, platelet function studies or blood clotting studies are done as an outpatient to evaluate the adequacy of therapy. If therapy is inadequate, the patient should be hospitalized for further studies. When the patient requires hospitalization, the anticoagulants are not withheld prior to admission. If hypertension is present, it should not be treated vigorously, if at all, in a suspected TIA, since this may decrease cerebral blood flow to ischemic brain tissue.

A variety of screening tests will be performed in the hospital. Cerebral or carotid arteriography is the only means of defining the anatomic location, extent, and character of an intra- or extra-cranial vascular lesion. The more recent the TIA, the sooner the arteriogram should be done. Arteriography is performed in patients who are potential candidates for carotid endarterectomy. Angiography is not performed in patients with vertebro-basilar TIAs unless the TIAs persist in spite of adequate medical treatment.

Long-term therapy of TIAs is beyond the scope of this text.

Strokes

The Clinical Manifestations of Strokes

Strokes are characterized by:

1. Etiology—thrombosis, embolism, or hemorrhage;
2. Location of the pathologic process in the brain.

Embolic and thrombotic strokes damage brain tissue supplied by a particular arterial system, producing well-defined syndromes. Clinical "stroke syndromes" corresponding to the vessels afflicted, are described in textbooks of Neurology. Hemorrhages may extend deeply into brain tissue and cross into territories supplied by more than one artery. Two problems occasionally associated with strokes and complicating the clinical picture are:

Table 9-7 Disorders mimicking cerebral vascular disease:

a. Mechanical compression of neck vessels
b. Postural hypotension
c. Cardiovascular syncope (including hypovolemia)
d. Cardiac dysrhythmias
e. Focal seizure disorders
f. Meniere's disease
g. Labyrinthitis
h. Migraine headaches
i. Cerebral tumor
j. Hypoglycemia

1. Generalized increase in intracranial pressure.
2. A mass effect on the brain resulting from accumulation of blood under pressure.

The clinical picture associated with occlusion of the common internal carotid arteries is widely varied. Complete occlusion can occur without accompanying symptoms if there is sufficient collateral blood flow.

The lacunar syndrome represents small thrombotic infarcts in the territories of the penetrating branches of major surface arteries of the brain. These infarcts usually involve the pons and deeper parts of the cerebral hemispheres. They produce recognizable syndromes, such as pure hemisensory loss, pure hemiplegia, a clumsy hand—dysarthria syndrome, or bilateral upper motor neuron signs (spasticity and paralysis). Lacunar infarcts are commonly seen in patients with hypertension. They represent small vessel disease and require no treatment, unless the patient's hypertension is poorly controlled.

Table 9-8 Clinical stroke syndromes—internal carotid artery

Specific Clinical Signs (Motor, sensory and vision)
a. Contralateral paralysis of one side of the body
b. Contralateral sensory loss of one side of the body
c. Contralateral loss of vision for one half the visual field of both eyes
d. Ipsilateral blindness (Transient or permanent)
e. Loss of all forms of communication (receptive aphasia and conductive aphasia)

Types of strokes

At some early point in the management of a patient with a stroke, an attempt should be made to clinically differentiate between the three general etiologies. This is done by evaluating:

1. The temporal profile of the event
2. The suspected precipitating cause
3. Predisposing factors

Thrombotic Strokes: Cerebral infarction caused by internal carotid artery thrombosis is the most common of all strokes (Table 9-8). Thrombotic strokes produce a clinical picture that is more variable than that of embolic strokes. In 80% of cases, the event is preceded by transient ischemic attacks. TIAs rarely precede other types of strokes. The attack can either have a sudden onset or evolve in a gradual or "stuttering" progression over a period of hours or days. Deficits can develop in various parts of the body in a serial fashion, occasionally with periods of partial improvement. Intermittency characterizes the thrombotic process. Cerebral edema may develop to varying degrees, depending on the size of the infarct.

Thrombotic strokes, being unrelated to activity, commonly occur during sleep or shortly after waking. Signs of generalized arteriosclerosis and peripheral vascular disease are often present in patients with thrombotic strokes. If a headache is present, it is rarely severe. Hypertension, which aggravates the atherosclerotic process, is present in 60% of cases. During hospitalization, arteriography is the most informative procedure that can be performed, demonstrating stenosis or total occlusion and collateral flow. It is useful when the presence of a vascular lesion is uncertain or when vascular surgery is contemplated.

Embolism: Embolic strokes occur suddenly, usually without warning, and immediately produce a maximum deficit. They tend to occur in the awake person but can occur during sleep. If emboli are responsible for multiple transient ischemic attacks, the patterns of neurologic deficit are different with each attack. Headache is usually not a major component of the clinical picture. An embolus lodging in the basilar artery can produce sudden coma and total paralysis. There is a danger of recurrence within the first few days in embolic strokes.

Cerebral embolus implies the existence of a source producing the embolus, which in most cases is the heart. An atheromatous plaque in an artery is another common source of emboli. Fat, tumor, and air emboli, emboli from pulmonary vein thrombosis, and paradoxical embolism associated with congenital heart disease are uncommon occurrences.

The careful search for the source of the embolus is best conducted during hospitalization. Chronic atrial fibrillation is the cause of embolism in 50% of all cases. Mitral stenosis secondary to rheumatic heart disease increases the probability of embolism seven-fold, and is a likely cause in a young person suffering a stroke. Additional cardiac conditions predisposing to embolism include other dysrhythmias, myocardial infarction (with mural thrombus formation), prosthetic valves, bacterial endocarditis and non-bacterial endocardial vegetations. Emboli may result from surgery of the heart, neck, or thorax. Upon recognizing a condition that can potentially produce emboli, the initial examiner might suspect that a stroke is embolic in nature.

Hemorrhage: Two distinct clinical pictures appear with intracranial hemorrhage, represented by hypertensive intracerebral hemorrhage and by subarachnoid hemorrhage. Each will be discussed.

Hypertensive Intracerebral Hemorrhage: This stroke syndrome, resulting from intraparenchymal hemorrhage, consists of an abrupt onset without warning symptoms and a steady evolution of deficits that reach a maximum usually within an hour but up to 24 hours. In most cases, the stroke develops while the patient is awake and active. A sudden, severe headache is common to this type of stroke. Other evidence of long-standing hypertension—cardiac and retinal manifestations—are present. The patient can rapidly deteriorate into a comatose state. Recurrence of the bleeding is not a problem in intracerebral hemorrhage.

Neurologic deficits are determined by the site and extent of hemorrhage. In some hemorrhages, death unavoidably follows in a matter of hours. Of all the syndromes of hemorrhage, cerebellar hemorrhage is the most important to recognize (Table 9-9). It can lead to dissection into the brain stem, rapid brainstem compression, brainstem herniation, or acute hydrocephalus by blockage of the fourth ventricle. Sudden stupor progressing to coma indicates that brainstem compression, and an irreversible state, has occurred. With cerebellar hemorrhage, unlike any of the other stroke syndromes, neurosurgical consultation is imperative, because evacuation of the clot can be life-saving.

Table 9-9 Cerebellar hemorrhage

a. Inability to walk or stand by normal strength
b. Occipital headache
c. Vomiting
d. Incoordination
e. Ipsilateral nystagmus
f. Weakness in looking toward the side of the lesion
g. Deviation of both eyes to the side opposite the lesion or ipsilateral sixth nerve palsy
h. Mild ipsilateral facial weakness
i. Dysarthyria, dysphagia
j. No motor or sensory loss

Subarachnoid Hemorrhage: This is probably the only intracranial lesion capable of producing almost instantaneous death in an otherwise healthy individual. The majority of subarachnoid hemorrhages are caused by rupture of intracranial aneurysms and bleeding from arteriovenous malformations. The hemorrhages occur suddenly, often during activity or exercise, and without any warning except for an excruciating headache. The patient may quickly lose consciousness or remain lucid. In mild cases, consciousness may be regained quickly, but confusion, vomiting, headache, neck stiffness and other meningeal signs remain. Hyporeflexia and bilateral extensor plantar responses can develop within an hour. Seizures may occur with the onset of the hemorrhage or soon thereafter. Ruptured aneurysms should be considered in a normotensive or young patient presenting with sudden unconsciousness or death. Exertion, hypertension, head trauma, and the Valsalva maneuver can cause rupture of aneurysms.

The neurological deficits are varied, and early in their course there are usually no

Table 9-10 Significance of blood pressure in TIAs or stroke

a. Extreme hypertension—consider hypertensive encephalopathy as well as intracranial hemorrhage
b. Hypotension—consider dysrhythmias, cardiovascular collapse, occult extracranial hemorrhage, or terminal brain stem injury.
c. Orthostatic changes in blood pressure (marked drop in blood pressure from supine to standing position)—consider extracranial hemorrhage
d. Discrepancy of ≥ 20 mm Hg pressure between arms—consider dissecting aortic aneurysm involving the brachocephalic vessel or left common carotid vessels

lateralizing signs. Later, on physical examination nuchal rigidity is usually present; retinal subhyaloid hemorrhages and papilledema are common. Fever can develop within hours. The presence of a bruit on auscultation of the skull suggests the possibility of an arteriovenous malformation. Major problems occurring after the bleed are recurrence of hemorrhage and vasospasm; both can cause more damage.

Management of Strokes: Initial management of a patient who suffers a stroke in the dental office is supportive and is identical for any of the stroke syndromes. The first step is to determine the respiratory status of the patient. If the patient is comatose, the airway should be secured by opening the patient's mouth, extending the neck, and if necessary, pulling the tongue forward. The patient should have dentures and packing removed and any secretions or vomitus suctioned. An oropharyngeal airway may be placed in the mouth if the gag reflex is absent. If respirations are shallow or if the rate is less than eight per minute, the patient's ventilations should be supported, using the mouth-to-mouth-technique or a bag-mask device. If there is any question of hypoxia, supplemental oxygen can be provided until arterial blood gases are obtained at the hospital. If there is any warning of an impending seizure and the teeth are not yet clenched, a padded object may be placed between the teeth to protect the tongue; the extremities should be protected from striking any object.

The vital signs are then determined—blood pressure, pulse, respiratory rate and pattern, and temperature. An intravenous line is secured, if possible. Any solution except 5% dextrose in water can be used prior to arrival at the hospital. The optimal solution is 2.5% dextrose 0.5% normal saline, infused at the slowest possible rate. Shock is uncommon in an acute stroke; its presence signifies either terminal brainstem compression or cardiovascular collapse secondary to myocardial infarction or dysrhythmia. Only the cardiac disorders are treatable (Table 9-10). A change in respiratory pattern is an important observation because it indicates that the level of neurologic deficit has changed.

A pertinent history and brief physical examination obtained by the dental practitioner in the office is invaluable to physicians subsequently caring for the patient. The history may later be unobtainable if the patient becomes comatose, and neurologic deficits observed initially may resolve or progress.

Another goal of the initial history and physical examination, in addition to providing information for later use, is to identify urgent conditions requiring immediate treatment. These conditions are:

1. Cerebellar hemorrhage
2. Brainstem herniation secondary to hemorrhage
3. Subarachnoid hemorrhage
4. Increased intracranial pressure
5. Evidence suggesting an etiology other than stroke.

The history used for patients experiencing TIA's is also useful for those patients suffering strokes. Additional historical data should include:

1. Subjective information—presence of headache, visual problems, sensory symptoms, dizziness, vertigo;
2. Present medication (especially anticoagulants);
3. Medical illnesses, including risk factors for stroke, previous TIAs, previous strokes and residual deficits;
4. Allergies.

A cardiac examination should be performed to detect dysrhythmias requiring urgent therapy. The important parts of a neurological examination that should be performed by the dental practitioner are:

1. Level of consciousness: describe the response to calling the patient's name, to commands, or to painful stimuli; note subsequent changes;
2. General posture of the body (decerebrate, decorticate);
3. Neck stiffness
4. Cranial nerves
   a) pupillary size and reaction to light
   b) direction of gaze
   c) voluntary ocular movements
   d) fundiscopic examination (to detect subhyaloid hemorrhages, vascular spasm, papilledema)
   e) droop of one half of the face
   f) presence of gag reflex;
5. Sensory—sensation of touch and/or pinprick symmetrical in the extremities, face;
6. Motor—comparative strength in upper and lower extremities in the awake patient; movement of each extremity in response to painful stimuli in comatose patients;
7. Deep tendon reflexes—asymmetry of response, plantar responses; (optional);
8. Cerebellar—clumsiness in upper or lower extremities, best demonstrated with finger-to-nose or heel-to-shin testing.

This abbreviated examination requires no more than a few minutes to perform yet provides enough information to allow early recognition of serious strokes (cerebellar hemorrhage, subarachnoid hemorrhage) or brainstem herniation.

The patient should be examined for evidence of head or neck injury. An electrocardiogram can be done before or after transporting a patient to the hospital. It is useful for:

1. Detecting dysrhythmias responsible for cerebral emboli or secondary to the intracerebral disorder.
2. Demonstrating an unsuspected acute or old myocardial infarction.

In the presence of subarachnoid hemorrhage, however, electrocardiographic abnormalities mimicking myocardial ischemia are common.

No drug altering the mental status of the patient should be given prior to transport to a hospital. One exception is a medication required to control a prolonged seizure. In stroke patients with elevated blood pressures, unless there is malignant hypertension, the blood pressure should not be reduced, because this may precipitate cerebral ischemia and cause further damage. The exception to this rule is the stroke secondary to subarachnoid hemorrhage. Some clinicians recommend using hypotensive agents to lower the blood pressure to 100 mm. Hg systolic pressure (or 160/100 mm Hg in chronically hypertensive patients) if subarachnoid hemorrhage has occurred. This may be deferred if the patient is to be immediately transported to a hospital facility. If severely increased intracranial pressure or brainstem herniation is present, 10% mannitol in a dose of one gram per kilogram may be administered intravenously to reduce intracranial pressure temporarily.

In transit to a hospital, if not being ventilated, the patient should be placed in the lateral decubitus position to prevent aspiration and to allow the tongue to fall forward. A pillow should not be placed under the patient's head. A written report of the initial examination and course should accompany the patient to the hospital.

Summary

Cerebrovascular disease is generally not thought of as a treatable disorder. On the contrary, when practitioners recognize early signs of cerebrovascular disease such as transient ischemic attacks and initiate appropriate medical care, many patients can be spared the disabling and often lethal consequences of stroke.

Once a patient has suffered a stroke, simple but important supportive measures begun immediately in the office will minimize or prevent the complications that kill most stroke victims.

Finally, it is crucial that the dental practitioner identify those unusual strokes, such as cerebellar hemorrhage, hemorrhage with brainstem herniation, or subarachnoid hemorrhage, that require urgent neurosurgical or pharmacologic management in order to preserve the patient's life.

References

1. Bannister, R. *Brains Clinical Neurology,* 4th Ed. Cambridge: Oxford Univ., 1973.
2. Burns, R.A. *Diagnosis and Management of Transient Ischemic Attacks, Current Topics,* Vol. 4, No. 3. The Medical College of Pennsylvania, 1979.
3. Caronna, J.J. "Transient Ischemic Attacks: Pathophysiology and Medical Management" (Symposium: Evaluation and Management of Stroke). *Postgraduate Medicine* 59:106-111. 1976.
4. Chusid, J.G. "Disorders Due to Vascular Disease of the Central Nervous System." *Correlative Neuroanatomy and Functional Neurology,* 11th Ed., Lange, 1973.
5. Committee on Cerebrovascular Disease. "A Classification and Outline of Cerebrovascular Diseases II." *Stroke* 6:564-593. 1976.
6. Conneally, P.M., et al. "Cooperative Study of Hospital Frequency and Character of Transient Ischemic Attacks: III Risk Factors." *The Journal of the American Medical Association* 240:742-746. 1978.
7. Gifford, R.W. *Hypertensive Crisis.* Schwartz, G.R., et al (Ed.). *Principles and Practice of Emergency Medicine.* Philadelphia: Saunders, 1978.
8. Gotshall, et al. "Cooperative Study of Hospital Frequency and Character of Transient Ischemic Attacks: Initial Diagnostic Evaluation." *The Journal of the American Medical Association* 239:2001-2003.
9. Leonberg, S.C., Elliott, F.A. "Preventing Stroke After TIA." *American Family Physician* 17:179-183. 1978.
10. Machleder, H.I. "Strokes, Transient Ischemic Attacks and Asymptomatic Bruits (Medical Progress)." *Western Journal of Medicine* 130:205-217. March 1979.
11. Mohr, J.P., Fisher, C.M., Adams, R.D. "Cerebrovascular Disease." Issenbacher, K.J., et al (Ed.). *Harrison's Principles of Internal Medicine,* 9th Ed. N.Y., McGraw-Hill 1911-1942. 1980.
12. Report of the Joint Committee for Stroke Facilities: VII. "Medical and Physical Management of Stroke." *Stroke* 4:270-320. 1973.
13. Samuels, M.A. *Neurologic Emergencies.* Cohen, A.S., Freiden, R.B., Samuel, M.A. (Ed.). *Medical Emergencies: Diagnostic and Management Procedures from Boston City Hospital.* Boston: Little, Brown, 1977.
14. Sandok, B.A., et. al. "Guidelines for the Management of Transient Ischemic Attacks." *Mayo Clinic Proceedings* 53:665-674. 1978.
15. The Canadian Cooperative Study Group. "A Randomized Trial of Aspirin and Sulfinpyrazone in Threatened Stroke." *New England Journal of Medicine* 299:53-59. 1978.
16. Toole, J.F., Patel, A.N. *Cerebrovascular Disorders,* 2nd Ed. New York: McGraw-Hill 1974. pp. 280-292.
17. Weiner, H.L., Levitt, L.P. *Neurology for the House Officer.* Baltimore, Williams and Wilkins, 1974.
18. Weintraub, B.M., McHenry, L.C. "Cardiac Abnormalities in Subarachnoid Hemorrhage: A Resume." *Stroke* 5:384-392. 1974.

Chapter 10

Drug Related Emergencies

Barry H. Hendler, D.D.S., M.D. and Louis F. Rose, D.D.S., M.D.

Introduction and general considerations

The use of any drug carries with it certain risks. In his therapeutic decisions the doctor must weigh these risks against the effectiveness of the drug and the need for its use. Hazards of drug therapy are reduced by regulations that make it difficult to market drugs without considerable critical scrutiny. However, the ultimate safety and effectiveness of drugs are determined to a great extent by the doctor's knowledge of pharmacology. With the expansion of drug therapy and the introduction of potent agents having complex effects and even more complex interaction with one another, it is increasingly necessary for the doctor to have a scientific attitude and considerable knowledge of drug evaluation.

The term "idiosyncrasy," has been used rather vaguely in medicine to cover drug reactions that are qualitively different from the usual effects obtained in the majority of patients. These idiosyncratic reactions cannot be attributed to drug allergy.

Drug allergy is an altered response to a drug resulting from a previous sensitizing exposure and an immunologic mechanism. It differs from drug toxicity in a number of respects: 1) the altered reaction occurs in only a fraction of the population, 2) its dose response is unusual in that a minute amount of an otherwise safe drug elicits severe reaction, 3) the manifestations of the reaction are different from the usual pharmacologic effects of the drug, 4) there is a primary sensitizing period before the individual responds with an unusual reaction to a further exposure. A presumptive diagnosis is made by obtaining a history of a similar reaction on previous exposure to the drug that was characterized by typically "allergic symptoms," such as skin rash, hives, bronchial asthma or hematologic disturbances. Differentiation of drug toxicity in allergy is most important. When dealing with drug toxicity a simple reduction of the dose of the drug may be sufficient to eliminate the adverse effect. In case of drug allergy, reinstitution of treatment with the same drug is always hazardous and may be catastrophic.

The terms "immediate" and "delayed reactions" originated from the observations of the rapidity with which positive skin test allergens become manifest. Thus, in anaphylactic hypersensitivity, skin tests are immediate, while in the delayed state such as tuberculin hypersensitivity, it takes many hours before there is a visible change in the skin where the antigen was injected. Among the many types of drug allergies, some are considered immediate, others delayed, and still others not classified at present. Contact dermatitis is a delayed allergy. Many other cutaneous reactions and some severe hematologic disturbances elicited by drugs most likely belong in the delayed category. Serum sickness reactions are characterized by a delay in the appearance of manifestations following the initial sensitization to a drug. This same delay is observed after the first administration of a foreign serum. On the other hand, anaphylaxis, urticaria, angioneurotic edema, drug fever and asthma are categorized as immediate reactions.

Acute anaphylaxis

Anaphylaxis is an acute, potentially fatal reaction most often due to parenteral drug administration. Penicillin, iodinated contrast media, and other drugs are frequently implicated. Atopic individuals are predisposed to anaphylaxis. A negative history of an adverse reaction to a drug does not preclude the occurrence of anaphylaxis. Symptoms begin between 5 and 60 minutes after parenteral drug administration. Laryngeal edema and hypotension are most often associated with a fatal outcome. Symptoms may respond rapidly to therapy or may last for a day or more. Cutaneous and respiratory manifestations are the most common, but cardiovascular dysfunction may supervene. Skin lesions include a generalized sensation of warmth or burning, diffuse urticaria and angioedema, especially of the face and tongue. Respiratory distress results from either laryngeal edema with strider or airway obstruction from bronchospasm which leads to tightness of the chest, tachypnea, cough, wheezes and occasional rales. Hypotension leads to tachycardia, dizziness and syncope. Anoxia due to respiratory tract involvement can potentiate vascular collapse and lead to cardiac arrythmias and cardiac arrest. Other symptoms such as nausea, vomiting, abdominal cramps and diarrhea may occur. Occasionally, respiratory or cardiovascular patterns may be noted without skin lesions. Early diagnosis and treatment are mandatory to avert death which can occur within 15 minutes. Constant attention must be given to an adequate airway. Any agent known to cause anaphylaxis should be injected below the deltoid area in the arm. Emergency equipment should be available and the following measures taken, if adverse reaction occurs:

1. Aqueous epinephrine 1:1,000, 0.3 to 0.5 cc IM usually improves urticaria, bronchospasm and hypotension. Epinephrine may be repeated in 5 to 15 minutes, if necessary. If profound hypotension occurs, the aqueous epinephrine dose can be diluted in 10 ml. of saline and given slowly intravenously, but this method may precipitate cardiac arrythmias.
2. To retard absorption of an injected drug, place a tourniquet proximal to the injection site and infiltrate the area with aqueous epinephrine 1:1,000, 0.3 cc. If laryngeal edema progresses, a cricothyroidotomy or tracheostomy may be necessary since an endotracheal tube may not pass through an edematous larynx. In any event, the maintenance of an airway and respiratory assist is essential. If bronchospasm persists after epinephrine therapy then aminophylline 500 mg. should be administered slowly IV. Aminophylline may increase hypotension and should only be used in patients not responding to epinephrine.
3. Oxygen assisted ventilation is helpful. A positive pressure breathing apparatus often helps relieve bronchospasm. Prolonged hypotension may respond to intravenous administration of vasoconstrictors or intravenous fluids.
4. Antihistamines are usually administered to block further histamine binding and target cells. Diphenhydramine (benadryl) 50 mg. IM should be given early in the course of treatment.
5. Corticosteroids do not act rapidly enough to reverse acute anaphylaxis. When prolonged anaphylaxis and persistent hypotension or bronchospasm are noted, hydrocortisone succinate 100-500 mg. IV is given every six hours.
6. Cardiorespiratory arrest should be managed by CPR and assisted ventilation (See chapter 8).

Serum sickness

Serum sickness is an allergic disorder characterized by skin lesions, fever, arthralgias, and lymphadenopathy that appear 7 to 12 days after initial drug exposure, but in a shorter period of time in a sensitized person. Although the reaction was originally reported to be due to horse serum, drugs are now the most common cause, notably penicillin.

Skin lesions are the most frequent findings. Edema and urticaria at a drug injection site may be the initial manifestations. Urticaria are the most common cutaneous lesions, although morbilliform rashes occur, and rare instances of erythema nodosum, erythema multiforma and vasculitic purpura have been observed. Angioedema usually involves the face but may affect the glottis and external genitalia. Low grade fever is frequently present, except in the more severe cases where it is markedly elevated. Arthritis and arthralgias, usually migatory polyarthritis of large joints, are common. Lymphadenopathy is noted in most patients, but may be mild or restricted to the lymph nodes draining the site of drug injection.

Often there is malaise, anorexia, headache, and myalgias. Although neurologic and cardiac involvement are rare, they are potentially lethal. There may be peripheral neuritis, polyneuritis, or meningoencephalitis in a minority of patients so affected. Angina pectoris and acute myocardial infarction from involvement of the coronary arteries are rare sequelae.

Laboratory findings are sparse. A mild leukocytosis occurs with the acute illness, and occasionally an eosinophilia is noted during recovery. The urine may reveal small amounts of protein and occasionally red and white blood cells, but renal function is maintained.

The illness is self-limiting and subsides in two to three weeks. Residua or death may follow the infrequent involvement of the nervous system and heart. Treatment is mainly directed at alleviating symptoms:

1. Urticaria and angioedema are quickly alleviated by subcutaneous injection of 0.2 to 0.3 cc of aqueous epinephrine 1:1000. Epinephrine also is effective in managing glottal edema, which, however, may be severe enough to require tracheostomy. Antihistamines such as diphenhydramine hydrochloride (Benadryl), 25 to 50 mg. orally every four to six hours, provide more prolonged relief of urticaria and angioedema.
2. Fever, discomfort, and joint pains are alleviated by aspirin 300 to 600 mg. every four hours.
3. Parenteral fluids may be needed to treat dehydration.
4. In severe cases, when symptoms are not relieved by the above measures, or if there is nervous system or coronary artery involvement, corticosteroids (e.g., prednisone, 60 mg. daily) should be used.

Drug overdose

Overdosage of drugs is responsible for an increasing number of medical emergency situations. Although such poisoning in children is usually accidental, in adults it is almost invariably deliberate and usually done in an effort to commit suicide or as an impulsive gesture to attract attention, or as a means of escaping from an awkward or unpleasant environmental situation.

It is important to understand certain basic principles in the handling of any patient with suspected drug overdose. As much information as possible should be obtained from all available sources at the time the patient is first seen for suspected overdose. A careful medical history must be taken and when necessary, next of kin or a close relative should be questioned about previous psychiatric and physical illnesses and the patient's present mental state.

Second-hand information is obviously necessary if the patient's level of consciousness is impaired, but even if he is fully conscious details which he volunteers in this particular situation may be quite unreliable and certainly need to be verified. The identity of the drug or drugs taken must be established as soon as possible. The drug containers may be labeled or it may be possible to recognize the remaining tablets on sight. If any difficulty is experienced, the doctor who prescribed the drugs or pharmacist who filled the prescription should be contacted. The use of a tablet or capsule identification guide should also be available and is commonly included in the Physician's Desk Reference (PDR).

Two points must be emphasized—first, specific antidotal therapy depends upon identification of the toxic agent; failure to identify the agent may limit the effect of therapy. Second, appropriate systematic and supportive therapy should not be withheld pending confirmation of the suspected diagnosis or the identification of the agent. Treatment of drug overdoses depends on:

1. Prevention of further absorption of the toxic agent,
2. Systematic and supportive therapy and
3. Specific antidotal therapy.

Management which includes the administration of specific antidotes—emesis, gastric lavage and the use of cathartics can generally be delayed until the patient has reached a hospital facility, however, the initiation of systematic and supportive therapy is of utmost importance in outpatient practice. Such problems as hypoxia and hypotension must be attacked directly. Hypoxia may be due to central respiratory depression. When signs of central nervous system depression are evident, 100% oxygen by mask should correct the problem. Ventilation must be either assisted or performed artificially. Hypoventilation and minor degrees of airway obstruction may result in abrupt respiratory arrest. Hence, these patients require constant scrutiny. The establishment of a patent airway along with ventilatory assistance is the first step in successful support of an overdosed patient.

Narcotics

Narcotic overdose can produce depressed or absent respirations, constricted pupils, coma and cyanosis. Shock and pulmonary edema may eventually occur. Meperidine (Demerol) or propoxyphene (Darvon) overdose can cause convulsions; meperidine usually produces dilated pupils.

Treatment

The narcotic antagonist, naloxone (Narcan) will reverse apnea and coma due to heroin, morphine, codeine, meperidine, propoxyphene, methadone, pentazocine (Talwin) and related drugs. Apnea due to barbiturates or other sedative drugs will not be made worse with naloxone. An initial dose of 0.4 mg. (1 ml) can be given intravenously or intramuscularly and can be repeated in three minutes. If respirations do not improve, opiate overdose is ruled out. Manual or mechanical artificial respiration with oxygen and an airway, along with the use of gastric lavage, vasopressor drugs, plasma expanders, cardiac massage or defibrillation (if cardiac arrest ensues) are among the other measures which may be required.

Central nervous system depressants

Acute Intoxication: sleeping pills and minor tranquilizers in large amounts produce a syndrome resembling acute intoxication with alcohol. As with alcohol, overdose induces coma, hypotension and impaired respirations. The pupils may be unchanged or somewhat constricted, but certain drugs such as glutethimide (Doriden), may cause pupilary dilatation. Overdosage with benzodiazopines e.g., flurazepam (Dalmane), diazepam (Valium) or chlordiazepoxide (Librium) will rarely cause serious effects when taken alone. CNS depressants are additive or potentiating in their effects. However, when used with alcohol or in combination with other depressants, these effects may become increasingly more serious. Methaqualone (Quaalude) overdosage is marked by hyperirritability, seizures and hyperactive reflexes, including hyperactive gag reflex, which can make the placement of an oral airway or endotracheal intubation difficult.

Treatment

The vital signs must be supported. If the patient is deeply unconscious the first essential, as mentioned previously, is to establish a clear airway. This can often be achieved by removing secretions, hyperextending the head and turning the patient into a semi-prone position, inserting an oropharyngeal airway to keep the tongue from the posterior pharyngeal wall, and administering oxygen in high concentration by face mask. Depressed or diminished respiration can be assisted with a ventilatory assist bag. After an unobstructed airway has been assured, the question of gastric lavage must be considered. If the ingestion has been within six hours gastric lavage may remove some of the depressant drug to be followed by the administration of activated charcoal. Hypotension and shock require appropriate management; cardiorespiratory assistance may be necessary. No antagonist can be recommended and stimulants are contraindicated. The patient, therefore, should be transferred to a hospital facility.

Barbiturates are essentially depressants of the central nervous system. This is manifest by: 1) depression of level of consciousness ranging from drowsiness to deep coma where there is no response to maximal painful stimulation, 2) depression of the respiratory center causing a decrease in the respiratory rate and reducing the depth of respirations. Severe barbituate poisoning may cause respiratory failure, 3) depression of the activity of the vasomotor center resulting in systemic hypotension, tachycardia and diminished arterial pulse, 4) depression of temperature regulatory mechanisms causing a fall in body temperature, and 5) depression of other reflex activity such as absent pupilary, corneal or tendon reflexes. Thus, the appearance of a patient who has taken an overdose of barbiturates may vary from being drowsy, but otherwise normal, to being deeply comatose, with low body temperature, pallor, hypotension and extremely shallow respirations. Although in theory all cases of impairment of consciousness must be considered, in practice, the diagnosis of barbiturate overdose is not difficult. It can usually be made clinically by consideration of certain clinical manifestations, as well as circumstantial evidence of drug overdosage. Many cases of barbiturate intoxication recover without specific treatment.

Salicylate intoxication

The clinical features of salicylate intoxication are dizziness, excitability, tinnitus, nausea and vomiting and hyperventilation. There is usually tachycardia, and a good pulse volume. Depression of the level of consciousness is a late feature of salicylate poisoning and therefore its absence does not necessarily mean that the patient is not seriously poisoned. When unconsciousness does occur, usually a short period elapses before circulatory collapse and cardiac arrest ensue. Clinical diagnosis is relatively easy although the condition could conceivably be confused with diabetic coma, in view of the patient's rapid breathing and hyperventilation. Confirmation of the diagnosis is obtained by history, and ultimately by measuring the serum salicylate level.

Treatment

Gastric lavage is a worthwhile measure in patients who have taken an overdose of salicylates regardless of the time interval between ingestion of the drug and the time the patient is initially seen. The patient is usually conscious, so the risk of inhalation of gastric contents does not arise. Mild cases can also be treated by insuring high oral intake of fluid; but if there is clinical evidence of severe salicylasism the technique of forced diuresis should be used.

Aspirin-induced asthma

Aspirin can cause severe wheezing in up to 10% of asthmatic patients by a poorly understood non-immunologic mechanism. Affected persons usually have a family history of asthma, rhinorrhea, nasal polyps, and chronic sinusitis that antedates the onset of aspirin sensitivity. A low incidence of atopy and negative skin tests are characteristic of affected persons.

Salicylates other than aspirin do not precipitate wheezing, but sensitivity to the following structurally dissimilar drugs also exists: indomethacin (Indocin), aminopyrine, mefanamic acid (Ponstel) and tartrazina, a yellow food dye.

In a few minutes to hours after ingestion of aspirin or the other drugs listed, severe, potentially fatal bronchospasm occurs. There may be accompanying rhinorrhea, flushing, pruritus, urticaria, or hypotension.

In order to prevent this reaction, a sensitive individual should be warned against taking any precipitating drugs or over the counter preparations that may contain aspirin.

Treatment

Treatment is the same for any asthmatic attack, except that wheezing is characteristically severe and often does not respond to the usual measures but requires corticosteroid therapy. Initial measures include:

1. Aqueous epinephrine 1:1000, 0.3 to 0.5 cc subtaneously, which can be repeated in 15 minutes if necessary.
2. Aminophylline, 250 to 500 mg. IV slowly over five to ten minutes.
3. Adequate hydration, which may require intravenous administration to loosen secretions.
4. If carbon dioxide retention and respiratory acidosis occur, they should be corrected with intravenously administered sodium bicarbonate, since a normal blood pH facilitates the effectiveness of drug therapy.
5. Corticosteroids are usually employed in conjunction with the above measures. If the patient is unable to take oral medicine, hydrocortisone succinate (Solu-Cortef), 100 mg. IV should be given every six hours. If oral medicines can be taken, prednisone, 15 mg. every six hours, is recommended. The dosage of corticosteroids should be tapered over a week as the attack subsides.

Stevens-Johnson syndrome

The Stevens-Johnson syndrome is an acute, severe form of erythema multiforme with skin and mucous membrane lesions. About 35% of cases are due to drugs, the most frequently implicated being penicillin, phenolphtalein, sulfonamides, barbiturates, and hydantoin anticonvulsants. Other causes include herpes and mycoplasma infections, vaccines, deep X-ray therapy, malignancies, pregnancy and foods.

Skin lesions tend to be symmetrical and are most numerous on the extensor areas of the distal parts of arms and legs, and often involve the palms and soles. The typical lesion begins as a red spot. Small bullae may develop in the center; these then become surrounded by concentric circles of deeper color, the so-called "iris" or target lesions. Although the iris lesion is characteristic, it is not always present. Vesicular and erosive lesions frequently occur in the mouth and on the gingiva and tongue. The lips are often swollen and encrusted. Conjunctival and genital lesions are noted in most patients. Other frequent findings are fever, toxemia, myalgias, arthralgias, and less often, cough with patchy pulmonary infiltrates.

Laboratory abnormalities are few. Mild anemia occurs in severe cases; occasionally a leukocytosis, due to secondary infection, is present.

Most cases abate in two weeks but severe forms may last up to six weeks. Skin lesions heal without scarring, though blindness may result from scarring of ocular lesions. Statistics have shown there is a low mortality rate.

Treatment

1. Discontinuing all suspected drugs.
2. Corticosteroids are beneficial in severe cases. If the patient is able to swallow, prednisone in divided daily doses of 60 to 100 mg. is given until improvement occurs and the dose is then tapered. If mouth lesions prevent swallowing, hydrocortisone succinate (Solu-Cortef), 100 mg. IV every six to eight hours may be used.
3. Fluid and electrolyte imbalances can occur in patients unable to take oral sustenance. This is corrected with intravenous fluid administration.
4. Mouth care is important for oral lesions. Raw areas should be cleaned with saline soaks and then covered with glycerine, or triamcinolone acetonide in emollient dental paste (Kenalog in Orabase).
5. Patients with eye involvement require care from an ophthalmologist. Conjunctival involvement plus drying and turning in of the lashes can lead to corneal abrasion with infection and later corneal opacification and, rarely, rupture of the globe.

Local anesthetics

Most adverse reactions related to local anesthetic injection are due to either toxic overdose of the local anesthetic or to vasoconstrictors used in combination with the local anesthetic agent. The resulting plasma level following injection of a drug into tissues depends upon the vascularity of the tissue, the concentration and total quantity at the injection site, and the rapidity of absorption and buildup of the plasma level. Ultimately, all of a drug injected at a particular site passes into the blood stream. The resulting plasma level will be determined by the balance between absorption and clearance from the blood.

The ester compounds which are readily hydrolized by plasma are cleared quickly and as a general rule, are not likely to cause reactions.

The liver hydrolizes that portion of the esters that is not hydrolized by the plasma, in the case of drugs which are totally hydrolized. Some esters are less rapidly hydrolized than others. For example, tetracaine is hydrolized less rapidly by plasma than procaine. The amides undergo metabolic transformation in the liver. The plasma levels decline more slowly than the level of procaine. In cases of inadvertent overdosage, the high plasma level persists and as a consequence, the adverse reactions persist for a longer time than they do with the drugs which are hydrolized. Drugs which are not readily hydrolized are inclined to be toxic and frequently cause reactions.

There are many other factors which can account for adverse reactions to local anesthetics: the age and general medical condition of the patient, along with the presence of any pre-existing organic pathology which may impair metabolism of the drug; the emotional and mental attitude of the patient; the concentration of the drug used, as well as its route of administration and rate of injection and the concentration or dosage of the drug in relation to the size and age of the patient.

The rapid absorption of any local anesthetic into the circulation is directly related to whether or not the drug is injected intravascularly.

Drugs used for local anesthesia

The Ester Compounds

Cocaine: This was the first local anesthetic introduced and is still employed in the form of the hydrochloride acid salt. It is used in 4-10% concentrations for topical anesthesia of the mucous membranes of the nose, pharynx, larynx, trachea and bronchi. No more than 200 mg. should be applied at a time. The local vasoconstrictor property of cocaine, unequalled by other local anesthetics, is useful for decreasing bleeding and shrinking congested mucous membranes. Vasoconstriction results from an action of cocaine which prevents re-uptake of norephinephrine of nerve endings. The high incidence of toxic reactions after injection of this drug, the liability to addiction and the difficulty in preparing sterile solutions, led to a search for a synthetic compound with fewer undesirable properties.

Procaine: Procaine has certain advantages over cocaine in that although it possesses no topical action, it is useful for all other forms of local or regional anesthesia. At the beginning of the twentieth century, procaine hydrochloride was prepared as an ester of diethylaminoethanol and paraaminobenzoic acid. When procaine is injected the onset of analgesia is almost immediate. When used for infiltration the latent period is less than one minute. The duration of anesthesia varies with the site of injection. The peak effect obtained in most cases is within several minutes. The maximum dose ordinarily should not exceed one gram. The use of 0.5, 1 and 2% solutions has been universally adopted for regional block in adults; the maximum dose of 0.5% solution should not exceed 200 cc., an average dose being 150 cc. With a 1% solution, the maximum dose should not exceed 100 cc, with an average dose being 75 cc. Of a 2% solution, the maximum dose should be 50 cc, with the average dose 25 cc.

Tetracaine (Pontocaine): Tetracaine is available in crystalline form or in solution. It is 10 times as potent and 10 times as toxic as procaine. Only 1/10th the strength of procaine is required, therefore, its relative toxicity is the same as that of procaine. Its duration of action is approximately twice that of procaine. Aqueous solutions are available for nerve blocking and topical use. Tetracaine is one of the most potent of the topical local anesthetics available.

The amides

The structure of the amide local anesthetic is essentially the same as for the ester compounds, except for the amide linkage. Because of the amide, these compounds are less readily metabolized and the liability of adverse reactions is greater. On the other hand, some have significant anti-arrhythmic affects on the heart.

Lidocaine (Xylocaine): Lidocaine is a potent local anesthetic which produces prompt, intense and extensive anesthesia, being far more effective than procaine. The drug is detoxified in the liver and is conjugated to a certain extent by the liver and excreted into the urine. Lidocaine lacks the vasoconstrictive property of cocaine, but is compatible with epinephrine, with which it must be combined in order to delay absorption. The ability to diffuse and penetrate tissues is much greater with lidocaine than with any of the other local anesthetics currently in use. Its major advantages are the more rapid onset of anesthesia and the freedom from local irritation. Lidocaine causes certain unusual systemic reactions not observed from other drugs. It often causes general drowsiness, lassitude and at times amnesia when it is used without epinephrine. The systemic effects due to high plasma levels are similar to those of procaine. Hypotension, pallor, sweating, nausea and vomiting, twitching and convulsions can occur, as may cardiac depression. The total dose injected should not exceed 500 mg. Since lidocaine is effec-

Table 10-1 Number of dental cartridges permissible based on MG dosage

%Solution	Mg/ml	Mg/Cartridges (1.8cc)	Number of cartridges permissible		
1	10	18	Lidocaine	Mepivacaine	Prilocaine
2	20	36	2%	3%	4%
3	30	54	8–13 cartridges	5 cartridges	8 cartridges
4	40	72	(Toxic Dose = 300–500 mg)	(Toxic Dose = 180–270 mg)	(Toxic Dose = 600 mg)

tive in low concentrations of small volume, dosages in excess of 500 mg. are never warranted. A 1.8 cc. dental local anesthetic carpule contains 36 mg. of lidocaine (Table 10-1). Lidocaine is an excellent substitute for procaine when allergic reactions to the latter have occurred.

Mepivacaine (Carbocaine): Mepivacaine is chemically allied to lidocaine, being an amide of similar configuration. Pharmacologically it possesses the same attributes as lidocaine. The drug is approximately twice as potent and twice as toxic as procaine and produces prompt and extensive anesthesia. It, too, undergoes bio-degradation in the liver by oxidation and demetholation. Mepivacaine appears to induce a longer duration of action than lidocaine. It is also alleged to manifest local vasoconstrictor effects on its own, differing in this regard from a majority of local anesthetics. It has a somewhat decreased ability to diffuse through the tissues when compared to lidocaine. The systemic reactions observed with mepivacaine are similar to those occuring with other local anesthetics. General drowsiness, lassitude and amnesia observed with lidocaine are not, however, observed with mepivacaine. The total dose should not exceed 270 mgm of a 3% solution or 180 mgm, if vasoconstrictor is added (Table 10-1).

Prilocaine (Citanest): Prilocaine is chemically allied to lidocaine and mepivacaine. It has one methyl group attached to the benzine ring instead of two. There is little demonstrable difference in effectiveness between 1 and 2% solutions of prilocaine and similar concentrations of lidocaine or mepivacaine. Toxic manifestations are similar to those of other local anesthetics. Convulsions and cardiac depression occur as they do with procaine and lidocaine. The impression, however, is that systemic toxicity is less, on a weight for weight basis, than with lidocaine and mepivacaine. Methemoglobinemia may occur after the use of a total of 0.05 gr. or more, even in the robust individual. Clinical reports indicate that it is longer lasting than lidocaine, but at higher concentrations. Epinephrine prolongs the action even more. A 2% solution of prilocaine is approximately equivalent to a 1% solution of lidocaine and mepivacaine. The maximum dose should not exceed 600 mgm at any one time of the usual 4% solution (Table 10-1).

Bupivacaine (Marcaine): Bupivacaine hydrochloride is a compound which differs from mepivacaine in that a butyl group is substituted for a methyl in the molecule. It is most potent, with a markedly longer duration of action, than lidocaine and mepivacaine, probably due to increased tissue protein binding. Epinephrine in concentrations usually of 1:200,000 is added to the solution when indicated. The total amount of the drug injected at any one time should not exceed 200-500 mg. since its toxicity approximates that of tetracaine. While onset of anesthesia may be slower than with lidocaine or mepivacaine, the duration is two to three times longer. Upon repeated injection, it accumulates in the blood stream, with arterial concentrations 20-40% higher than venous concentrations.

Prevention and treatment of adverse reactions to local anesthetic drugs

The management of any local anesthetic overdose is directly related to the severity of the reaction which results. In many cases the reaction may be mild and last for a short period of time, requiring virtually no treatment. Local support, with establishment of an airway and the administration of oxygen by face mask, usually is sufficient until the reaction terminates.

Local anesthetic reactions are generally characterized by two phases—an excitatory phase and a depressive phase. (These phases can occur independently, or the depressive phase can follow excitation which will thus require concurrent treatment of both phases.) Systemic manifestations of local anesthetics differ markedly from local effects in their direct action on the central nervous system, respiratory and cardiovascular systems. The actual concentration required locally, to stabilize the membrane of a nerve fiber and produce blockade, is several times greater than the concentration in the blood that is necessary to produce unwanted or hazardous systemic effects. Exceedingly high plasma levels of local anesthetics can cause systemic effects which may be fatal.

At first, high circulating plasma levels precipitate excitation of the central nervous system. This is manifested primarily by cortical stimulation. Apprehension, excitement, and disorientation are usual symptoms. Nausea and vomiting may occur but are rare. These symptoms vary with the rate of uptake. If the plasma level rises slowly, reaches a peak and then falls, the symptoms subside. If a constant level is maintained the symptoms persist. As the blood level increases and the cells are profused with more of the drug, twitching of small muscles appears, which progressively increases in intensity. These then merge into generalized convulsions. It is strongly emphasized that the plasma level capable of causing these symptoms is only a fraction of the concentration necessary to block a nerve fiber. If the plasma level rises excessively, the excitation subsides and depression of the central nervous system then follows. These drugs, therefore, follow a general pharmacologic pattern: that any drug which stimulates an organ eventually depresses that system if given in excess. Coma and respiratory failure are usual manifestations of a depressed nervous system.

The other system adversely affected is the cardiovascular system. High plasma levels of local anesthetics directly depress the myocardium and reduce myocardial contractability. They also depress the conduction system producing an antiarrythmic affect. Slow intravenous influsions have been used for this purpose in therapy for ventricular arrythmias. As an additional complication, local anesthetics may cause dilatation of the vascular bed and may further aggravate the circulatory effects. In either case, hypotension ensues, accompanied by bradycardia, and a shock-like state develops, which requires institution of immediate treatment. The reaction can terminate fatally if there is any delay in treatment. Both the central nervous system and cardiovascular effects are untoward and often unanticipated. Hence, one cannot be too cautious in the administration of any local anesthetic drug. Inasmuch as reactions resulting from local anesthetics are severe, it is prudent to take all precautions possible to avoid these reactions. The following are fundamental principles to be observed:

1. Use the smallest volume of a dilute solution which is effective. No more than eight dental carpules of any local anesthetic should be used at any time.
2. The use of a vasoconstrictor to retard absorption may be extremely effective. Untoward effects of these drugs can occur and will be discussed in the next section.
3. Keep a mental record of the total dose or volume of solution used. Many operators inject ad lib and are often unaware of the acceptable limits.
4. Allow sufficient time for absorption before re-injection.
5. Always aspirate in several planes before injecting solution, particularly intraorally, in areas around the facial bones, or any highly vascular tissue.
6. Allow sufficient time for the drug to take effect. Important point to remember—if excessive blocks have been performed then the doctor should observe the patient closely and record vital signs of respiration, pulse and blood pressure which may harbinger a potential adverse reaction.

Treatment

Treatment of reactions to local anesthetics is based on symptoms. The majority of reactions, as previously stated, are due to high plasma levels and overdosage. Convulsions, respiratory failure, hypotension and cardiac arrest are extreme manifestations of systemic toxicity and are rare; however, one should be prepared to treat all these symptoms:

1. Respiratory Support—when using local anesthetics, doctors should be prepared to artificially assist respiration using oxygen or air, with high inspired oxygen concentrations, if pure oxygen is not available. As the patient begins the excitation phase, he should be reassured and placed in the Trendelenburg position. A face mask with an Ambu assist bag should be placed, for administration of oxygen. This permits inflation of the lungs in the apneic patient. If the doctor is unprepared to cope with respiratory failure, then mouth-to-mouth resuscitation must be instituted.

2. Convulsions from local anesthetics are usually transitory, particularly when drugs are rapidly hydrolized by plasma esters, e.g., procaine. Convulsions may persist, however, when drugs are used which are not as rapidly detoxified, e.g., lidocaine.
   The convulsions in and of themselves are not the most serious aspect of the reaction, but merely portend the most ominous sequelae which occur when there is further systemic response to high plasma levels. The cardiovascular effects, and respiratory depression due to impaired ventilation from the convulsions can cause death. For this reason, the convulsion should be treated. Diazepam (Valium) has been shown to be highly effective in the therapy of local anesthetic toxic convulsions, as well as generalized convulsions from other sources. Slow injection of 10-15 mgs in the average adult, intravenously, will be adequate therapy for such convulsive disorders. Ultra-short-acting barbiturates, such as thiopental (Pentothal) and methohexatol (Brevital) have also been used for treatment of these convulsive disorders, because of their relatively short latent period and rapidity of action. Barbiturates, however, like other central nervous system depressants, can depress heart muscle when used in excessive quantities. The possible additive effects on the myocardium of the barbiturates, coupled with local anesthetics, must not be overlooked.

3. Cardiovascular manifestations of local anesthetic toxic overdose should be treated, based on symptoms. Bradycardia is treated with atropine in doses of 1 mgm intravenously. Hypotension is corrected by the use of vasoconstrictors which act directly on the heart muscle and the vascular bed. Ephedrine is a myocardial stimulant as well as a vasoconstrictor, which is given intravenously in small increments of 15 or 20 mg. until the blood pressure is restored to the desired level. Asystole or failure to obtain a palpable pulse should be treated promptly by external cardiac compression and CPR.

Vasoconstrictors in local anesthetic solutions

Vasoconstrictors are an integral part of most local anesthetic solutions used in dentistry. There are certain advantages to their use in local or regional anesthesia. Vasoconstrictors cause a retardation of local anesthetic absorption, thereby reducing toxicity and increasing duration. This, therefore, increases the overall efficiency of the local anesthetic solution and permits smaller volumes of the anesthetic to be used. Toxic reactions to these drugs occur primarily when an intravascular injection occurs and when the volume of the drug given is at toxic or near toxic levels. The concentration can be varied to give the anesthetic agent a greater range of usefulness, for optimum patient satisfaction and treatment result.

The vasopressor drugs are adrenergic and act directly upon affector cells. Their constricting effects are their only action when used in therapeutic doses. In extremely small amounts, organ systems should not be markedly affected. On the other hand, increased volumes and concentrations, with inadvertent intravascular injections, may produce toxic manifestations which are: tachycardia, hypertension, palpation, headache, tremors and pallor. These drugs exhibit both excitatory and inhibitory activity and may produce vasodilation and vasoconstriction, depending upon existing conditions.

The overall dosages of vasoconstrictors should be carefully computed. It should be kept in mind that with additional injections the vasoconstrictor volume is increased, until systemic manifestations may be exhibited. Furthermore, the endogoneous adrenalin released under the stress or excitement of the procedure is a factor to be considered.

Epinephrine (Adrenalin): Epinephrine is available from the synthetic as well as the natural source and there is very little, if any, difference in their actions. Epinephrine is an alkaloid secreted by the adrenal medulla and it is important in the use of steroids in the maintenance of body function, especially in the stress state. Its effect on the cardiovascular system is complex, with the response in individual patients varying greatly. It is even possible for some patients to develop tolerance to the drug.

Epinephrine is the most potent and efficient of the vasoconstrictor drugs used in anesthetic solutions. Concentrations of from 1:50,000 to 1:200,000 are commonly used; concentrations greater than 1:50,000 are usually unnecessary. Epinephrine in the concentration used in dental practice exhibits extremely low systemic toxicity. The most minute amount of the drug, particularly in susceptible individuals, may give rise to exaggerated side-effects, such as, 1) marked elevations in blood pressure, 2) tachycardia, 3) cardiac arrythmias, 4) severe headache and 5) light-headedness and dizziness. The severity of the effects of the drug depends upon the dosage and the method of administration. Epinephrine stimulates the heart by direct action upon the myocardium, increasing the cardiac rate and output. Epinephrine should not be used in the hyperthyroid patient; these patients are particularly susceptible to the drug. The action of epinephrine is of short duration and it is relatively unstable, being

Table 10-2 Number of dental cartridges permissable when epinephrine is utilized

Drug	Dilution	Mg/1.8 ml cartridge	Number of cartridges in non-cardiac patients (maximum 0.2 mg)
Epinephrine	1:1000 (used therapeutically)		
Epinephrine	1:10,000 (used therapeutically)		
Epinephrine	1:50,000	0.036	5
Epinephrine	1:100,000	0.018	10
Epinephrine	1:200.000	0.009	20

destroyed by oxidation rather than by any specific enzyme. The vasoconstricting effect of this drug which slows its absorption and its short duration are factors in reducing its overall systemic toxicity.

Dosage: It should be noted that 0.3 mg. to 0.5 mg. is the therapeutic dose for epinephrine when used for such conditions as acute bronchial asthma, and anaphylaxis. This dosage should be used with caution in patients with pre-existing hypertension, generalized cardiovascular, or arteriosclerotic heart disease since the direct systemic effects previously noted are often seen in therapeutic dosage. A solution containing 1:50,000 epinephrine is equivalent to 200ths of a milligram per ml. 10 ml of the solutions therefore will contain approximately 0.2 mg. and will approximate the therapeutic dose. This amounts to approximately five local anesthetic carpules. A solution containing 1:100,000 epinephrine is equivalent to 100th ml. per milliliter, so this concentration permits 20 ml. or approximately 11 local anesthetic carpules in order to reach the 0.2 mg. maximum dosage (Table 10-2). It would be safe to assume that any dosage less than 0.2 mg. could be used in patients without pre-existing cardiovascular disease. It should be used with caution in others. It is interesting to note that gingival retraction cord is responsible for the achievement of much higher levels of epinephrine than local anesthetics and are contraindicated in patients with cardiovascular disease.

Levonordefrin (Neo-Cobefrin): Neo-cobefrin is one of the newer vasoconstrictors used in dental anesthesia. The dextroisomer is essentially inert as most of the biologic activity of nordefrin resides in the levoisomer. Levonordefrin is approximately one-half as active in pressor activity as epinephrine, being used in 1:20,000 concentrations. The compound is readily soluble in acid and practically insoluble in distilled water or common organic solids. It should be remembered, however, that there is a great difference in activity of many of the vasopressor drugs. The systemic toxicity of neo-cobefrin is well within usable ranges with a 1:20,000 concentration per ml being commonly employed.
Remember that toxic reactions can be caused by any of the drugs commonly used as vasoconstrictors in local anesthetics. These reactions are manifested by palpations, headaches, tremors, restlessness and hypertension with tachycardia, or in some cases, bradycardia. The toxic manifestations may in some respect resemble those experienced with the local anesthet-

ic itself. One of the main points of differences with vasoconstrictors is restlessness and apprehension displaying cortical stimulations usually followed by palpation, tremors and perhaps headache. With the local anesthetic solutions, the first toxic manifestations are cortical stimulation exhibited by restlessness, talkativeness and apprehension. Fortunately, the treatment for both is similar.

Treatment

In most instances epinephrine and neocobefrin overdose reactions are of short duration and little or no management is required aside from reassuring the patient. It is important that the conscious patient be placed in a comfortable position and in the absence of hypotension, the semi-fowler (semi sitting) position, or 45° upright position is satisfactory. The patient should be reassured to decrease the patient's anxiety and restlessness. Vital signs should be monitored and oxygen administered. These signs, such as blood pressure and heart rate should be recorded every 3 to 5 minutes. Rather large elevations can be initially recorded, but these seem to return to normal baseline levels over a short period of time, usually within 5 to 10 minutes.

References

1. Adatia, A.K. "Intravascular Injection of Local Anesthetics." *Br. Dent. J.* 138:328. 1975.
2. American Medical Association, Council on Drugs. "The Misuse of Pentazocine: Its Dependence Producing Potential." *J.A.M.A.* 209:1518. 1969.
3. Beeson, P.B. and McDermott, W. Eds. *Textbook of Medicine,* Ed. 14. Philadelphia: Saunders, 1975.
4. Broughton, P.M.G., Higgins, G. and O'Brien, J.R.P. *Acute Barbiturate Poisoning.* Lancet 270:180, 1956.
5. Conn, H.F. and Conn. R.B. Eds. *Current Diagnosis 5.* Philadelphia: Saunders, 1977.
6. Crampton, R.S. and Oriscello, R.G. "Petit and Grand Mal Convulsions During Lidocaine Hydrochloride Treatment of Ventricular Tachycardia." *J.A.M.A.* 204:201. 1968.
7. Eckenhoff, J.E. and Oech, S.R. "The Effects of Narcotics and Antagonists Upon Respiration and Circulation in Man." *Clin. Pharmacol. Ther.* 1:483. 1960.
8. Foldes, F.F., Molloy, R., McNall, P.G. and others. "Comparison of Toxicity of Intravenously Given Local Anesthetic Agents in Man." *J.A.M.A.* 172:1493. 1960.
9. Girwood, R.H. "Death After Taking Medicaments." *Br. Med. J.* 1:501. 1974.
10. Hadden, J., Harris, R.S., Katz, R.I. and others. "Acute Barbiturate Intoxication and Concepts of Management." *J.A.M.A.* 209:893. 1969.
11. Hendler, B.H. and Rose, L.F. "Common Medical Emergencies: A Dilemma in Dental Evaluation." *J. Am. Dent. Assoc.* 91:575-582. 1975.
12. Irey, N.S. "Adverse Drug Reactions and Death." *J.A.M.A.* 236:575. 1976.
13. Kelly, J.F. and Patterson, R. "Anaphylaxis." *J.A.M.A.* 227:1431. 1974.
14. Klein, S.W., Sutherland, R.I.L. and Morch, J.E. "Hemodynamic Effects of Intravenous Lidocaine in Man." *Can. Med. Assoc. J.* 99:472. 1968.
15. Kramer, H.S. and Mitton, V.A. "Complications of Local Anesthesia." *Dent. Clin. North Am.* 17:443. 1973.
16. Malamed, Stanley, F. *Handbook of Medical Emergencies in the Dental Office.* St. Louis: Mosby, 1978.
17. McCarthy, F.M. *Emergencies in Dental Practice,* Ed. 2. Philadelphia: Saunders, 1972.
18. *Merck Manual of Diagnosis and Therapy,* Ed. 11, West Point, Pa.: Merck, Sharp and Dohme Research Laboratories, 1966.
19. Rose, L.F. *Diagnosis and Management of Medical Emergencies in the Dental Office, Continuing Education Manual.* University of Pa.: School of Dental Medicine, vol. 1, no. 3, 1977.
20. Salvaggio, J. and Crane, E. "Severe Allergic Reaction After Ingestion of Acetylsalicylic Acid Compounds." *J. La. State Med. Soc.* 113:292. 1961.
21. Schiano, A.M. and Strambi, R.C. "Frequency of Accidental Intravascular Injection of Local Anesthetic in Dental Practice." *Oral Surg.* 17:178. 1964.
22. Speer, F. "Aspirin Allergy: A Clinical Study." *South. Med. J.* 68:314. 1975.
23. Stetler, C.J. "Drug-Induced Illness." *J.A.M.A.* 229:1403. 1974.
24. Verrill, P.J. "Adverse Reactions to Local Anesthetics and Vasoconstrictor Drugs." *Practitioner* 214:380. 1975.

Chapter 11

Office Emergency Protocol

B. Kyle DeMartino, D.D.S., F.A.D.S.A. and Barbara J. Steinberg, D.D.S.

The ability of the individual dental practitioner to successfully manage a patient experiencing a catastrophic event is at present not easily estimated. There are few if any profession-wide standards; with the exception of voluntary peer evaluation by oral surgeons who employ general anesthesia. To date little has been done to provide convenient and understandable emergency protocol guidelines for the office.

Unfortunately, though numerous articles have been written that explore dental emergency management, the academic journals have as yet failed to appreciate the need for a *simplified* and holistic approach to the difficult task of advising the profession regarding available equipment, staff education and practical emergency pharmacology.

The following chapter is structured so that the interested practitioner may equip himself and his staff with sufficient information and hardware to develop an emergency management regimen. The state of "emergency" will be defined and causes explored. Various emergency management products (kits) will be discussed and a list of medications—their principal effects and side-effects, dosages and routes of administration—will be presented. Finally, an office-evaluation questionnaire will be presented.

It has been the authors' experience that the average dental practitioner tends to equate the term "emergency" with catastrophic events such as cardiac arrest rather than to recognize it as encompassing a spectrum of events ranging from the relatively benign (i.e. dizziness) to the extremely serious (i.e. unconsciousness and sudden death). So-called syncope is often accepted as a more or less normal, if unusual, dental office event; whereas, our medical colleagues might view this transient loss of consciousness as a potentially serious symptom until proven otherwise.

When one accepts the broader interpretation of the word, (accepting the premise that *any* deviation from the patient's normal state may be a symptom of serious consequence) it becomes relatively simple to devise a program that can maintain life until the patient is turned over to the appropriate medical personnel.

Emergency management

Within the context of the dental office, emergency management will be acute in nature designed to support life until the patient is transferred to a medical center or hospital. Because of this single fact the dentist may view emergency management from the vantage point of being geared to support of the cardiovascular and respiratory systems. All other chronic components of the emergency event will be deferred for ultimate treatment by the physician(s) responsible for the patient's long-term management.

The definition of what should be considered an "emergency" is fairly simple: The rapid onset of alterations in the patient's condition that, if unchecked, could lead to collapse and death. Interestingly, the actual cause of the event is not of prime importance in the acute phase of treatment and therefore being prepared becomes a situation in which we must have consummate mastery of certain physical skills (i.e. cardiopulmonary resuscitation) and knowledge of emergency pharmacology. Additionally, one must be capable of recognizing shifts from so-called normal that are signals.

As stated above the actual initiating cause of an emergency event is of less importance than one might assume. What *is* of importance is the physiologic cause of the symptoms by which we may recognize impending disaster—by this we mean, for example, that loss of consciousness is probably related to inadequate perfusion of the brain with oxygenated blood. If it is determined that the brain is not being properly oxygenated (and as stated unconsciousness strongly suggests exactly this situation) then steps must be taken immediately to rectify this. Two systems are implicated, the cardiovascular system and the respiratory system. In acute management *all* of our efforts will be concentrated in efforts to restore the integrity of these two systems.

Recognition

It goes without saying that if one fails to recognize that the patient is in distress very little will be done until conditions deteriorate, possibly to the point of hopelessness. Therefore, it becomes important that one be acutely sensitive to the patient's total condition during his time in the office. With the increasing popularity of inhalation analgesia, supine operating position and extensive draping the dentist is substantially removed from the patient and his attention is focused on the operating field. Rather than ignoring the patient's totality it must become the reponsibility of someone in the operating team to stay in touch with the patient's physical condition and monitor his moment-to-moment status so that any untoward event may be identitied as rapidly as possible and corrected (See chapter 2). This sort of rapport will frequently help one to abort "emergency" circumstances before they progress beyond being a minor event.

As a first step in preparing oneself and one's staff to handle emergencies, certification in Cardio-Pulmonary Resuscitation is essential.

As a second preparatory step, members of the operating team should be able to identify the outward signs that often accompany impending emergencies so they may be brought to the attention of the dentist.

Signs to watch for include:

1. Rapid or slow respiratory rate—more than 20 or less than 10 breaths per minute,
2. Rapid or slow pulse—generally speaking if the patient normally has a pulse of 72 then increases beyond 120 and decreases below 55 might warrant attention,
3. Hyper or hypotension—shifts in blood pressure greater than 25% may be symptomatic of impending problems,
4. Dyspnea—labored or difficult breathing, shortness of breath,
5. Wheezing,
6. Crowing—an audible, high-pitched sound of partial airway obstruction,
7. Diaphoresis—profuse sweating, wet clammy skin,
8. Pallor—pale, white or gray complexion,
9. Cyanosis—a blue color of lips, nail beds, tongue—rather than the usual pink,
10. Rash, flush or swelling,
11. Edema—swelling of the extremities or in the laryngeal area,
12. Unexplained pain—particularly in the chest or
13. Agitation or tremors.

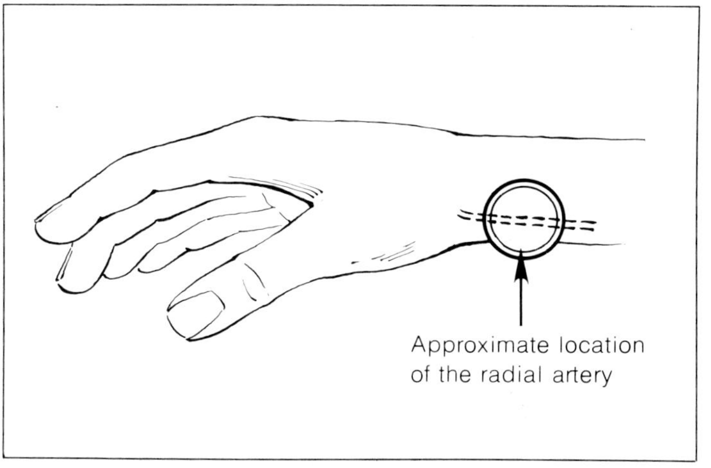

Fig. 11-1 Wrist showing location of pulse.

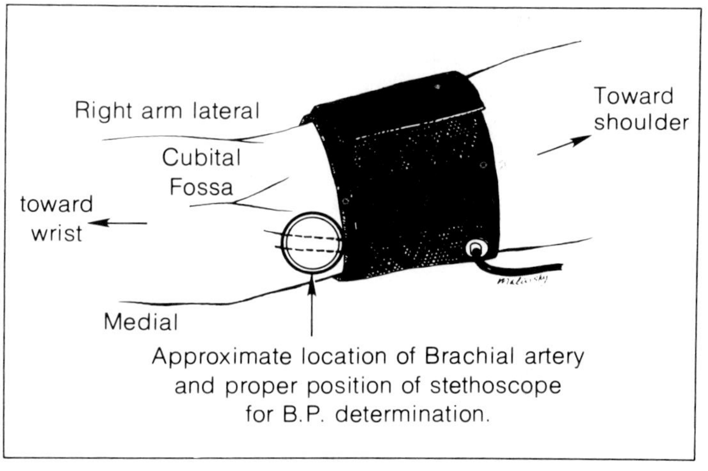

Fig. 11-2 Blood pressure cuff and location of brachial artery.

Obviously, there may be other indications that all is not right with a particular patient and an astute dental auxiliary may sense difficulty before any of the above occurs; however, as a training list the preceeding covers the major symptoms of mild to serious respiratory and cardiovascular emergencies.

In addition to being able to recognize outward physical changes, all members of the operating team should be taught to palpate and count the pulse and to place and use a blood pressure cuff (See chapter 1). The most convenient pulse point for routine evaluations is at the wrist and it is a good practice to encourage the auxiliary staff to routinely take a pulse until they are completely comfortable doing this simple procedure (Fig. 11-1).

Blood pressure determinations are equally simple once one learns the proper placement of the cuff and stethoscope. (The semi-automated electronic blood pressure cuffs are *not* recommended for the inexperienced, as they tend to complicate situations when they fail to function.) Placement of the cuff should be above the elbow and snugly wrapped. The stethoscope should be above the cubital fossa and medial. This places it over the brachial artery which can

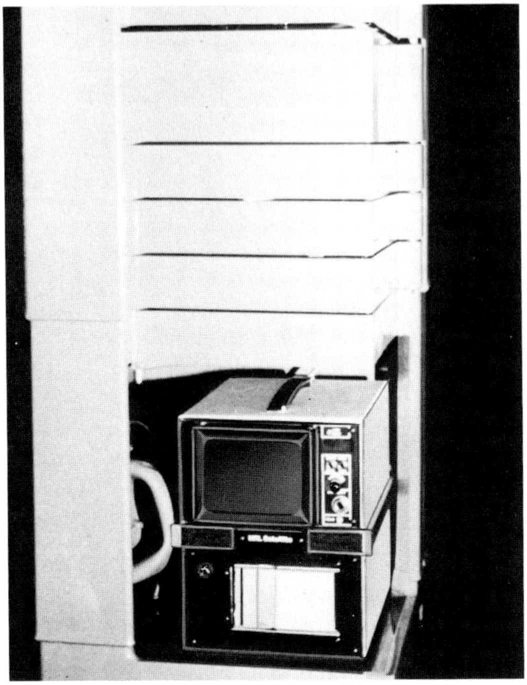

Fig. 11-3 Ideal dental emergency cart.

be located by palpation of the pulse prior to placement of the cuff (Fig. 11-2).

Routine vital sign determination (pulse and blood pressure) is a wise addition to office procedures both as a screening measure and as a teaching tool for the auxiliary staff. The last place one wants to be teaching is during an actual emergency.

The third step in proper preparation of the office and staff for emergency procedures would be the acquisition of sufficient equipment either in kit form or as individual items. A general criticism of the kit approach is that far too many dentists tend to rely on the mere possession of a "kit" as a talisman against disaster, and never actually go through the items contained in the kit to evaluate whether there is enough medication and appropriate equipment. Another problem is that kits often are relegated to a back space in a closet and for one reason or another the medications are not kept up to date.

We think the very best way of equipping oneself is to construct an emergency cart from scratch. Use one of the inexpensive plastic dental cabinet-carts, and then equip it with medications, monitoring instruments, airway management equipment, intravenous fluids, administration sets and so forth. Fig. 11-3 shows an ideal emergency cart for the dental office fully equipped, including an electrocardiograph. This particular emergency cart is used by a dental anesthesiologist and is the most sophisticated we have been able to locate. For the average dental office it is not necessary to have large quantities of medications in this unit; however, a complete kit will contain virtually everything in the one pictured but in smaller quantities.

When either purchasing or building an emergency kit, one should have an idea of what would be included in the way of equipment and medications in the "ideal" example. This will enable the dentist to select one of the kits discussed later in the chapter that best fits the individual needs of his office, or to augment one of the more basic kits with separately purchased items.

Resuscitation Equipment:
- Positive pressure manual resuscitator—such as an Ambu bag
- An emergency oxygen source and equipment for delivering oxygen under pressure
- Adult and child size masks

Airway Equipment:
- Laryngoscope with light source
- Oropharyngeal airways
- Nasal airways
- Endotracheal tubes (three sizes)
- Stylet

Monitoring Equipment:
- Sphygmomanometer
- Stethoscope

Additional Hardware:
- IV solutions (Dextrose 5% and water)
- IV administration sets
- Intravenous catheters
  - Scalpel
  - Scissors
  - Alcohol sponges
  - Tape
  - Tourniquet
  - Hemostats
- Magill Forceps (a special forcep that can reach to the larynx)
- Syringes (an assortment) 3cc, 5cc, 10cc, 20cc
- Needles (18 gauge)
- Tonsilar suction tips

Prevention of drug effects

The opportunity to prevent a given emergency situation from becoming irreversible often depends upon the ability to administer not only appropriate supportive therapy in the form of cardiopulmonary resuscitation but also the wise selection and rapid administration of pharmaceuticals. Obviously, a good emergency set-up will include a comprehensive array of drugs. The following is a list of medications which will provide the dentist with a nucleus to which may be added other drugs at the discretion of the individual. Also noted are the major effects and side-effects and the route of administration for each drug.

Amyl Nitrite: a potent vasodilator which relaxes the coronary vessels and has specific application in angina pectoris. Packed in vaporules it is snapped in the fingers and wafted under the patient's nose until inhaled—it is very rapidly absorbed from the lungs and relief from anginal pain is rapid. Side effects include transient dizziness, weakness, a flush to the skin, a pulsating headache and decreases in systemic blood pressure.

Aminophylline: Available as an intravenous solution, oral tablet or suppositories, this drug is usually most efficacious in the intravenous form and will effect bronchial smooth muscle. It is a potent bronchial relaxant and has application for the patient suffering from asthma. Usually given in a drip (250 mg diluted in 250cc of sterile water) it may also stimulate the heart. Side effects include headache, dizziness, palpitations or nausea.

Atropine: Given intravenously to allow the heart to return to a more rapid rate by blocking the effects of the vagus nerve. Dosage ranges from 0.2 mg to 1.0 mg. Side effects include dryness of the mouth and a reduction of secretions.

Benadryl: An antihistamine, this drug is highly effective in treating the systemic effects associated with histamine release. It is included for the specific purpose of halting the classic symptoms associated with allergic reactions (rash, hives, etc.) It is given intravenously or intramuscularly, generally in doses of 25 to 50 mg. Side-effects include drowsiness, dizziness, nervousness and nausea, but they are generally mild.

Calcium Gluconate: Much lower in calcium content than Calcium Chloride, this preparation is also less irritating. It is used as is the chloride preparation but onset is slower. It has been said that calcium and the cardiac glycosides (such as digitalis) may have similar effects on cardiac muscle and in circumstances of cardiac arrest one might consider administering 250 mg, slowly, in an attempt to augment contractility.

Demerol: A potent narcotic analgesic, this preparation can be administered either intravenously or intramuscularly. The significant side-effects include respiratory depression or arrest. Dosage is 50 to 100 mg when given intramuscularly or 20 mg if given intravenously.

Epinephrine: Generally considered the most potent of the class of drugs known as catacholamines, this drug has a host of applications. It will increase contractility of the heart, heart rate, and blood pressure as well as dilate the bronchioles in asthmatic states and will help reverse allergic manifestations. It may be given intravenously, intramuscularly, subcutaneously, by inhalation or intracardiac although each route is not effective for all problems. Dosage ranges from 0.1 mg to 1.0 mg.

Ephedrine Sulfate: Less potent than epinephrine this is a good first line drug for use in hypotensive states. It will increase blood pressure and enhance contractility of the heart without increasing the rate. Dosage is 25 to 50 mg intravenously or intramuscularly.

Naloxone: This drug has the trade name Narcan. It is the drug of choice for reversing narcotic overdose. Dosage is 0.4 mg intravenously or intramuscularly. Results are highly predictable and very dramatic. It does not contribute depressant effects of its own.

Nitroglycerine: This drug is virtually standard therapy for patients suffering from angina pectoris. Highly effective and rapidly absorbed from the oral mucosa, it is given under the tongue in tablet form to abort an attack of angina.

Steroids: Adrenocorticosteroids are complex substances synthesized from cholesterol by the adrenal glands. They are responsible for many diverse physiological functions. In an emergency situation their application can very generally be described as being associated with ameliorating the disastrous effects of a near death state including cerebral edema. Given in single administration dosage depends upon the specific product selected. Solucortef and/or Solu medrol may be given in dose ranges of 15 to 30 mg per Kg intravenously. This quantity is usually from 1 to 3 grams for the adult.

Sodium Bicarbonate: In serious cardiovascular crises the waste products of metabolism are not eliminated through the usual mechanisms and acidosis becomes a prominent feature in the problem of resuscitating the patient. In order to maintain an acid-base balance compatible with life, exogenous bicarbonate is given to neutralize the acidosis present. Dosage in cardiac arrest is usually 1 meg/Kg or 50 to 100 milliequivalents given intravenously; and another 50 milliequivalents given at ten minute intervals until spontaneous cardiac activity is reestablished.

Valium: Used for the management of convulsions and seizure states, the dosage range depends upon individual response and is given in small increments of 2.5 mg intravenously until the seizure stops. Side effects include drowsiness, amnesia and unconsciousness.

Xylocaine: Lidocaine has a specific application in the control of cardiac arrythmias. The drug helps to soothe an irritable heart muscle and helps avoid the progression from an occasional ventricular premature beat to more complex and dangerous ventricular arrhythmias. Administration is by bolus; dose is 50 mg if given intravenously. Side-effects include bradycardia and convulsions, both of which are treatable.

Additional drugs may be available in commercially available kits or the dentist may wish to have alternate preparations. Whatever the situation he must have a thorough working knowledge of all drugs to be used in a given medical emergency. There is no solution to the need for each dentist to familiarize himself with the pharmacology of the drugs in his emergency kit other than re-reading the description of the major actions of each drug in the kit at periodic intervals.
Additionally, he or she must also be knowledgable in administering parenteral injections and starting an IV line. It is usually possible to arrange to gain experience in venipuncture at local community hospitals in the medical laboratory.

Venipuncture techniques

The successful orchestration of an office medical emergency may depend upon the ability to quickly achieve intravenous access. Regrettably there is no way to teach venipuncture technique from the printed page. However, there are guidelines that can be extremely helpful to the beginner. Ultimately, only practice will enable one to overcome ineptitude and fear.
The recommended equipment for starting an IV line includes the following:

1. A bottle of sterile solution. 250 cc of dextrose 5% in water is convenient. Saline or one of the other salt solutions such as Lactated Ringer's is acceptable though the salt solutions can under some circumstances complicate the event.
2. An administration set. This, of course, is the plastic tubing through which the solution will travel. Tubings come in all sorts of configurations, but one suitable for emergencies can be of sufficient length (48 inches or longer); it will have one or more injection ports—these are the locations on the tubing where drugs may be injected into the line; it must be compatible with the fluid container—this refers to the fact that some administration sets will not function with different brand fluid containers (Travenol sets do not work with Abbott bottles); and it should be sterile.
3. A catheter of appropriate size. One of 18 gauge is probably the smallest catheter through which one can expect to move significant volumes of drug or fluids; additionally it is somewhat less difficult to insert than the larger bore units. Conventional metal needles are not recommended because of difficulties associated with avoiding infiltration of the vein under the stress of emergency conditions. The flexible plastic catheter is much less likely to fail once it is in place.
4. A tourniquet. The simplest to use is one of the heavy gauge rubber types with a Velcro insert, however, a piece of rubber drain tube or similar item will work.
5. Alcohol sponges for cleansing the skin.
6. Tape for securing the catheter and line, once they are in place.

The technique of locating a suitable vein requires secure placement of the tourniquet medial to the area where one wished to place the catheter. It should be tight enough to allow the entry of blood into the limb but restrict its return to the central circulation. Then one attempts to locate a vessel large enough to accept the catheter. It should be easily palpated and preferably seen as well. A good simulation can be prepared by taking several lengths of rubber tubing and inserting them into a feather pillow, then attempting to feel for them through the substance of the pillow itself.
When the vein has been selected, the area is cleansed with antiseptic and traction is placed on the skin distal to the planned point of entry. This helps immobilize the

vein, puts the skin under tension which makes insertion of the catheter easier, and generally gives the operator greater control. The catheter is grasped in the opposite hand in such as way as to brace all parts of the device and insure the integrity of the catheter itself (which is the outer layer) and the introducer (which is the metal needle-like inner portion). Then with the bevel up, and the unit held at an angle between 25 and 45 degrees to the surface of the limb, the catheter is inserted at the selected target point and advanced until there is blood return in the plastic chamber attached to the end of the introducer. When blood is noted, you may conclude that the wall of the vein has been breeched. The entire catheter must then be advanced an additional one or two millimeters so that the flexible outer portion is fully within the lumen of the vein. At this point the two parts of the device may be separated and the catheter is advanced bit by bit further into the vein—threaded into place—as the metal introducer is gradually withdrawn. At this point the tourniquet may be released.

When the catheter is fully in place, one may, by placing one's fingers approximately over the point where the tip of the catheter lies in the vein, stop the leakage of blood by pressing very firmly. Then attach the end of the administration set which has been previously placed in the bottle of solution and purged of air. One may then tape all parts securely to prevent the catheter from being pulled out.

There are no rules regarding the setting of the drip rate other than to note that an IV line, in an emergency, is a route through which other drugs can be administered. If one is attempting to administer drugs rapidly then the drip rate will be rapid to expedite the entry of the drug into the vein. By contrast if one merely wishes to keep the vein open, a slow drip rate is appropriate.

There is nothing mystical about venipuncture, but many dentists who are quite competent with intraoral injections find insertion of a needle or catheter into a vein, a disturbing and difficult task. Fortunately, little permanent injury can be done with intravenous line placement. Accidental intraarterial injection can be avoided by avoiding the areas where arteries are common. Additionally, one would anticipate a spurting of blood from the catheter after removal of the introducer and prior to connection of the adminstration set, if one were in an artery.

However, the best teacher is practice and any opportunity to attempt venipuncture under non-emergency circumstances should be seized.

Office armamentarium

There are numerous commercial emergency kits available ranging in price from under $50 to almost $600. The only criticism that can be lodged against any of the kits offered is that the practitioner may be lulled into a sense of false security when he purchases one of the simpler products, assuming that he has the necessary drugs and equipment to definitively handle an emergency, when in fact he may be woefully underprepared.

Without question one of the most sophisticated and best equipped kits available is produced by the Banyan Company as the "Emergency-I-Kit" and the Banyan CPR Kit (Fig. 11-4). The CPR Kit is virtually a complete emergency cart in a suitcase and provides all the necessary hardware and drugs and includes a thirty-minute supply of oxygen as well as a system for delivering it under pressure (Fig. 11-5). As one moves down to the less expensive Banyan products various pieces of hardware are deleted (e.g., oxygen adminstration system) and the packaging is different—the top of the line kits offer a number of drugs in prefilled syringes and the case is a bit more deluxe (Fig. 11-6). However, with the possible exception of sodium bicarbonate, of which only one ampoule is provided, the suggested drugs are all represented in quantities sufficient to manage one emergency confidently.

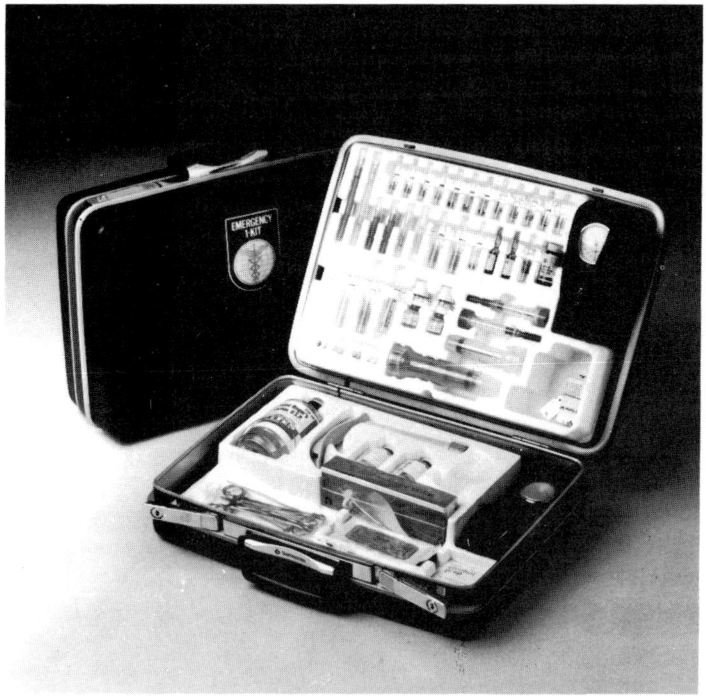

Fig. 11-4 Banyan Emergency-1 kit model E-100.

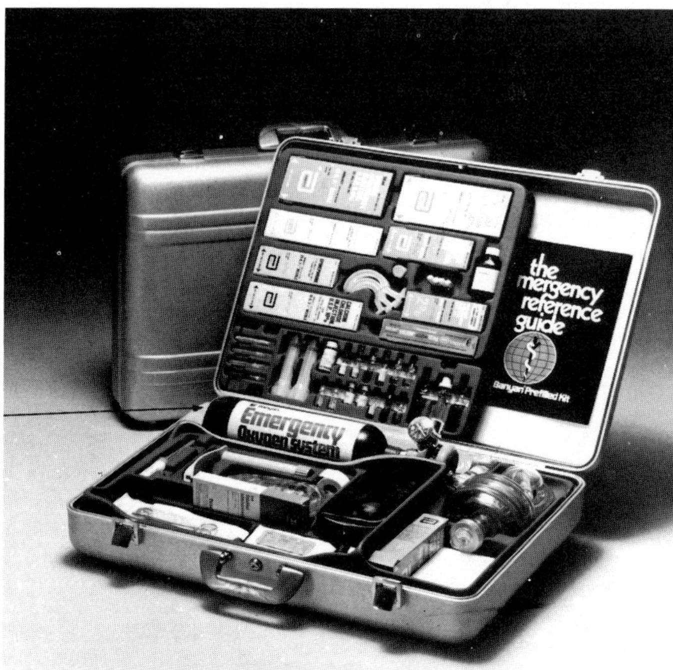

Fig. 11-5 Banyan prefilled CPR kit model E-260.

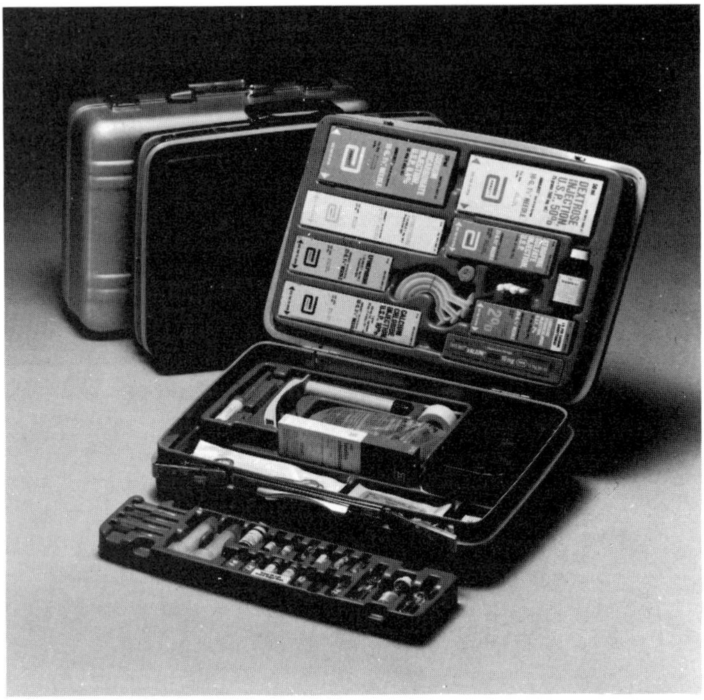

Fig. 11-6 Banyan prefilled kit model E-110.

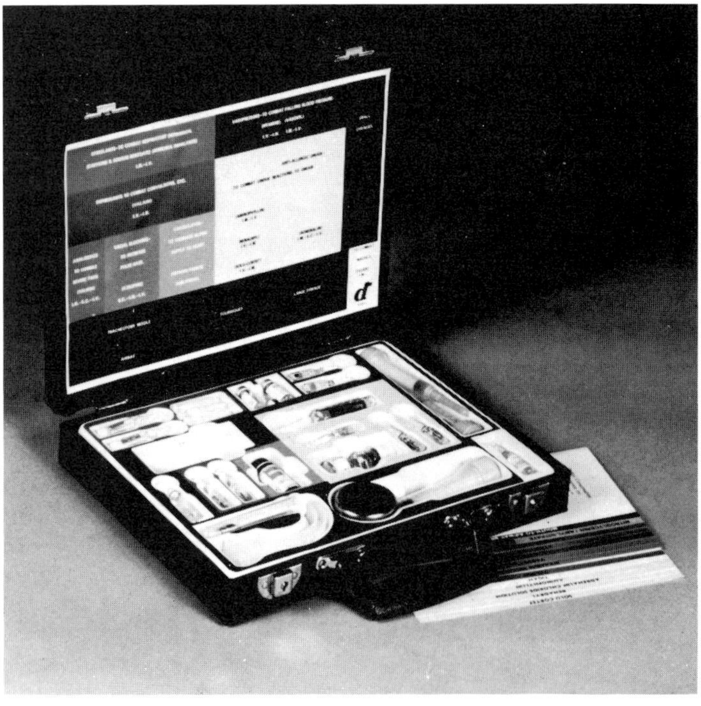

Fig. 11-7 Dencoa color kit.

The Dencoa company markets emergency kits which are color-coded, in an attempt to help relate the symptoms to drugs that might be effective in treating the problem (Fig. 11-7). These kits are significantly less expensive than Banyan's and require substantial augmentation.

Hoyt laboratories also markets kits that are packaged in sealed containers which are labeled either "Anaphylactic Shock" or "Cardio-Pulmonary Resuscitation." These kits supply only drugs and can not be considered complete. Their main advantage is that they provide the drugs in prefilled MIN-I-JET syringe and needle sets in a sealed container. One presumes that when the seal is broken on a canister the wise practitioner will then order a fresh replacement.

Each of these products has a place; however, as stated above, with the exception of the most costly none of them provide all the medications and tools necessary to manage an emergency and therefore must be viewed with a very critical eye prior to purchase.

The dentist has a moral obligation to his patient to have the appropriate equipment, drugs and knowledge to prevent, recognize, evaluate and treat the common medical emergencies which may arise in the dental office.

As previously discussed many emergency situations can be prevented by obtaining a thorough medical history, and follow-up consultation with the patient's physician where indicated. If, however, an emergency does occur, the dentist must try to prevent it from becoming fatal. Because of the need for expedient sure-footed action one must be completely organized. It has been said that one cannot prepare for an emergency during the emergency.

In addition to having the appropriate equipment and sufficient drugs, as well as being competent in C.P.R. and able to recognize the outward signs of impending crises, it is also the dentist's responsibility to be confident of the skill of his auxiliary staff. This will involve periodic study of the causes, signs, symptoms and treatment for common emergencies. A quick reference on emergency therapy should be readily available in the office at all times and the auxiliaries should be encouraged to read it and re-read it at regular intervals.

Teamwork is the key to success in the treatment of a medical crisis. Once all members of an office staff have had minimum formal training (certification in C.P.R.; exposure to and tested competence with support equipment—such as assembling IV bottles and sets; use of the manual resuscitation equipment and monitoring equipment) the next step is assignment of specific responsibilities to each member of the team in the event of catastrophe.

Initial responsibilities in an emergency would be for the attending assistant to calmly and quickly inform another assistant and the receptionist of the situation. While the dentist is beginning emergency treatment the receptionist can notify the ambulance, rescue squad or hospital. The first assistant should be getting oxygen and ventilation equipment ready as well as blood pressure cuff and stethoscope while the second assistant produces and sets up the emergency drug kit. All assistants should be able to monitor vital signs (i.e., pulse blood pressure and respiratory rate), know how to set up an intravenous administration line (bottle of solution and administration set) and be knowledgeable in the simple act of drawing drugs from an emergency ampoule into a syringe. Additionally, they should be able to deliver positive pressure oxygen with a manual resuscitation bag (Ambu bag). These skills are easily learned through regularly scheduled practice sessions on a monthly basis, for each new employee. The sessions can be brief. They serve to remind employees of their exact function. Drugs and equipment should be inspected at these times, and those drugs which have expired should be replaced. Inspection dates should be recorded. Ambulance, rescue squad and hospital numbers should be posted at each telephone.

Time	T.	P.	R.	B.P.	Therapy	Drugs		Comments
						dose	route	

Fig. 11-8 Record of emergency treatment.

In the absence of a municipal rescue service the dentist might find it helpful to make an arrangement with one or two physicians in his vicinity to assist if summoned in the event of an emergency. The aid of qualified persons is invaluable; however, one must be certain that these additional members of the team are also adequately prepared. The office plan for treating the medical emergencies including drugs, equipment and personnel should be made known to the physician prior to a crises situation. Furthermore it must be ascertained that the physician has been adequately trained in emergency management. The mere possession of a medical degree does not automatically endow an individual with expertise in emergency management skills.

For medico-legal purposes a written record of the emergency treatment must be maintained. This record as shown in Fig. 11-8 should include the following:

1. Time of onset
2. Serial vital signs—sequential recordings of blood pressure and pulse
3. Drugs given, time given, dosage and route of administration
4. Comments including effects of the drugs given or initiation of adjunctive therapy such as CPR.

It must be kept in mind that the dentist is responsible for the emergency care rendered to the patient until a more qualified therapist assumes responsibility.

Ideally, when planning a dental operatory there should be a chairside emergency-alert-system which would signal staff throughout the office of an impending problem and its location. This can save precious minutes which may be desperately needed in a crisis. Also if the dentist is working alone in the operatory at the time of the catastrophe he would not have to leave the patient unattended to summon assistance.

Unfortunately, there is no kit available which can insure success in emergency treatment. The only way to improve the chances of patient survival is through hard work and complete preparation.

As concern within the profession grows,

more and more continuing education programs are being made available that deal with basic and advanced life support. Truly comprehensive preparedness involves a total practice philosophy, starting with the detailed medical history. There is no substitute for knowing where a patient's weaknesses lie and being prepared in advance.

The following self evaluation test will assist you in discovering the weak areas in your own emergency protocol.

Self Evaluation Check List

This checklist is of value in determining how well you and your staff are prepared to deal with a medical emergency should it occur in your office. Each question will be assigned points. At the end count up your points and see in which category your numerical score places you.

1. Are you and your staff trained and certified in Cardiopulmonary Resuscitation? (Score 2 points for each. Maximum 10 pts.)

   _____ a. Self

   _____ b. Associate

   _____ c. Assistant

   _____ d. Hygienist

   _____ e. Receptionist

   _____ f. Other

2. Do you have appropriate emergency equipment, including the following? (Score 2 points for each. Maximum 20 pts.)

   _____ a. Ability to ventilate the patient with O_2 under pressure?

   _____ b. Manual resuscitation device—Ambu bag?

   _____ c. Orophyaryngeal/nasopharyngeal airways?

   _____ d. Laryngoscope?

   _____ e. Tonsillar suction?

   _____ f. Magill Forceps?

   _____ g. I.V. set-up (tourniquet, I.V. solution, catheters, administration sets)?

   _____ h. Blood pressure cuff?

   _____ i. Stethoscope?

   _____ j. Adequate selection of sterile syringes (more than ½ dozen of 3 cc, 5 cc and 10 cc)?

3. Do you have a comprehensive selection of emergency drugs? (Score 1 point for each of the following that you have that is within its expiration date)

    _____ a. Aminophylline
    _____ b. Amyl Nitrite
    _____ c. Atropine
    _____ d. Benadryl (Dephenhydramine)
    _____ e. Calcium Chloride or Calcium Gluconate
    _____ f. Demerol
    _____ g. Ephedrine Sulfate
    _____ h. Epinephrine
    _____ i. Morphine Sulfate
    _____ j. Narcan (Naloxone Hydrochloride)
    _____ k. Nitroglycerine
    _____ l. Sodium Bicarbonate
    _____ m. Solu Medrol (Steroids)
    _____ n. Valium (Diazepam)
    _____ o. Xylocaine Hydrochloride 2%

4. In the event of an emergency how rapidly could you produce the appropriate equipment and drugs required to treat the patient?

	(Score)
a. less than 4 minutes	5 pts.
b. less than 10 minutes	0 pts.
c. greater than 10 minutes	−5 pts.

5. Are emergency drills part of your office routine?

	(Score)
a. 1 every month	5 pts
b. 1 every 6 months	2 pts.
c. 1 every year	1 pt.
d. no regular drills	−5 pts.

6. Are new members of the staff required to know the following? (Score 2 points for each).

    _____ a. Their specific role in a medical emergency in your office?
    _____ b. Location of emergency drugs?
    _____ c. Cardiopulmonary resuscitation?
    _____ d. Location of emergency equipment?
    _____ e. How to set up an I.V.?
    _____ f. How to draw up drugs in a syringe?
    _____ g. How emergency equipment functions?
    _____ h. How to monitor vital signs?
    _____ i. How to inform the other staff of an emergency situation?
    _____ j. Location of rescue squad/ambulance and hospital numbers?

7. Medico-legal responsibility dictates the dentist's role as head of the emergency team. Therefore, each practitioner must be skilled in the following. Are you knowledgeable—(Score 2 points for each).

    ____ a. in closed chest cardiac massage?

    ____ b. in manual respiratory support (mouth to mouth or via an Ambu bag?)

    ____ c. in venipuncture technique?

    ____ d. in vital sign monitoring?

    ____ e. in setting up an I.V. infusion (Administration set, solution, etc.)?

    ____ f. in the use of a laryngoscope?

    ____ g. in the use of sterile syringes in drawing up and administering solutions?

    ____ h. in emergency pharmacology (drugs listed in chapter)?

    ____ i. as to the extent of your medical legal responsibility in an emergency situation?

    ____ j. as to the best emergency transport mechanism in your community (i.e., rescue squad, ambulance, etc.) and are their numbers posted in your office?

8. Are you competent in taking a good medical history and physically evaluating your patient as a preventive emergency measure? (Score 5 points if you are and 0 points if you are not).

Total Points:

95-100	Excellently prepared to deal with office catastrophies
85-95	Partially prepared with possibility of emergency mismanagement present
75-85	Poorly prepared with significant preparation required to know how to deal with emergencies
below 75	Substandard—Medico-legally considered negligent

Chapter 12

Summary: Common Medical Emergencies

Louis F. Rose, D.D.S., M.D. and Barry H. Hendler, D.D.S., M.D.

In the majority of emergencies occurring in dental practice, the medical history is the key to accurate evaluation, diagnosis and treatment. No matter what the emergency, attention is first given to the patient's cardiovascular and respiratory status. The clinician must first determine:

1. respiration rate,
2. pulse, and
3. pupillary dilation.

It is most important to maintain adequate perfusion to all vital organs of the body, especially the brain. The ABCD's (airway, breathing, circulation and drugs) of emergency care must always be considered when treating the medical emergency.

Four basic categories of common medical emergencies will be discussed:

1. Cardiovascular emergencies,
2. Emergencies involving transient unconsciousness,
3. Respiratory emergencies and
4. Toxic reactions to local anesthesia (i.e., Xylocaine).

Cardiovascular emergencies

It is estimated that approximately twelve million people in the United States have some form of cardiovascular disease. One of the most common types of cardiovascular disease is *coronary heart disease,* a category which includes angina pectoris, and myocardial infarction. Coronary heart disease has reached enormous proportions and ranks second highest in mortality rates for young adults and middle-aged men.

The medical evaluation should reveal any predisposition for coronary heart disease. Major risk factors which frequently contribute to coronary heart disease include: 1) a positive family history, 2) the modern diet which is excessively high in carbohydrates and total fat (contributing to obesity, hypertension, hyperuricemia, and hyperglycemia), 3) a sedentary mode of living (contributing to poor cardiopulmonary fitness), 4) societal pressures, such as financial success (contributing to anxiety and stress) and 5) cigarette smoking.

It is clear that individuals who have a predilection for (or already have) coronary heart disease require special evaluation and management prior to and during dental treatment, since as a group, they have a decreased ability to recover from a stressful situation.

Angina pectoris

Angina pectoris is characterized by a discomfort located in the retrosternal area that may radiate across the chest, down the left arm, possibly between the shoulder blades and occasionally to the side of the neck, mandible, and face. Pain duration is measured in minutes; it is constricting or crushing in nature. Any situation — physical or psychological — that may increase the demands of the myocardium beyond the capacity of the coronary circulation may initiate such pain.

Usually the patient will have a history of cardiovascular disease. If an inadequate history has been obtained, an anginal attack would be difficult to diagnose. The differential considerations in angina pectoris may be anxiety states, esophageal or gastric spasm or distention, acid reflux into the esophagus, and myocardial infarction.

A patient who is experiencing anginal pain will usually have a rapid pulse rate, a slightly elevated blood pressure, shortness of breath, tachypnea, and pallor of the skin.

Treatment

The administration of oxygen and sublingual nitroglycerine (0.4mg), usually relieves chest pain within one to two minutes. However, if the pain does not subside within this period of time, the dosage should be repeated. Meperidine hydrochloride (Demerol, 50 mg. intramuscularly) is often effective in alleviating the pain. In any case, the patient should be transferred to a hospital for further evaluation, monitoring, and treatment.

Since angina may be precipitated by the stress associated with dental procedures, it is important to decrease anxiety and instill confidence in the patient. This may be accomplished by premedicating the patient with mild tranquilizers, such as valium, and using profound local anesthesia in order to decrease any possibility of pain during treatment. Stressful, extensive dental procedures should be avoided; visits should be as short and atraumatic as possible. If an anginal attack does occur during dental treatment, the patient's physician should be consulted in order to discuss subsequent treatment of the patient.

Myocardial infarction

Acute coronary occlusion with myocardial infarction usually causes severe discomfort in the retrosternal area. However, *unlike angina pectoris:* 1) the pain is frequently more intense, 2) the pain persists for a number of hours (not minutes, or until it is relieved by drug therapy), and 3) the pain does not subside with rest, or the ingestion of nitroglycerine.

Although pain is a symptom which may be helpful in diagnosis, it should be remembered that 20 to 25 percent of all myocardial infarctions are silent in nature, i.e., *occurring with no pain.*

Although retrosternal pain may be the only symptom of myocardial infarction, the attack is usually associated with diaphoresis, dizziness, nausea, indigestion, vomiting, palpitations and a feeling of faintness and mental confusion.

The pulse rate is rapid and may be irregular if an arrhythmia is present; bradycardia may ensue. Blood pressure is usually below normal. Respiratory signs include shortness of breath and dyspnea accompanied by cyanosis or pallor of the skin. The patient may eventually lose consciousness.

The most severe complication in myocardial infarction is the occurrence of arrhythmias (especially during the first and second day after the infarction). Mortality is highest during the first few hours. The weakened heart may be unable to maintain its output; this may result in cardiogenic shock, pulmonary edema, or cardiac arrest.

Treatment

The administration of oxygen is the first step in treatment. For relief of pain morphine (10 mg, intramuscularly) should be used. If respiratory depression ensues as a result of the morphine, the depression can be reversed with naloxone hydrochloride (Narcan, 0.2 mg, intravenously). The objective of treatment in the dental office is essentially to maintain the life of the patient until he can be placed in a hospital where he can be properly monitored and definitively treated.

Precautions to be observed following a

myocardial infarction include avoidance of any dental procedures for six months and all precautions that were noted under angina pectoris. Any medications which may have been prescribed for the cardiac disorder, such as anticoagulants, should be noted and recorded in the patient's medical history.

Cardiac arrest

The term "cardiac arrest" implies a sudden cessation of the heart's pumping function due to either ventricular asystole (electrical or mechanical) or ventricular fibrillation. There are many causes of reversible cardiac arrest, including acute hypoxemia, drug toxicity (e.g., digatalis, quinidine), advanced heart block and cardiac trauma; however, the most frequent cause in adults is coronary artery disease. Cardiac arrest may refer to *cardiovascular collapse, ventricular fibrillation* or *cardiac standstill.* In cardiovascular collapse the heart is still beating but its action is so weak that the blood is not being circulated through the vascular system to the brain and other body tissues. This condition may result from severe hemorrhage, shock, or various drugs. In ventricular fibrillation the individual muscle fascicles of the heart beat independently rather than in the normal coordinated manner. This condition sometimes occurs following myocardial infarction. In cardiac standstill the heart has stopped beating completely. This condition may be terminal and is usually caused by anoxia of the heart muscle.

Although it may be helpful to know the various types of cardiac arrest in an emergency situation, it is not necessary to determine which type of cardiac arrest is present in order to treat the condition. All three types can be recognized by *absent respiration* (although the patient may experience periods of agonal breathing) and *absent pulse* (carotid pulses must be used since they are more readily available) in an *unconscious* patient with a deathlike appearance. The patient may be cyanotic or ashen gray. The pupils are dialated, centric and fixed.

Treatment

Without rapid treatment, permanent brain damage or death is imminent. Basic life support measures, that is, cardiopulmonary resuscitation (CPR), must be started immediately and continued until 1) effective respiration and pulse are restored, 2) the rescuer or team of rescuers are completely exhausted and cannot continue resuscitative therapy, 3) trained personnel arrive, or 4) the patient is pronounced dead.

Life support can be divided into two categories: basic and advanced life support.

Basic Life Support (ABC's):
- Airway Patent
- Breathing Restored
- Circulation Restored

Advanced Life Support:
- Definitive Therapy
  - Drugs
  - Defibrillation
- Accurate Diagnosis
- Cardiac Monitoring
- Transportation
- Communication

In order to assist the immediate basic needs of the dentist, only *basic life support* (ABC's) will be discussed in this program.

Airway

The most important factor for successful resuscitation is a patent airway. In the unconscious patient lying in the supine position, the relaxed muscles allow the mandible to drop backward causing oropharyngeal obstruction by the tongue. This can be corrected quickly and easily by tilting the head backward as far as possible. To perform the head tilt:

1. Place the patient in a supine position.
2. With one hand placed under the patient's neck, lift the head upward while

simultaneously tilting the head backward with the other hand by exerting pressure on the forehead (Fig. 12-1).

The head must be maintained in this position at all times. It should be noted that sometimes this simple maneuver is all that is required for breathing to resume spontaneously.

Once the patient is resting in the supine position with the head tilted back, it should be determined if spontaneous respirations have returned. If there is no evidence of spontaneous respirations, artificial respiration should be instituted.

Breathing

To perform mouth-to-mouth resuscitation (Fig. 12–2):

1. Perform the head tilt as described previously.
2. Continue to exert pressure on the patient's forehead while rotating the hand positioned on the forehead so that the patient's nostrils can be occluded (use your thumb and index finger).
3. Open your mouth wide, take a deep breath, make a tight seal with your mouth around the patient's mouth and blow forcefully into the patient's mouth in order to inflate the lungs.
4. Remove your mouth and allow the patient to exhale passively making sure that the patient's chest falls.

This cycle should be repeated *once every five seconds* as long as respiratory inadequacy persists. The initial ventilatory maneuver consists of four quick, consecutive full breaths.

Circulation

External cardiac compression is effective in providing artificial circulation because the heart lies between the non-resistant sternum and vertebral column (Fig. 12-3). When the lower portion of the sternum is depressed, the right and left ventricles are squeezed, forcing the blood into the pulmonary artery to the lungs, and into the aorta to the brain and other organs of the body. To perform external cardiac compression:

1. Place the patient in a horizontal position on a firm surface, such as the ground or floor.
2. Position yourself close to the side of the victim's chest and place the long axis of the heel of your hand over the long axis of the lower half of the sternum.
3. Since great care must be exercised not to place the hand on the xiphoid process, first palpate the xiphoid process and then measure two finger breadths up from this point (about one to one and a half inches) before positioning your hand.
4. Place the other hand on top of the first, bringing your shoulders directly over the patient's sternum.
5. Arms straight, exert pressure almost vertically downward to depress the lower sternum one and a half to two inches.
6. For optimal pressure, keep the fingers of the hands off the chest wall at all times (Fig. 12-4).

CPR is best performed by two individuals. One positions himself at the patient's side performing external cardiac compression while the other remains at the patient's head, keeping it tilted back and continuing artificial respiration. When there are two resuscitators, the rate is 60 compressions per minute. This rate facilitates timing (one compression per second). Maximum ventilation and circulation is achieved by interposing one quick inflation after each five chest compressions (5:1 or 60:12 ratio). While inflating the lungs, *cardiac compressions should not be interrupted*—interposing breaths without any compressions would result in the precipitous drop of both blood pressure and blood flow. When there is only one resuscitator, both artificial respiration and artificial circulation are accomplished by using a 15:2 ratio, i.e., 15 chest compressions followed by two very quick inflations.

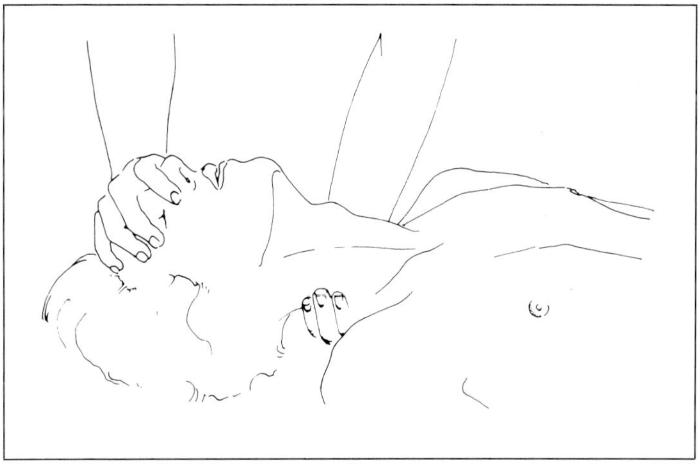

Fig. 12-1 (Airway) Head tilt is performed to keep airway patent and prevent oropharyngeal obstruction.

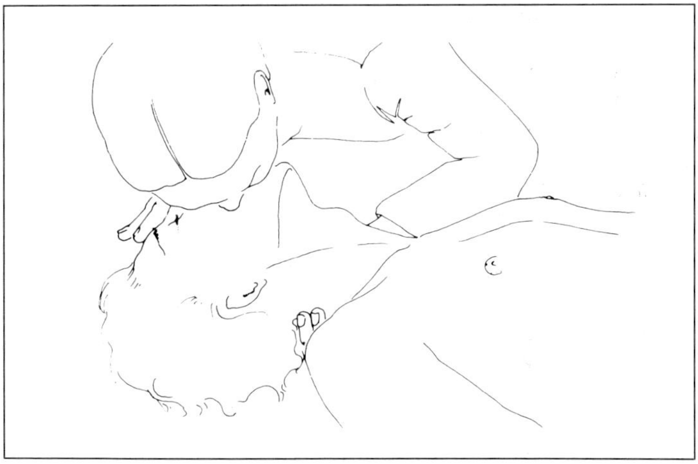

Fig. 12-2 (Breathing) Head tilted back with mouth-to-mouth resuscitation.

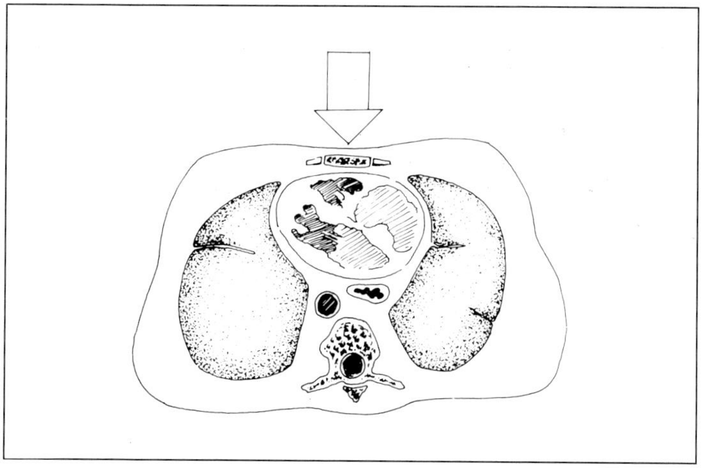

Fig. 12-3 (Cross Section of Chest) Sternum is depressed one and a half to two inches to compress the heart between vertebral column and sternum during external cardiac massage.

Precordial thump

In the *witnessed cardiac arrest* that is, a situation in which the dentist actually sees the arrest occur the precordial thump may be performed prior to the ABC's (Fig. 12-5). This procedure is accomplished by placing the clenched fist eight to ten inches above the chest and delivering a quick, firm blow over the midsternum. In order for the precordial thump to be effective, however, the rescuer must deliver the blow to a heart that is oxygenated. Therefore, the precordial thump should be executed as soon as cardiac arrest has been witnessed.

Evaluating the effectiveness of CPR
The reaction of the pupils should be checked periodically during cardiopulmonary resuscitation. This provides the best indication of delivery of oxygenated blood to the patient's brain. *Pupils that constrict when exposed to light indicate adequate oxygenation and blood flow to the brain.* If the pupils remain widely dilated and do not react to light, serious brain damage is imminent or has already occurred.
In addition, the carotid pulse should be palpated (Fig. 12-6) after the first minute of CPR and every few minutes thereafter to determine whether a spontaneous heartbeat has returned.
The objective of cardiopulmonary resuscitation is to provide sufficient circulation of oxygenated blood to maintain the brain and vital organs until spontaneous respirations and circulation resume. The administration of drugs and other advanced techniques of monitoring are indicated when support personnel have arrived, or when the patient has been transported to an appropriate facility.

Transient unconsciousness

In dental practice, the most common medical emergency is the transient loss of consciousness. Although usually due to the "common faint" or vasovagal syncope, there are other causes of transient loss of consciousness, such as grand mal seizures and hypoglycemia.

Common faint

The most frequent cause of syncope is the decrease in cerebral blood flow due to a vasovagal response. The reaction is fairly simple. Through neurogenic mechanisms, there is a pooling of capillary blood and dilation of the vascular bed that lead to decreased cerebral perfusion.
Syncope is almost always preceded by a prodrome which lasts for seconds to minutes. The prodrome is characterized by a feeling of weakness, nausea, dizziness, sweating and a sensation of warmth. The skin assumes a pale or ashen gray color and becomes cold and clammy.
Evaluation of the patient's vital signs reveal the following: shallow respirations, a sudden fall in blood pressure accompanied by a severe bradycardia with a pulse rate of 40 to 60 beats per minute. The patient experiences a light-headedness which can lead to a loss of consciousness (lasting for a few seconds to several minutes).
Since the actual occurrence of the "faint" is usually observed as it occurs, syncope is easily diagnosed. In addition, a carefully taken medical history (recording previous syncopal episodes or lack thereof) will help immensely in arriving at an accurate diagnosis.

Treatment
1. Place the patient in Trendelenburg's position. An upright position in the chair may cause prolonged cerbral anoxia, which can precipitate convulsions, nausea, etc.
2. Administer oxygen.

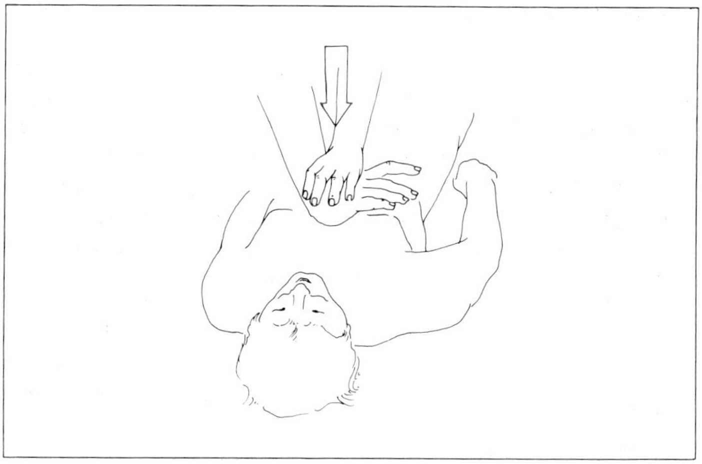

Fig. 12-4 (Circulation) Heel of hand is placed over long axis of lower half of sternum (two finger breadths above xiphoid process). Second hand is placed on top of first and pressure is exerted vertically downward. Fingers of hand must be kept off chest in order to achieve optimal pressure.

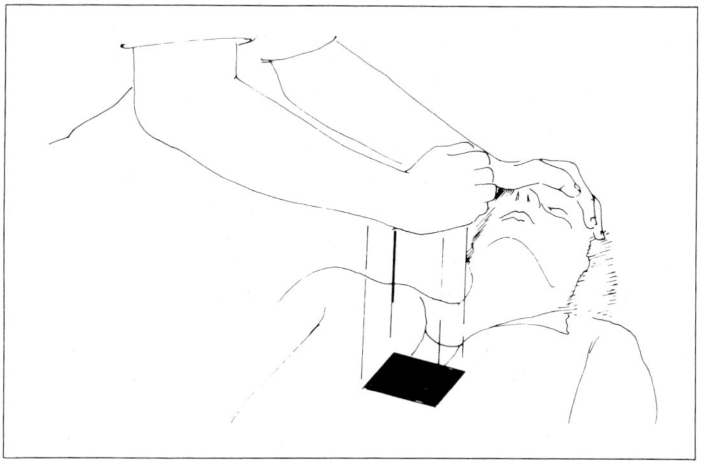

Fig. 12-5 (Precordial thump) Performed only in the *witnessed cardiac arrest.*

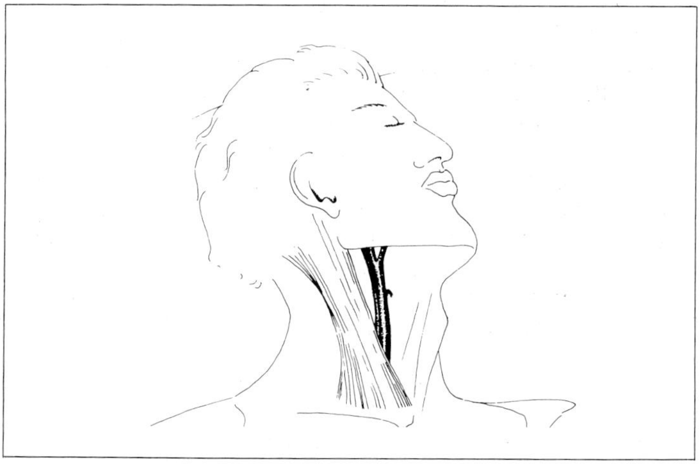

Fig. 12-6 (Carotid pulse) Palpated along the anterior border of the sternocleidomastoid muscle.

3. Use stimulants, such as spirits of ammonia.

The administration of a vasodepressor for syncope is rarely indicated, although atropine, 0.4 mg IM/IV, may be used for sustained bradycardia.

In the post-syncopal period, the patient may experience mental confusion and still complain of weakness, dizziness, and perspiration.

Epilepsy

The term epilepsy refers to many types of recurrent seizures produced by excessive paroxysmal neuronal discharges. Epilepsy is usually divided into two categories: *idiopathic* and *symptomatic.* Idiopathic epilepsy is not caused by a detectable, specific brain disease, or by a metabolic disorder. In the vast majority of patients, the onset of idiopathic epileptic seizures occurs prior to age 30. Symptomatic epilepsy, on the other hand, is due to a structural cerebral lesion or metabolic abnormality, such as hypoglycemia or hypocalcemia. With advancing age and onset of seizures, the incidence of symptomatic epilepsy rises steadily.

Of all the different types of epileptic seizures, it is the grand mal seizure which poses the greatest danger to an individual and will be the only one discussed.

Grand mal is the most conspicuous and severe of all seizure types, affecting more people than any other form of epilepsy. Loss of consciousness, its hallmark, is sudden in onset and brief in duration. Frequently the patient has a history of seizures and may experience an aura (e.g., a disagreeable odor or taste, irritable feeling, or sensation of flashing lights) which often precedes the seizure.

The grand mal seizure can be loosely divided into two phases: *tonic* and *clonic.* During both phases the pulse rate is usually rapid: blood pressure (often difficult to obtain), normal or slightly increased. Respirations may be irregular with periods of apnea, and the patient becoming progressively cyanotic.

The tonic (muscle tension) phase begins when the patient loses consciousness and collapses. At the same time, a massive tonic spasm racks the body, often accompanied by a loud cry or scream. The back arches and the face grimaces. The limbs are rigidly extended; the ankles and wrists sharply flexed. The head is hyperextended and may rotate from one side to the other.

In a fully-developed major motor convulsion, a sequence of catatonic movements is very characteristic. The entire body may twist and turn if the tonic spasm is not symmetrical. The tonic phase seldom lasts more than 10 to 15 seconds.

The tonic phase is followed by the clonic phase, characterized by rhythmic, jerking movements which at first are barely perceptible.

Within seconds, however, the movements mount in magnitude and intensity but become slower and more distinct.

The patient will usually experience a post-ictal period of sleep or confusion after one to five minutes of convulsing.

It is during the seizure activity that the tongue may be bitten and caught between the teeth. There may be blood-tinged saliva frothing from the mouth. In addition, the patient may be incontinent of urine and feces.

Treatment

1. Establish an adequate airway.
2. A mouth prop may be inserted to prevent the patient from traumatizing the tongue and to prevent the development of airway obstruction.
3. Administer oxygen.
4. Turn the patient's head to the side to prevent aspiration.

In the majority of cases, the seizure activity is self-limiting. If it continues, or is repetitive, the administration of diazepam (10 mg, intravenously) is indicated. Inject the diazepam *slowly* and stop when the seizure activity has abated. (A word of caution: respiratory depression or apnea may occur in the postictal phase if diazepam has been given, especially in older individuals.)

Hypoglycemia

The term hypoglycemia usually refers to those clinical signs and symptoms resulting from a marked decrease in blood glucose. The most common etiology of hypoglycemia is intake of hypolycemic agents, especially insulin. Conditions which may be associated with, or may be responsible for hypoglycemia due to hypoglycemic drugs include: dietary change or nutritional inadequacy, weight reduction, exercise, termination of pregnancy, removal or decrease in stress, and onset of diseases associated with hypoglycemia (e.g., hypoadrenalism, pituitary insufficency, liver disease).

Hypoglycemia associated with the use of insulin may be due to an error in the technique of injection, a reduction of insulin required as a result of a change in the course of diabetes, the chronic use of an excessive dosage, or dietary alterations.

Although the clinical manifestations of hypoglycemia are highly variable, the condition will almost always affect both the autonomic and central nervous systems. The pulse rate is rapid; blood pressure is usually decreased, although it may be normal. Respirations are shallow and rapid. Other findings include lethargy, mental confusion, diaphoresis, excessive appetite, nausea, dizziness, severe tremors and possible convulsions.

Treatment

Since the hypoglycemic patient will usually have a history of diabetes mellitus, it is most important that you have recorded in the medical history the status of the disease as well as data regarding dietary habits and insulin requirements. The management of a patient experiencing a hypoglycemic episode will be dictated by the patient's state of consciousness.

Conscious Patient

The treatment of choice for the conscious patient is the administration of oral carbohydrate (e.g., high-carbohydrate beverages such as orange juice, cola, ginger ale or a glucose drink, such as Glucola). The patient should respond almost immediately.

Unconscious Patient

In the unconsciousness individual, 50% dextrose in water (30 to 50 ml, intravenously) is administered at once. Within three to five minutes after glucose injection, the patient should regain consciousness. It should be noted that a patent airway must be maintained.

Respiratory emergencies

Respiratory emergencies are divided into three categories: allergic reactions (mild and severe), asthma, and aspiration of a foreign body.

Allergic reactions

Both mild and severe allergic reactions have common initial signs and symptoms (e.g., sneezing with rhinorrhea, itching of the eyes, ears, nose). However, they may be differentiated by the progression and severity of these clinical manifestations.

Mild allergic reactions may be drug-induced or secondary to exposure to allergens. Clinical manifestations include nasal obstruction with rhinorrhea and sneezing, skin rash or hives with intense itching or swelling of hands, face, and eyelids. More serious reactions may lead to respiratory difficulty caused by intraoral or laryngeal edema. Since the patient may have a history of allergy to a particular drug, caution is required before administering or prescribing any medications.

An important criterion in evaluating the

severity of an allergic reaction is the period of time between the administration of the drug and manifestation of the signs and symptoms. Although a severe allergic reaction (anaphylactic shock) is *usually* rapid in onset (occurring within *minutes* after ingestion of or exposure to the sensitizing substance), it may take *hours* for the signs and symptoms to become manifest. Generally, the longer it takes for the clinical findings to appear, the milder the reaction will be.

Anaphylactic shock is a life-threatening emergency which commonly occurs in patients who have been previously sensitized to a particular drug or other allergic substance. It is associated with a rapid and weak pulse, as well as profound hypotension.

Respiration is characterized by dyspnea with severe bronchial constriction or laryngeal edema. The skin may exhibit urticaria and occasionally petechiae. The reaction may also be accompanied by abdominal pain and nausea. In general, there will be a rapid progression in the severity of the clinical manifestations associated with the mild allergic reaction.

Without prompt treatment the patient will experience complete circulatory and respiratory collapse, with death ensuing within 10 to 15 minutes.

Treatment of the Mild Allergic Reaction

A mild allergic reaction is treated with diphenhydramine hydrochloride (Benadryl, 50 mg, intramuscularly). If the reaction is accompanied by wheezing, epinephrine may also be given (the dosage is similar to that for asthma). To treat severe respiratory distress, a good airway should be maintained and the procedure for anaphylactic shock followed.

Treatment of the Severe Allergic Reaction (Anaphylactic Shock):

1. Make sure the airway is patent.
2. Establish an intravenous route.
3. Administer the following triad of drugs:
   a) Epinephrine 1:1,000 (0.5 to 1.0 mg, intravenously) to alleviate the bronchial constriction.
   b) Benadryl (50 mg, intramuscularly) for long-term antihistamine effect.
   c) Hydrocortisone (0.5 to 1 gm, intravenously), a drug believed to maintain and stabilize lysosomes, increase venous circulation, and improve heart contractility.

If the patient continues to experience severe hypotension, the use of a vasopressor, such as Wyamine (15 to 30 mg, intramuscularly or intravenously) is recommended. Hospitalization of the patient is indicated, since reoccurrence is a likely sequel.

Asthma

Bronchial asthma, which affects an estimated six to eight million Americans, is a clinical state of heightened reactivity of the tracheobronchial tree. An asthmatic attack may be caused by an allergic reaction, or by anxiety or apprehension. It is associated with factors indicative of airway obstruction, such as dyspnea, and coughing (with or without the production of tenancious sputum). These symptoms are caused by bronchospasms, bronchial wall edema, and hypersecretion by mucous glands. The asthmatic attack may be continuous or paroxysmal and may range from a mild episode to life-threatening asphyxiation, as in status asthmaticus. Asthma is usually reversible, either spontaneously or through treatment. For patients with a history of asthma, it is helpful to know the precipitating factors and management of previous attacks. For example, since many asthmatic attacks may be stimulated by anxiety, it may be possible to obviate an episode by the use of premedication.

Treatment

The patient experiencing a severe episode of asthma requires prompt treatment. The patient should be seated upright in the chair. Oxygen should be administered and epinephrine 1:1000 (0.2 to 0.5 ml, subcutaneously) injected. *If the patient has a history of hypertension, hyperthyroidism or cardiac disease, epinephrine must be used with extreme caution.* In these patients, it is recommended that aminophilline (250 to 500 mg, intravenously) be administered. This drug must be injected *very slowly*—over a 10 to 15 minute period—in order to avoid severe hypotension. If the attack is prolonged and the patient is unresponsive to treatment, he should be moved to a hospital for further evaluation and therapy.

Aspiration of a foreign body

An aspirated foreign body will produce either *partial* or *total* obstruction. If partial obstruction has occurred, the patient will usually be able to talk (or make "crow-like" sounds) and cough effectively; therefore, do not interfere with his attempts to clear his throat.

If there is total obstruction, in which case the patient is unable to breathe or make a sound, intervention would then be indicated.

Treatment

Conscious Patient: With the heel of your hand, strike the patient between the shoulder blades several times in rapid succession. If this technique is not successful, the *Heimlich maneuver* (Fig. 12-7) should be performed:

1. Position yourself behind the patient, wrapping your arms around his waist.
2. Form a fist and place it so the thumb-side is against his abdomen (between the navel and rib cage).
3. With the other hand, grasp your fist and quickly apply pressure in an inward and upward direction.
4. If necessary, repeat this procedure several times.

The objective of the Heimlich maneuver is to elevate the diaphragm in order to compress the lungs. This will increase air pressure within the tracheobronchial tree, expelling the aspirated object.

Unconscious Patient: If the patient is unconscious and breathing has ceased, it is imperative to first ascertain whether the individual has in fact aspirated a foreign object, or whether he is the victim of *another type of medical emergency* (e.g., cardiac arrest). In order to determine whether an object is occluding the airway:

1. Position the patient on his back.
2. Maintain an airway.
3. Attempt to restore breathing by using mouth-to-mouth resuscitation (Figs. 12-1 and 12-2).

If the chest does not rise as a result of assisted breathing, it may be assumed that there is occlusion of the airway secondary to aspiration of a foreign object. The resuscitator should check the mouth for any foreign objects and continue to treat the patient for aspiration. This should be accomplished in the following manner (Fig. 12-8):

1. Position the patient on his side.
2. Brace his chest against your legs.
3. With the heel of your hand, strike him between the shoulder blades several times in rapid succession.
4. Once the foreign object has been removed, initiate assisted breathing.

If this technique is unsuccessful, the *abdominal thrust* should be performed (Fig. 12-9):

1. Kneel next to the patient.
2. Place the heel of one hand in the middle of the abdomen (between the navel and rib cage).
3. Grasp this hand with your free hand and apply pressure in an inward and upward direction.
4. If necessary, repeat this procedure several times.

A patient who has aspirated a foreign body

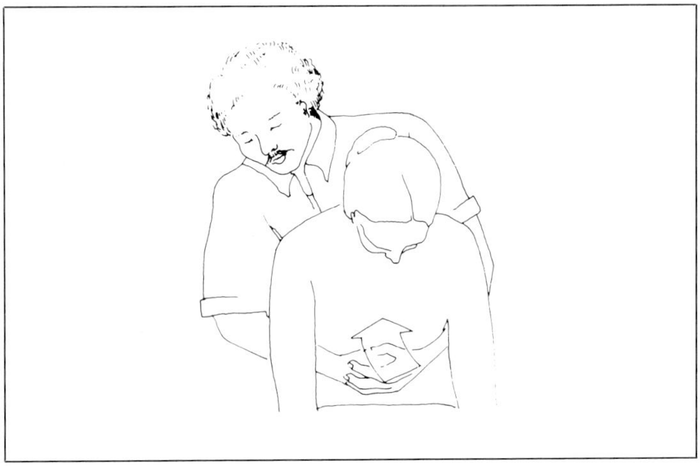

Fig. 12-7 (Heimlich maneuver) Treatment for aspiration of a foreign body in a conscious patient. Pressure is applied against abdomen (between navel and rib cage) in an inward and upward direction.

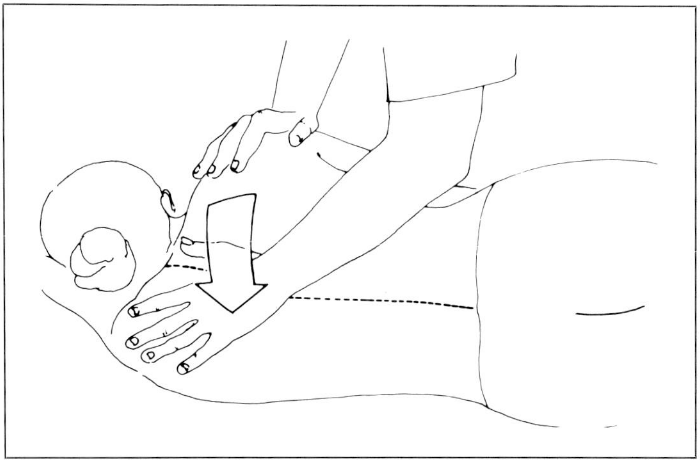

Fig. 12-8 (Treatment of aspiration of a foreign body in an unconscious patient) Position patient on his side and strike him between shoulder blades with the heel of your hand.

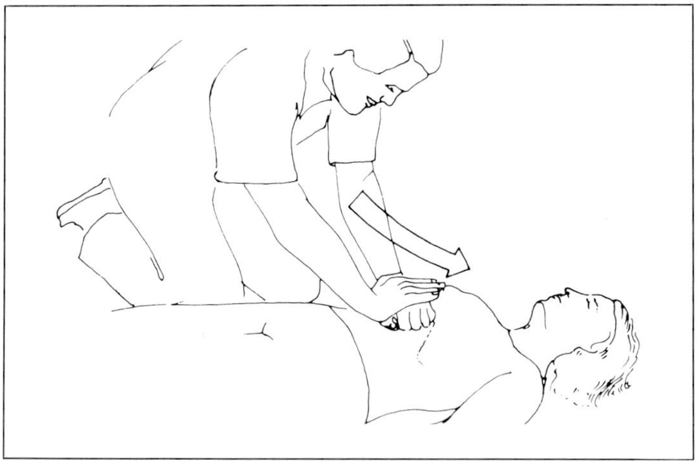

Fig. 12-9 (Abdominal thrust) Treatment of aspiration of a foreign body in an unconscious patient. Place your hands against patient's abdomen (between navel and rib cage) and apply pressure in an inward and upward direction.

and was treated with any of the procedures described should be examined by a physician for any complications.

Toxic reactions to local anesthesia

(Xylocaine)

The toxic dose of lidocaine hydrochloride (Xylocaine) for a normal, healthy 70 kg, adult male is 300 to 500 mg. This is equivalent to approximately 10 to 14, 1.8 ml cartridges of 2% Xylocaine. The toxic dose is lower for a child, small individual, or an elderly or medically-compromised patient. Adverse reactions may be a result of high plasma levels due to excessive dosage, rapid absorption, inadvertent intravenous injection, or allergic hypersensitivity. If the reaction is caused by an allergic hypersensitivity, the patient should be managed accordingly. If the reaction occurs as a result of excessive dosage, rapid absorption, or inadvertent intravenous injection, it would involve primarily the central nervous system or the cardiovascular system, or both.

The toxic reaction to Xylocaine is usually characterized by an *excitatory* and *depressive* phase. During both phases, there is central nervous system as well as cardiovascular system involvement.

In the excitatory phase, the patient may become restless, anxious, and mentally confused. Tremors are common and convulsions may ensue. The pulse rate is rapid; blood pressure is increased, but may be normal.

If the depressive phase follows, however, both blood pressure and pulse rate will drop precipitously. Unconsciousness and respiratory arrest are not unusual sequelae.

Treatment—Excitatory Phase

1. Establish and maintain an airway.
2. Administer oxygen.
3. Establish and maintain an intravenous route for the possible administration of drugs.
4. If the reaction precipitates convulsions, administer diazepam (10 to 15 mg, intravenously).
5. Observe for signs of the depressive phase.

Treatment—Depressive Phase

1. Establish and maintain an airway.
2. Administer oxygen.
3. If hypotension occurs, inject a vasopressor (Ephedrine 25 mg IV).
4. For severe bradycardia, administer atropine (1 mg, intravenously).

Reference

1. Rose, L.F. "Diagnosis and Management of Medical Emergencies in the Dental Office." *Continuing Dental Education,* University of Pa., Vol. 1, No. 3, December 1977.

Index

A

B

C

F

G

H

I

K

L

Q

R

S

T

Kenneth A. Freedman

Management of the Geriatric Dental Patient

People are living longer; this is inevitably reflected in the composition of the dental practice population. Senior citizens have some oral health problems similar to those of the general population, and other problems that reflect their age and their general health status.

The dentist sees such patients in several settings: his office, homes for the elderly, and—occasionally—in the patient's own home. Each of the settings requires some adaptation if the older patient is to receive care under optimal conditions.

Management of the older patient requires some adjustment on the part of the dentist as well. He must be particularly careful to recognize dental problems associated with long-term use of certain drugs, and he must learn to understand that older patients require special attention. This book will help the concerned dentist to provide optimal care to a growing segment of the population, with minimal disruption of his normal routines.

148 pages, 76 illustrations with 58 in color, size 17.5 × 24.5 cm, linen bound with gold stamping and protective cover.

ISBN 0-931386-05-5 Order MGP $42.00

Takao Fusayama

New Concepts in Operative Dentistry

Differentiating Two Layers of Carious Dentin and Using an Adhesive Resin

Local application of a dye permits differentiation of demineralized and remineralizable dentin, a step that makes non-retentive cavity shapes possible for durable restorations.

Chemical adhesion of the restorative resin material is assured when the Clearfil-F restorative system is used as described and illustrated.

The absence of pain for the patient throughout the restoration procedure is an unusual but desirable characteristic.

180 pages, 333 illustrations with 265 in color, size 17.5 × 24.5 cm, linen bound with gold stamping and protective cover.

ISBN 0-931386-34-9 Order TF $58.00

David A. Pyner

Simplified Painless Endodontics for the General Dentist: The Alternative to N2

Careful preparation, attention to detail, and meticulous execution assure patient cooperation and successful treatment of endodontic problems in the general dental office.

Dr. Pyner's book describes his new approach to simplified endodontics, and offers the clinician an alternative to disputed mummification procedures. The technique proposed is illustrated with photographs and line drawings to assure clear understanding.

176 pages, 384 illustrations with 128 in color, size 17.5 × 24.5 cm, linen bound with gold stamping and protective cover.

ISBN 0-931386-12-8 Order PY $48.00

Harold L. Hamburg

Sedation

"Everything you've always wanted to know but didn't know whom to ask" about sedation techniques in the dental operatory is provided in this illustrated, casually written introduction to the subject.

The information is given in a practical manner: how to use sedation techniques and which techniques are appropriate to specific conditions. Inhalation sedation, intravenous sedation, and other methods as well are described in clear terms.

This book will help the busy clinician by showing him what can be done with sedation techniques and how to make the most of them.

200 pages, 89 illustrations, pocket book.

ISBN 0-931386-07-1 Order HS $16.00